UNIVERSITY OF STRATHCLYDE
30125 00542106 9

D1761297

ANDERSONIAN LIBRARY
WITHDRAWN
FROM
LIBRARY
STOCK
UNIVERSITY OF STRATHCLYDE

TECHNIQUES FOR ANALYZING FOOD AROMA

FOOD SCIENCE AND TECHNOLOGY

A Series of Monographs, Textbooks, and Reference Books

1. Flavor Research: Principles and Techniques, *R. Teranishi, I. Hornstein, P. Issenberg, and E. L. Wick*
2. Principles of Enzymology for the Food Sciences, *John R. Whitaker*
3. Low-Temperature Preservation of Foods and Living Matter, *Owen R. Fennema, William D. Powrie, and Elmer H. Marth*
4. Principles of Food Science
   Part I: Food Chemistry, *edited by Owen R. Fennema*
   Part II: Physical Methods of Food Preservation, *Marcus Karel, Owen R. Fennema, and Daryl B. Lund*
5. Food Emulsions, *edited by Stig E. Friberg*
6. Nutritional and Safety Aspects of Food Processing, *edited by Steven R. Tannenbaum*
7. Flavor Research: Recent Advances, *edited by R. Teranishi, Robert A. Flath, and Hiroshi Sugisawa*
8. Computer-Aided Techniques in Food Technology, *edited by Israel Saguy*
9. Handbook of Tropical Foods, *edited by Harvey T. Chan*
10. Antimicrobials in Foods, *edited by Alfred Larry Branen and P. Michael Davidson*
11. Food Constituents and Food Residues: Their Chromatographic Determination, *edited by James F. Lawrence*
12. Aspartame: Physiology and Biochemistry, *edited by Lewis D. Stegink and L. J. Filer, Jr.*
13. Handbook of Vitamins: Nutritional, Biochemical, and Clinical Aspects, *edited by Lawrence J. Machlin*
14. Starch Conversion Technology, *edited by G. M. A. van Beynum and J. A. Roels*

15. Food Chemistry: Second Edition, Revised and Expanded, *edited by Owen R. Fennema*
16. Sensory Evaluation of Food: Statistical Methods and Procedures, *Michael O'Mahony*
17. Alternative Sweetners, *edited by Lyn O'Brien Nabors and Robert C. Gelardi*
18. Citrus Fruits and Their Products: Analysis and Technology, *S. V. Ting and Russell L. Rouseff*
19. Engineering Properties of Foods, *edited by M. A. Rao and S. S. H. Rizvi*
20. Umami: A Basic Taste, *edited by Yojiro Kawamura and Morley R. Kare*
21. Food Biotechnology, *edited by Dietrich Knorr*
22. Food Texture: Instrumental and Sensory Measurement, *edited by Howard R. Moskowitz*
23. Seafoods and Fish Oils in Human Health and Disease, *John E. Kinsella*
24. Postharvest Physiology of Vegetables, *edited by J. Weichmann*
25. Handbook of Dietary Fiber: An Applied Approach, *Mark L. Dreher*
26. Food Toxicology, Parts A and B, *Jose M. Concon*
27. Modern Carbohydrate Chemistry, *Roger W. Binkley*
28. Trace Minerals in Foods, *edited by Kenneth T. Smith*
29. Protein Quality and the Effects of Processing, *edited by R. Dixon Phillips and John W. Finley*
30. Adulteration of Fruit Juice Beverages, *edited by Steven Nagy, John A. Attaway, and Martha E. Rhodes*
31. Foodborne Bacterial Pathogens, *edited by Michael P. Doyle*
32. Legumes: Chemistry, Technology, and Human Nutrition, *edited by Ruth H. Matthews*
33. Industrialization of Indigenous Fermented Foods, *edited by Keith H. Steinkraus*
34. International Food Regulation Handbook: Policy • Science • Law, *edited by Roger D. Middlekauff and Philippe Shubik*
35. Food Additives, *edited by A. Larry Branen, P. Michael Davidson, and Seppo Salminen*
36. Safety of Irradiated Foods, *J. F. Diehl*
37. Omega-3 Fatty Acids in Health and Disease, *edited by Robert S. Lees and Marcus Karel*
38. Food Emulsions: Second Edition, Revised and Expanded, *edited by Kåre Larsson and Stig E. Friberg*
39. Seafood: Effects of Technology on Nutrition, *George M. Pigott and Barbee W. Tucker*
40. Handbook of Vitamins: Second Edition, Revised and Expanded, *edited by Lawrence J. Machlin*
41. Handbook of Cereal Science and Technology, *Klaus J. Lorenz and Karel Kulp*

42. Food Processing Operations and Scale-Up, *Kenneth J. Valentas, Leon Levine, and J. Peter Clark*
43. Fish Quality Control by Computer Vision, *edited by L. F. Pau and R. Olafsson*
44. Volatile Compounds in Foods and Beverages, *edited by Henk Maarse*
45. Instrumental Methods for Quality Assurance in Foods, *edited by Daniel Y. C. Fung and Richard F. Matthews*
46. Listeria, Listeriosis, and Food Safety, *Elliot T. Ryser and Elmer H. Marth*
47. Acesulfame-K, *edited by D. G. Mayer and F. H. Kemper*
48. Alternative Sweeteners: Second Edition, Revised and Expanded, *edited by Lyn O'Brien Nabors and Robert C. Gelardi*
49. Food Extrusion Science and Technology, *edited by Jozef L. Kokini, Chi-Tang Ho, and Mukund V. Karwe*
50. Surimi Technology, *edited by Tyre C. Lanier and Chong M. Lee*
51. Handbook of Food Engineering, *edited by Dennis R. Heldman and Daryl B. Lund*
52. Food Analysis by HPLC, *edited by Leo M. L. Nollet*
53. Fatty Acids in Foods and Their Health Implications, *edited by Ching Kuang Chow*
54. *Clostridium botulinum*: Ecology and Control in Foods, *edited by Andreas H. W. Hauschild and Karen L. Dodds*
55. Cereals in Breadmaking: A Molecular Colloidal Approach, *Ann-Charlotte Eliasson and Kåre Larsson*
56. Low-Calorie Foods Handbook, *edited by Aaron M. Altschul*
57. Antimicrobials in Foods: Second Edition, Revised and Expanded, *edited by P. Michael Davidson and Alfred Larry Branen*
58. Lactic Acid Bacteria, *edited by Seppo Salminen and Atte von Wright*
59. Rice Science and Technology, *edited by Wayne E. Marshall and James I. Wadsworth*
60. Food Biosensor Analysis, *edited by Gabriele Wagner and George G. Guilbault*
61. Principles of Enzymology for the Food Sciences: Second Edition, *John R. Whitaker*
62. Carbohydrate Polyesters as Fat Substitutes, *edited by Casimir C. Akoh and Barry G. Swanson*
63. Engineering Properties of Foods: Second Edition, Revised and Expanded, *edited by M. A. Rao and S. S. H. Rizvi*
64. Handbook of Brewing, *edited by William A. Hardwick*
65. Analyzing Food for Nutrition Labeling and Hazardous Contaminants, *edited by Ike J. Jeon and William G. Ikins*
66. Ingredient Interactions: Effects on Food Quality, *edited by Anilkumar G. Gaonkar*

67. Food Polysaccharides and Their Applications, *edited by Alistair M. Stephen*
68. Safety of Irradiated Foods: Second Edition, Revised and Expanded, *J. F. Diehl*
69. Nutrition Labeling Handbook, *edited by Ralph Shapiro*
70. Handbook of Fruit Science and Technology: Production, Composition, Storage, and Processing, *edited by D. K. Salunkhe and S. S. Kadam*
71. Food Antioxidants: Technological, Toxicological, and Health Perspectives, *edited by D. L. Madhavi, S. S. Deshpande, and D. K. Salunkhe*
72. Freezing Effects on Food Quality, *edited by Lester E. Jeremiah*
73. Handbook of Indigenous Fermented Foods: Second Edition, Revised and Expanded, *edited by Keith H. Steinkraus*
74. Carbohydrates in Food, *edited by Ann-Charlotte Eliasson*
75. Baked Goods Freshness: Technology, Evaluation, and Inhibition of Staling, *edited by Ronald E. Hebeda and Henry F. Zobel*
76. Food Chemistry: Third Edition, *edited by Owen R. Fennema*
77. Handbook of Food Analysis: Volumes 1 and 2, *edited by Leo M. L. Nollet*
78. Computerized Control Systems in the Food Industry, *edited by Gauri S. Mittal*
79. Techniques for Analyzing Food Aroma, *edited by Ray Marsili*

Additional Volumes in Preparation

Food Proteins and Their Applications, *edited by Srinivasan Damodaran and A. Paraf*

TECHNIQUES FOR ANALYZING FOOD AROMA

EDITED BY
RAY MARSILI
Dean Foods Company
Rockford, Illinois

Marcel Dekker, Inc. New York•Basel•Hong Kong

Library of Congress Cataloging-in-Publication Data

Techniques for analyzing food aroma / edited by Ray Marsili.
p. cm.— (Food science and technology ; 79)
Includes index.
ISBN 0-8247-9788-4 (hardcover : alk. paper)
1. Food—Sensory evaluation. I. Marsili, Ray.
II. Series: Food science and technology (Marcel Dekker, Inc.) ; 79.
TX546.T43 1997
664'.07—dc20

96-36593
CIP

The publisher offers discounts on this book when ordered in bulk quantities. For more information, write to Special Sales/Professional Marketing at the address below.

This book is printed on acid-free paper.

Marcel Dekker, Inc.
270 Madison Avenue, New York, New York 10016

Current printing (last digit):
10 9 8 7 6 5 4 3 2 1

PRINTED IN THE UNITED STATES OF AMERICA

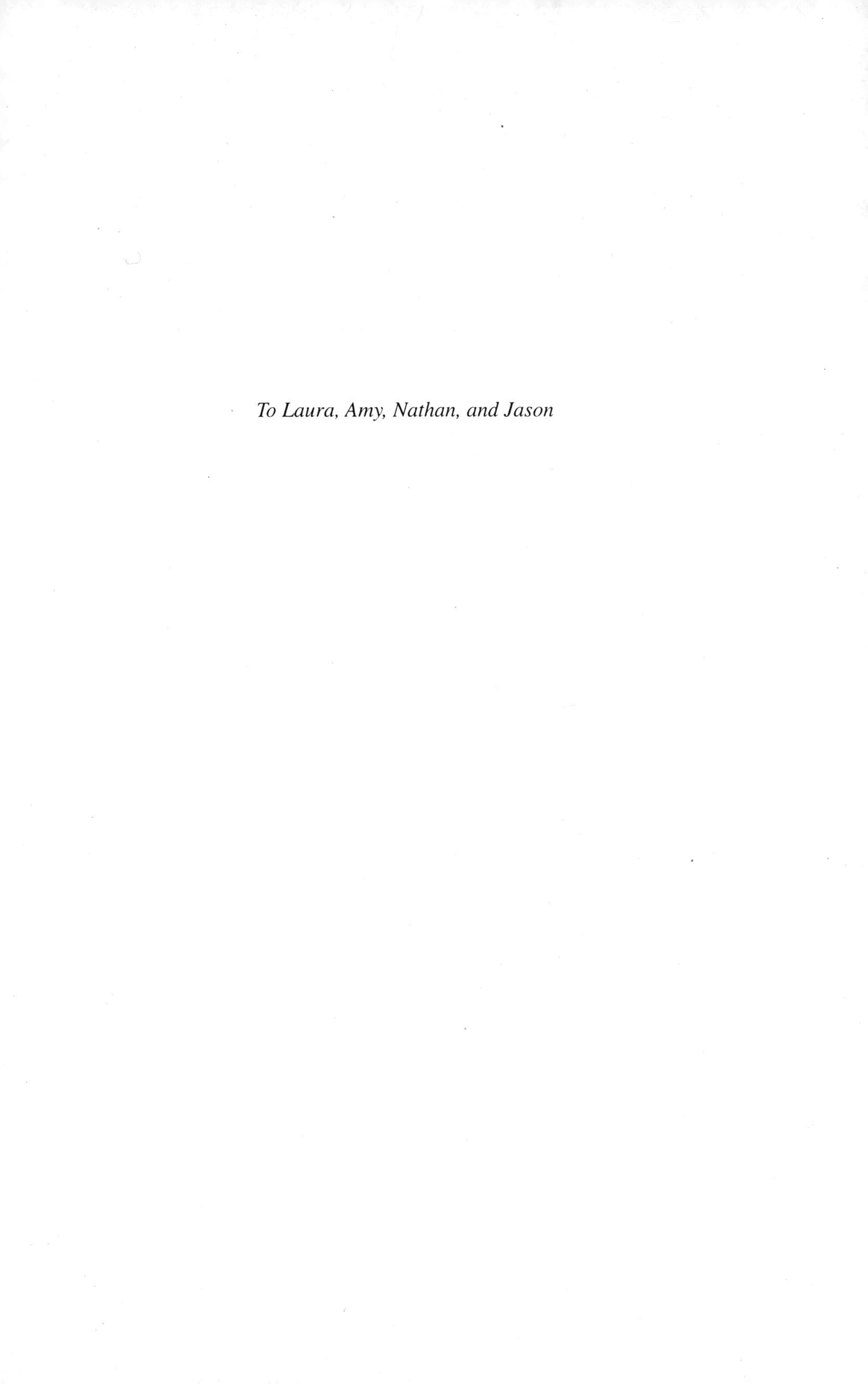

To Laura, Amy, Nathan, and Jason

The search for Truth is in one way hard and in another way easy. For it is evident that no one can master it fully nor miss it completely. But each adds a little to our knowledge of Nature, and from all the facts assembled there arises a certain grandeur.

Aristotle

Preface

Flavor is of major concern to food scientists because it is a significant factor influencing the public's food-buying decisions and its perception of food quality. Analyzing the volatile and semivolatile organic compounds that impact the flavor and aroma of foods can be a daunting task, and obtaining useful information from such measurements can be even more challenging.

It is the intention of the authors to describe analytical techniques that can be applied to the detection and quantitation of volatile aroma chemicals in foods and to explain how the sense of smell (olfactory detection) can be incorporated with these techniques to resolve important, practical problems related to food aromas. Advantages, disadvantages, and biases of each technique are discussed, as well as when and why specific techniques should be selected or avoided.

The chapters contain dozens of examples of applications showing how real food aroma problems have been resolved through the use of modern analytical instruments and olfactometry. Specifically, the book discusses various sample preparation techniques for isolating and concentrating food aroma compounds prior to gas chromatographic (GC) analysis; how GC column technology, column manipulation techniques, and GC/MS detection can be used to maximize resolution, discrimination, identification, and sensitivity for detecting important aroma-influencing components; and how sensory techniques, including the use of an olfactometry detector, can be combined with instrumental methods to create powerful systems for problem solving. Included in several chapters are discussions that critically review CharmAnalysis and aroma extraction dilution analysis (AEDA), two useful techniques for interpreting GC-olfactometry results. Valuable suggestions and ancillary techniques for supplementing CharmAnalysis and AEDA studies are presented.

Also included is a chapter discussing the operation and application of the "electronic nose," a new chemical sensor array–based instrument that emulates the human nose. While some excellent flavor work has been done with HPLC, supercritical fluid extraction (SFE), supercritical fluid chromatography (SFC), and other analytical methods, GC techniques are emphasized in this work since they are generally more applicable to the analysis of volatile organic polar compounds, which are frequently the most important contributors to food aroma.

The dedication, persistence, and splendid cooperation of all contributing authors, as well as the quality of information they have presented, are to be commended. Also, I would like to acknowledge my indebtedness to my associates, Gregory J. Kilmer, Nadine Miller, and Ronald E. Simmons, and to my supervisor, Dr. Scott Rambo, for their advice, encouragement, and continual support. Special thanks go to my wife, Deborah, for reviewing the chapters and for her patience and words of encouragement.

Ray Marsili

Contents

Contributors

Alexander Bernreuther Joint Research Center, Environment Institute, Ispra, Italy

Imre Blank Research Centre, Nestec Ltd., Lausanne, Switzerland

Ulrich Epperlein University of Tübingen, Tübingen, Germany

Casey C. Grimm Southern Regional Research Center, Agricultural Research Service, United States Department of Agriculture, New Orleans, Louisiana

Alan D. Harmon Research and Technical Development, McCormick & Co., Inc., Hunt Valley, Maryland

Diana Hodgins Wheathampstead, Hertfordshire, England

Charles K. Huston Varian Chromatography Systems, Walnut Creek, California

Berhard Koppenhoefer Institut für Organische Chemie der Universität, University of Tübingen, Tübingen, Germany

Steven W. Lloyd Southern Regional Research Center, Agricultural Research Service, United States Department of Agriculture, New Orleans, Louisiana

Ray Marsili Dean Foods Company, Rockford, Illinois

James A. Miller Southern Regional Research Center, Agricultural Research Service, United States Department of Agriculture, New Orleans, Louisiana

Behroze S. Mistry Aspen Research Corporation, St. Paul, Minnesota

Linda K. Olson Aspen Research Corporation, St. Paul, Minnesota

Thomas H. Parliment Kraft Foods, White Plains, New York

Terry Reineccius Aspen Research Corporation, St. Paul, Minnesota

Arthur M. Spanier Southern Regional Research Center, Agricultural Research Service, United States Department of Agriculture, New Orleans, Louisiana

Thomas P. Wampler CDS Analytical, Inc., Oxford, Pennsylvania

Donald W. Wright Microanalytics Instrumentation Corporation, Round Rock, Texas

1

Solvent Extraction and Distillation Techniques

Thomas H. Parliment
Kraft Foods, White Plains, New York

I. INTRODUCTION

The purpose of this chapter is to review techniques that have been published in the technical literature and developed in our laboratory for the isolation and concentration of samples prior to analysis by gas chromatography. It is our goal to emphasize those techniques that are easy to employ, require minimal equipment, and produce reproducible, meaningful results. In a number of cases, examples of the results will be presented.

As has been described previously (1), sample preparation is complicated by a number of factors:

1. Concentration Level: Aromatics levels are generally low, typically in the ppm, ppb, or ppt range. Thus it is not only necessary to isolate the components, but also to concentrate them by several orders of magnitude.

TABLE 1 Classes of Aroma Compounds in Coffee

Chemical class	Number of compounds
Hydrocarbons	74
Alcohols	20
Aldehydes	30
Ketones	73
Acids	25
Esters	31
Lactones	3
Phenols (and ethers)	48
Furans	127
Thiophenes	26
Pyrroles	71
Oxazoles	35
Thiazoles	27
Pyridines	19
Pyrazines	86
Amines and miscellaneous nitrogen compounds	32
Sulfur compounds	47
Miscellaneous	17
Total	*791*

Source: Ref. 2

2. Matrix: The volatiles are frequently intracellular and must be liberated by disruption. The sample frequently contains nonvolatile components such as lipids, proteins, or carbohydrates, which complicates the isolation process. These components may create problems of foaming and emulsification during isolation procedures and will create artifacts if injected into a hot gas chromatography injector port.
3. Complexities of Aromas: The aromatic composition of foods are frequently very complex. For example, coffee currently has almost 800 identified components, as shown in Table 1. Complicating the picture is the fact that the classes of compounds present cover the range of polarities, solubilities, and pHs.
4. Variation of Volatility: The components possess boiling points ranging from well below room temperature to those that are solids, such as vanillin (mp 81°C).
5. Instability: Many components in an aroma are unstable and may be oxidized by air or degraded by heat or extremes of pH.

Regardless of which sample preparation technique is employed, it is critically important to assess the organoleptic quality of the isolate. No single technique will prove optimal for every sample, and evaluations should be made to ensure that decomposition and loss of desired components do not occur. A very significant paper published by Jennings et al. (3) compared various sample preparation techniques, including porous polymer trapping and distillation-extraction. Their conclusion was that no isolation technique produced results that duplicated the original neat sample, but that distillation-extraction most nearly agreed (Fig. 1).

This is particularly important since current flavor research seems to be less directed to identification for the sake of adding to the numbers of the compounds in the knowledge base, and more to alternative reasons. At the present time it appears one purpose is characterization of components of organoleptic importance. Three techniques for gas chromatographic individual component assessment are in vogue: aroma extraction dilution analysis (AEDA), calculation of odor units, and CharmAnalysis (see Chapter 9). Another purpose of flavor research is to analyze products and to perform flavor stability studies.

At the present time, the two most common procedures reported in the literature for the isolation of the aromatics are headspace methods and extraction. The former will be covered in the next chapter. The purpose of this chapter is to review techniques for isolating and concentrating aromatics, which include various distillation and extraction procedures.

A number of references exist on the topic of flavor isolation, and these provide a different perspective on the topic (4–8). To quote Schreier (9): "It must be emphasized that sample preparation is the most critical step in the entire analytical process of the investigation of volatiles."

II. DIRECT INJECTION OF THE SAMPLE

A. Essential Oils

Direct injection is by far the most convenient technique and works particularly well for essential oils. The sample may have to be diluted with a solvent to obtain response within the limits of the detector.

B. Aqueous Samples

When concentrated aqueous samples are available, direct injection techniques can be employed. In industry, aqueous materials are frequently available from industrial operations. Examples of this would be condensates from coffee

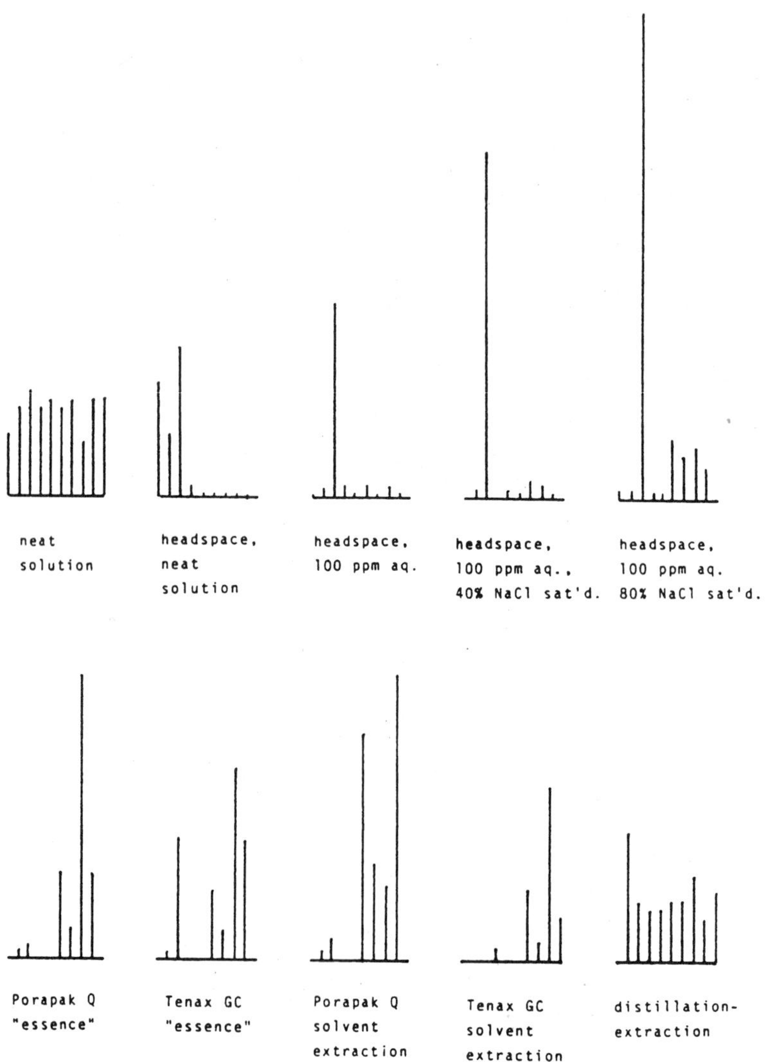

Figure 1 Relative integrator response for various sample preparation techniques. (From Ref. 3.)

grinders, vapors from chocolate conching operations, and aqueous materials from citrus juice concentrators.

The aqueous phase may be injected if the sample is sufficiently concentrated. A number of problems may be encountered under these circumstances. When water is converted to steam, the volume increases dramatically; 1 μl of water becomes more than 1000 μl of steam. This is larger than the injector volume of many current gas chromatographs, and the steam may degrade the performance of the system. Polar gas chromatography liquid phases such as Carbowax and PEG will degrade in the presence of steam unless they are bonded to the column.

If the aqueous sample contains dissolved solutes such as carbohydrates or proteins, additional problems will arise when the sample is injected. The nonvolatiles may decompose, leaving a nonvolatile residue in the injector and at the head of the column. Many researchers use a guard column of deactivated fused silica tubing between the injector and the analytical column. The guard column can be replaced periodically when it becomes contaminated. The tubing contains no liquid phase, thus it does not affect separation or retention time. The guard column can be connected to the analytical column with various types of press-tight connectors (10).

If the aqueous phase is too dilute, concentration techniques as described in the next section may be employed.

III. DIRECT SOLVENT EXTRACTION OF AQUEOUS SAMPLES

Aqueous samples are available from a number of sources. Industrial plant operations may yield such products. Carbonated beverages, fruit juices, and caffeinated beverages can often be extracted directly. Fruits and vegetables can be homogenized with water, treated with a pectinase enzyme to destroy the pectins, and filtered through a bed of diatomaceous earth to remove particulates.

A. Extraction

When relatively large amounts of aqueous samples are available, then separatory funnels or commercial liquid-liquid extractors may be employed. A large number of solvents have been summarized by Weurman (4) and reviewed by Teranishi et al. (5).

The solvents most commonly used today are diethyl ether, diethyl ether/pentane mixtures, hydrocarbons, Freons, and methylene chloride. The latter two have the advantage of being nonflammable. Solvent selection is an important factor to consider, and the current status has been summarized by Leahy and Reineccius (11). In general, the following suggestions can be made. Nonpolar solvents such as Freons and hydrocarbons should be used when the sample contains alcohol. Diethyl ether and methylene chloride are good general purpose solvents. Ether can form explosive peroxides, and for that reason contains inhibitors (e.g., BHT), which will show up in gas chromatography/mass spectroscopy (GC/MS) analysis. We find that methylene chloride is a satisfactory general purpose solvent, particularly for flavor compounds with an enolone structure (e.g., Maltol and Furaneol). It is somewhat toxic and is an animal carcinogen. To aid in extraction, sodium chloride may be added to the aqueous phase to salt out the organics when low-density solvents are employed.

If the sample contains any particulates, it should be filtered. A convenient way to filter samples is through a syringe filter (e.g., Gelman Sciences, Ann Arbor, Mich.) of the type recommended for HPLC sample preparation. These filters have a pore size of 0.45 μm and are solvent resistant. Microtypes with low solvent hold-up are available.

Figure 2 shows the total ion chromatogram of a coffee extract. In this case a decaffeinated roast and ground coffee was brewed in a commercial system. The brew was filtered through a Gelman 0.45 μm GHP Acrodisc to remove particulates, and the aqueous phase was extracted with methylene chloride. A highly complex chromatogram is evident. The large peak eluting at 25 minutes is caffeine.

Continuous extractors have been described in the literature for solvents more dense and less dense than water (e.g., Ref. 4) and are available commercially (e.g., ACE Glass, Vineland, NJ; Supelco, Inc, Bellefonte, Pa) for $200–600 (Fig. 3). These are a pleasure to use (providing there is no solvent loss and that emulsions don't occur) since they will operate relatively unattended. They are normally operated for 2–4 hours, but may be operated overnight.

Liquid carbon dioxide was recommended as an extracton solvent as early as 1970 (12). It has the advantages of being nontoxic and inexpensive. Liquid carbon dioxide is reported to have solvent properties similar to diethyl ether (12) and to be particularly selective for esters, aldehydes, ketones, and alcohols. If water is present, it will be removed also.

A commercial liquid carbon dioxide Soxhlet extractor is commercially available (J&W Scientific, Folsom, CA). The vessel holds a sample of 2.5 g. This apparatus seems to have achieved only limited use, perhaps because of its cost ($1500 plus accessories) and limited sample size. Moyler (13) dis-

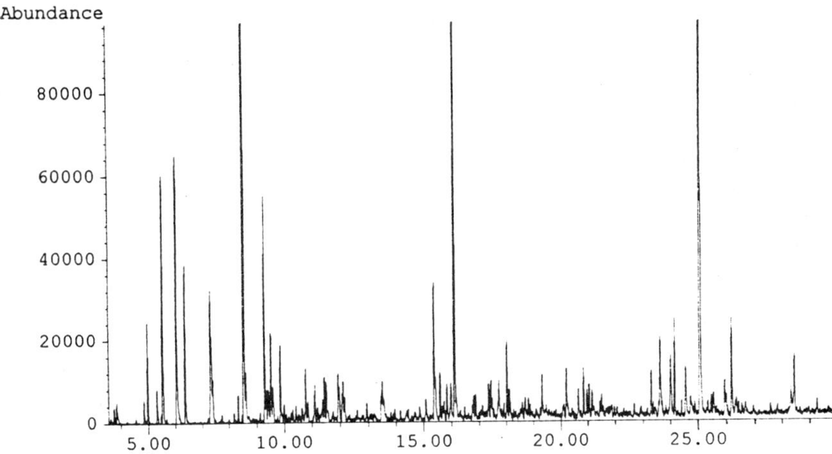

FIGURE 2 Total ion chromatogram (TIC) of brewed R&G coffee extracted with methylene chloride

cussed a commercial liquid carbon dioxide system and reported such extracts to be more concentrated than the steam distillates or solvent extracts. More important, he reported that the character was "finer."

Supercritical carbon dioxide has been employed recently as an extraction solvent. When using supercritical carbon dioxide, it is necessary to balance temperature, pressure, and flow rate, which requires complex instrumentation. Several instrument vendors produce supercritical fluid extractors in the price range of $25,000–90,000. Again, sample capacity is relatively limited.

B. Emulsions

Emulsions can be a problem, particularly if nonvolatile solutes are present. To prevent emulsions, the following methods can be employed:

Use gentle shaking
Filter the sample if particulates are present
Keep the system cool
Be patient
Adjust the pH of the aqueous phase

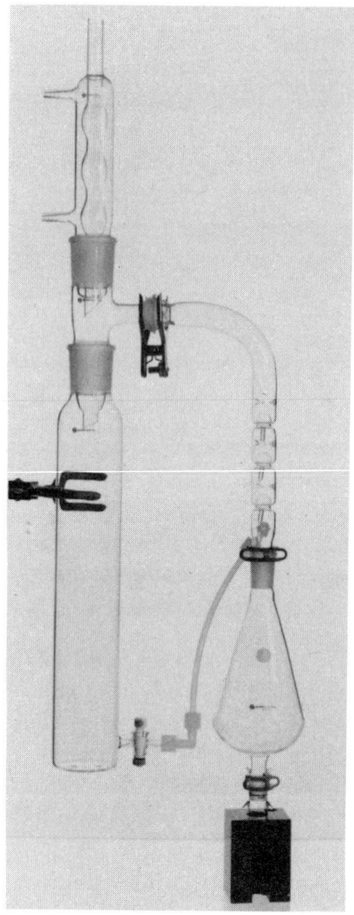

FIGURE 3 Liquid/liquid extractor concentrator apparatus. (Courtesy Supelco, Inc, Bellefonte, PA.)

The latter technique is particularly effective if organic acid, basic, or amphoteric compounds are present. If emulsions occur, centrifugation may be employed (but only for nonflammable solvents).

C. Concentration

The final step is concentration of the solvent. We usually dry the solvent over sodium sulfate or magnesium sulfate and then carefully concentrate it on a steam bath using a Vigreux column. A convenient method to concentrate large volumes of solvent is by use of a Kuderna-Danish Evaporative Concentrator, which is available in both macro (up to 1000 ml) and micro (1–4 ml) capacities for less than $100.

D. Impurities

High-boiling impurities both in solvent and sample will also be concentrated along with the desired analytes. Thus, solvent blanks should be prepared. If the sample was a direct extract, the solvent will contain nonvolatile components such as natural and Maillard pigments, lipids, alkaloids, etc. These may crystallize or precipitate on concentration and will leave a residue in the injector of the gas chromatograph.

For additional suggestions on extracting aqueous samples, see Sections IV and V.

IV. STEAM DISTILLATION OF SAMPLES FOLLOWED BY SOLVENT EXTRACTION

One of the most common sample-preparation techniques employed today involves steam distillation followed by solvent extraction. The primary advantage is that the distillation step separates the volatiles from the nonvolatiles. Other reasons for this include simplicity of operation, no need for complex apparatus, reproducibility, rapidity, and the range of samples that can be handled. Steam distillation works best for compounds that are slightly volatile and water insoluble. In addition, compounds with boiling points of less than 100°C will also pass over.

A. Direct Distillation

The sample is normally placed in a round-bottom flask and dispersed in water. The aqueous slurry can be heated directly (with continuous stirring) to carry over the steam-distillable components. Problems can be encountered due to scorching of the sample if too much heat is applied, and in addition bumping may occur when the sample contains particulates. Stirring may prevent these problems. Foaming is another potential problem. Many food products contain surface-active agents and will foam during distillation; addition of antifoams (e.g., DC polydimethyl siloxanes) may prevent this problem, but these silicones usually end up in the distillate, as evidenced by GC-MS peaks at m/z = 73, 147, 207, 221, 281, and 341.

B. Indirect Steam Distillation

Indirect steam distillation has many advantages over the direct technique. It is more rapid and less decomposition of the sample occurs since the sample is not heated directly. The steam may be generated in an external electrically heated steam generator or in a round-bottom flask heated by a mantle. It is even possible to use laboratory house steam, in which case the steam must be passed through a trap that allows removal of condensate and any particulates that may come out of the line. It is imperative that blank samples be run, since house steam may be highly contaminated. Even so, this technique has the great advantage of being rapid and easy. The steam and volatiles are usually condensed in a series of traps cooled with a succession of coolants ranging from ice water to dry ice/acetone or methanol.

C. Vacuum Steam Distillation

If sample decomposition remains a concern, then the steam distillation may be operated under vacuum. In this case inert gas should be bled into the system to aid in agitation. A number of cooled traps should be in line to protect the pump from water vapor and the sample from pump oil vapors. Another simple method to generate a condensate under vacuum is by use of a rotary evaporator. Bumping is normally not a problem in this case. The higher-boiling components do not distill as efficiently as they do under atmospheric pressure.

Once the vapors have been condensed, it remains to extract the sample, which is normally very dilute. Techniques described in Section III may be employed. In addition, there are two semi-micro extraction techniques that have value.

D. Extraction

Use of the Mixxor has been described by Parliment (14) and its utility described in a number of publications (15,16). Such a device is shown in Figure 4. These extractors are available with sample volumes ranging from 2ml to 100ml. The 10-ml capacity extractor is particularly convenient capacity for flavor research. Briefly, approximately 8ml of aqueous condensate is placed in receiver B and saturated with sodium chloride. The whole assembly is cooled and then a quantity of diethyl ether (typically 0.5–0.8ml) is added. The ether may contain an internal standard. The system is extracted by moving chamber A up and down a number of times. After phase separation occurs, the solvent D is forced into an axial chamber C, where it can be removed with a syringe

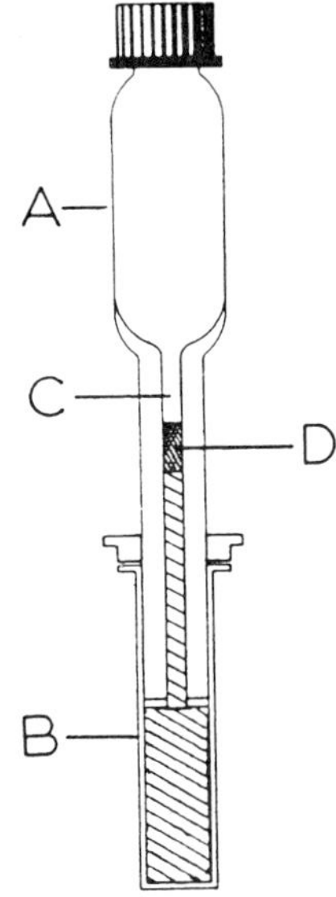

FIGURE 4 Mixxor apparatus for the extraction of aqueous samples. (From Ref. 14.)

for analysis. Percent recoveries for a series of ethyl esters from an aqueous solution were essentially quantitative even at the sub-ppm level. Unfortunately, these extractors were imported from Europe, and they are becoming difficult to procure.

A less sophisticated alternative exists. The sample may be placed in a screw-capped centrifuge tube and a small amount of dense solvent added. After exhaustive shaking, the tube can be centrifuged to break the emulsion and separate the layers. The organic phase can be sampled from the bottom of the tube with a syringe. Methylene chloride works well in this application.

Figure 5 compares the total ion chromatograms of two samples. Roasted and ground coffee was indirectly steam distilled at atmospheric pressure and a condensate collected. The upper curve in the figure represents the ethereal concentrate prepared via the Mixxor technique; the lower curve is the methylene chloride extract. Pattern differences are apparent. The largest peak in the ethereal extract (Rt = 6.0) is furfuryl alcohol; the largest peak in the lower curve (Rt = 8.5) is 5-methyl furfural.

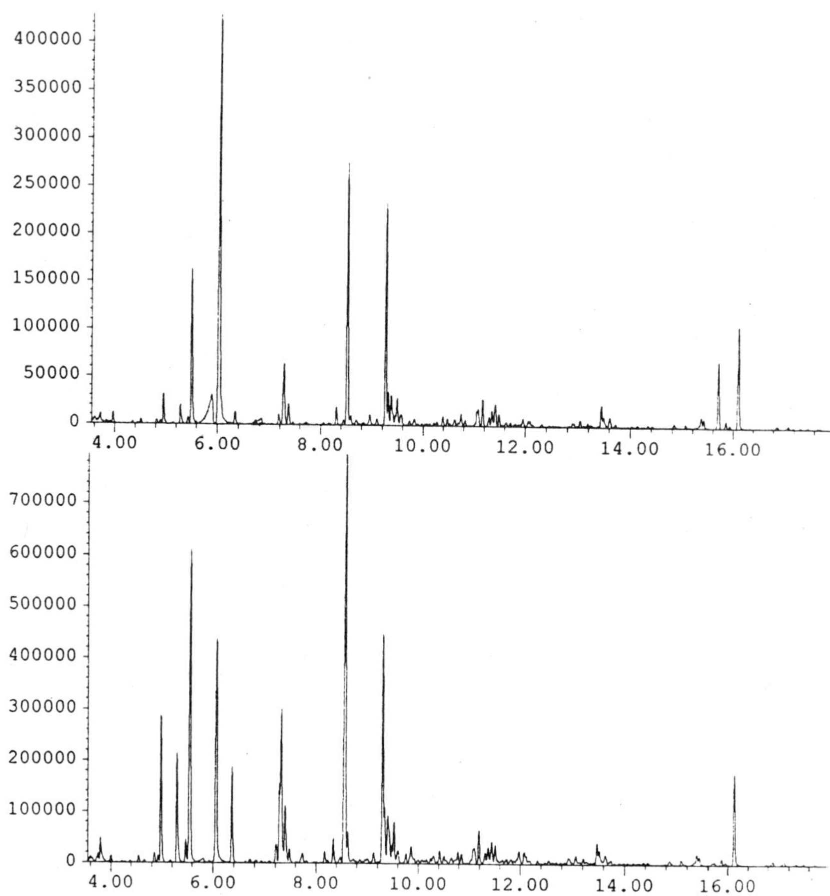

FIGURE 5 Comparison of chromatograms of etheral (upper) and methylene chloride (lower) extract of R&G coffee

E. Manipulation of the Aqueous Phase

Adjustment of the pH of the aqueous phase before extraction may accomplish two goals. First, emulsions may be broken, permitting phase separation to take place rapidly. Second, class separation will take place, which may simplify the gas chromatographic pattern. This is less necessary today since contemporary gas chromatography columns have high resolving power; however, frequently small peaks are concealed under larger ones, and the smaller ones may be revealed for organoleptic evaluation or identification.

This chemical manipulation of the aqueous phase can be carried even further. Many food aromatics contain carbonyl compounds. By adding sodium bisulfite to the aqueous phase, it is possible to selectively remove the aldehydes and the methyl ketones by forming their water-soluble bisulfate addition complexes. Thus, this analysis produces a carbonyl-free sample.

Figure 6 shows an example of such a manipulation. In this case the upper curve is the ethereal extract of a steam distillate of coffee at pH 3.6. The larger asymmetrical peaks at Rt = 5.8 and 6.8 represent fatty acids. These are eliminated at pH 10.0 (middle curve). The large peak at Rt = 3.8 in the latter is pyridine, a decomposition product of trigonilline. The lower curve in this figure is the material that remains after bisulfite extraction. It is immediately apparent that many of the lower boiling components of coffee are carbonyl in nature. For example, the peak at Rt = 5.5 is furfural. In this manner it is possible to simplify the gas chromatographic pattern.

If the aqueous phase is limited in quantity, the analyst can perform an interesting set of sequential experiments. The sample is placed in the Mixxor Chamber B, the pH adjusted to about 3 with acid, and the sample extracted with diethyl ether. Sufficient sample is removed for gas chromatographic analysis, e.g., 1 μl. The aqueous phase is made alkaline and the sample reextracted with the same diethyl ether and gas chromatographic analysis repeated. Finally, the sample is made neutral and saturated with sodium bisulfite and reextracted. The ethereal phase is reanalyzed. In this case three different analyses can be made from the same sample in a short period of time and subjected to GC-MS and organoleptic analysis.

V. SIMULTANEOUS STEAM DISTILLATION/EXTRACTION

One of the most popular and valuable techniques in the flavor analysis field is the simultaneous steam distillation/extraction (SDE) apparatus first described by Likens and Nickerson (17). The apparatus provides for the simultaneous condensation of the steam distillate and an immiscible organic solvent. Both liquids are continuously recycled, and thus the steam distillable-solvent soluble compounds are transferred from the aqueous phase to the solvent. The advantages of this system include the following:

1. A single operation removes the volatile aromas and concentrates them.
2. A small volume of solvent is required, reducing problems of artifact buildup as solvents are concentrated.

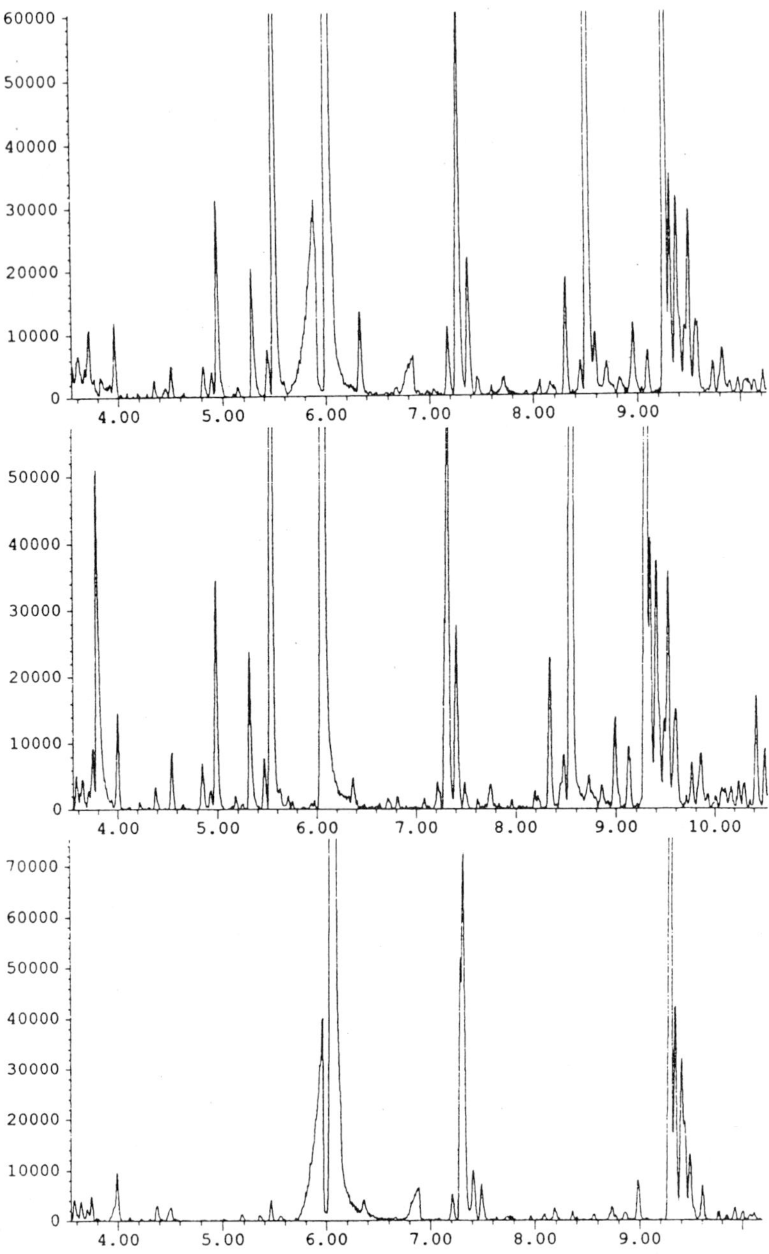

FIGURE 6 Comparison of chromatograms of R&G coffee extracted at pH 3.6 (upper curve), pH 10.0 (middle curve), and with bisulfite (lower curve).

3. Recoveries of aroma compounds are generally high.
4. The system may be operated under reduced pressure to reduce thermal decomposition.

A number of refinements have been made to the basic apparatus, some of which are shown in Figure 7a–d (9). One version is commercially available for less than $300 (J&W Scientific, Folsom, Ca); a diagram of it is shown in Figure 7e.

Typically the sample flask has a 500 ml to 5 liter capacity and contains the sample dissolved or dispersed in water so that the flask is less than half filled. Agitation is advisable if suspended materials are present to prevent bumping. As with all distillations, the pH of the sample should be recorded (and adjusted if necessary) prior to distillation. Heat may be supplied by a heating mantle or (better if solids are present) a heated oil bath with stirrer. The solvent is normally contained in a pear-shaped flask of 10–50ml capacity. Many solvents have been employed. In one model system study, Schultz et al. (18) compared various solvents as the extractant. They reported that hexane was an excellent solvent except for lower-boiling water-soluble compounds, where diethyl ether was considerably better. Use of methylene chloride has been recommended in a modified Likens-Nickerson extractor (19). Currently, most researchers appear to be using pentane-diethyl ether mixtures.

Regardless of which solvents are used, boiling chips should be added to both flasks to ensure smooth boiling. The distillation is generally performed for 1–3 hours. After the distillation is completed, the system is cooled and the solvent from the central extracting U tube is combined with that of the solvent flask. The solvent is dried over an agent such as sodium sulfate and concentrated by slow distillation.

An impressive example of the use of a Likens-Nickerson extractor is shown in Figure 8. This figure shows the gas chromatogram of a green and a roasted Kenyan coffee and shows how aromatic compounds are generated in the roasting process (W. Holscher, personal communication).

Vacuum versions of the SDE system have been described. These have the advantage of reducing the thermal decomposition of the analyte. Leahy and Reineccius report (11) that vacuum operation had a slightly negative effect upon recovery compared to atmospheric operation. Our experience is that operation under vacuum is quite complex since one must balance the boiling of two flasks, keep the solvent from evaporating, and hold the pressure constant.

Table 2 presents results of a series of experiments wherein typical flavor compounds in a model mixture were isolated by various SDE techniques. In

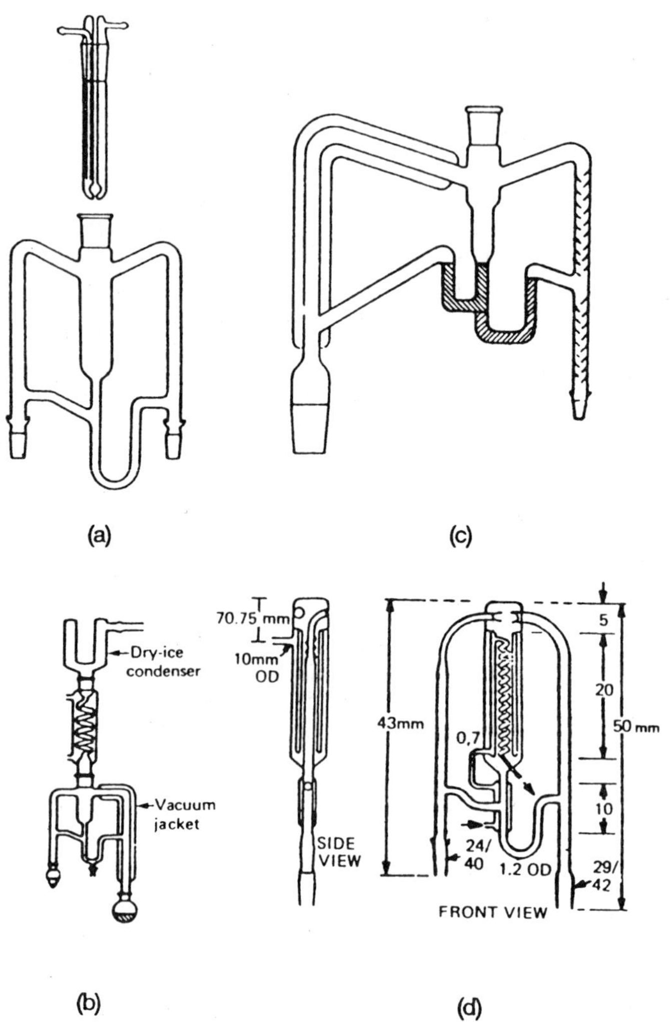

FIGURE 7 Various modificatins to SDE apparatus. (a,b,c,d from Ref. 9; e Courtesy J&W Scientific, Folsom, CA.)

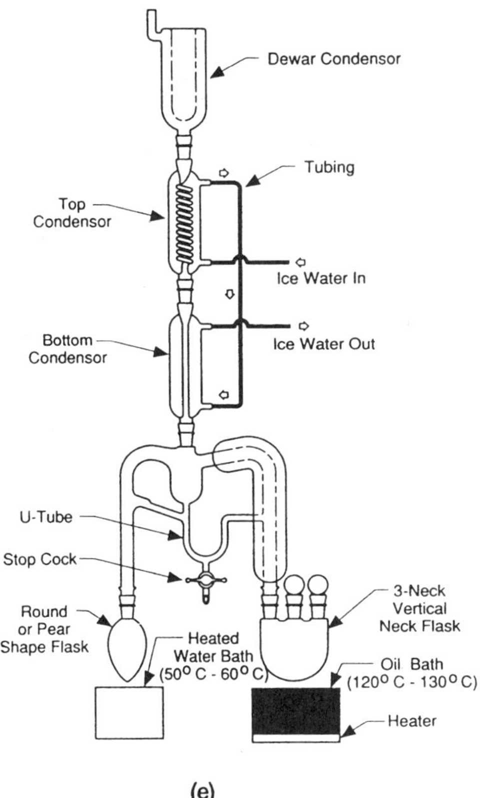

Figure 7 Continued

general, ether is a better solvent than hydrocarbons, and atmospheric pressure better than reduced pressure.

VI. DIRECT SOLVENT EXTRACTION OF SOLID SAMPLES

An entirely different process of sample-preparation technique involves direct solvent extraction, which is a very simple and convenient technique. Probably the easiest way to do such an extraction is with a Soxhlet extractor. A dried sample such as a spice, chocolate nib, R&G coffee, or a grain can be ground finely and placed in a Soxhlet thimble and extracted with an organic solvent. Either diethyl ether or methylene chloride may be used in such a system. After a number

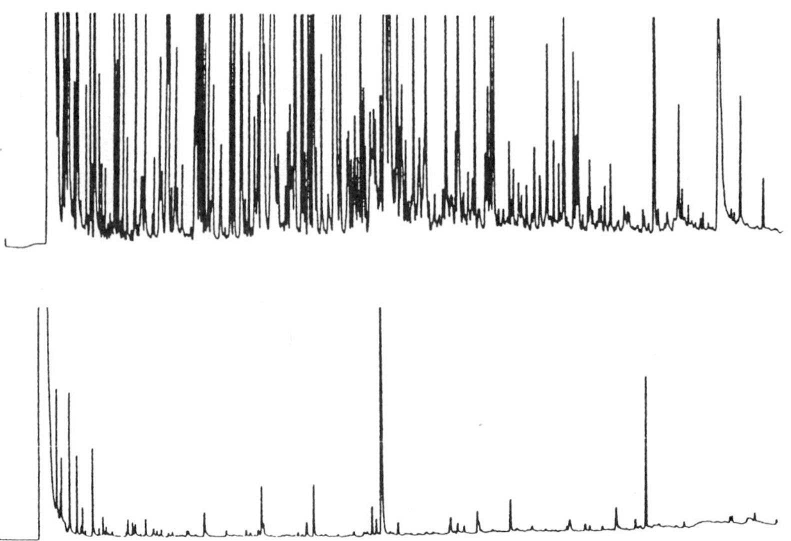

FIGURE 8 Chromatographic comparison of green and roasted coffee. (W. Holscher, personal communication.)

of cycles, the solvent can be combined and concentrated. Nonvolatile organic materials such as lipids, alkaloids such as caffeine and theobromine, and pigments will also be concentrated. The sample may be analyzed directly (with trepidation) or it may be treated as described in the section below, after removal of the solvent. If the sample contained large amounts of lipids (e.g., coffee, chocolate), then the volatiles may be removed by subsequent steam distillation or by a high vacuum stripping technique as described in Section VII.

Figure 9 is the GC-MS of a roast and ground coffee sample, which was moistened with water and extracted with methylene chloride in a Soxhlet extractor. The large component eluting at 26 minutes is caffeine.

VII. HIGH VACUUM DISTILLATION OF LIPIDS

A number of the procedures described in Section VI will yield a material that is primarily lipid in nature. In addition, many samples available to the researcher are themselves lipids. A few materials that one may encounter are coffee oil, vegetable and nut oils, cocoa butter, lard, butter oil, lipids used for deep fat frying, and lipids used as the solvent for Maillard reaction systems.

TABLE 2 Recovery of Components by SDE from the Model Mixture at a Concentration of 165 ppm (w/v) for Each Compound (Recovery as Percentage of Initial Amount)

Times of SDE	1 hr									4 hr
Pressure	Atmospheric pressure							100 mm Atm		
Vol. of solvent	125 ml							10 ml[a]	125 ml	125 ml
Solvent	Hexane					Pentane	Ether	Hexane	Hexane	Hexane
pH	3.4	5.0	6.5	7.8	5.0[b]	5.0	5.0	5.0	5.0	5.0
Ethyl acetate	0	0	0	0	0	59	89	19	0	0
Ethyl butyrate	98	99	99	91	99	101	97	84	100	98
Ethyl hexanoate	100	101	101	95	101	102	99	97	103	99
Ethyl octanoate	99	99	100	95	100	102	100	99	100	99
Ethyl 3-hydroxy-hexanoate	41	41	41	19	42	44	49	30	6	90
Ethanol	0	0	0	0	0	0	58	0	0	0
1-Hexanol	101	101	103	98	100	102	100	96	98	100
Linalool	73	99	100	96	99	99	97	97	99	98
Octanol	102	102	103	98	102	103	101	99	103	101
Citronellal	59	78	98	94	81	81	79	77	95	80
Carvone	98	97	98	95	98	99	97	97	92	99

[a]For this run, additional hexane (13 ml) was added through the vent to fill the overflow arm before the distillation was started, and the extract was not concentrated after SDE.

[b]1.0 ml of glacial acetic acid, titrated in solution to pH 5 with sodium hydroxide, was also present in this run in addition to the usual citrate buffer at 0.05 M.

Source: Ref. 18.

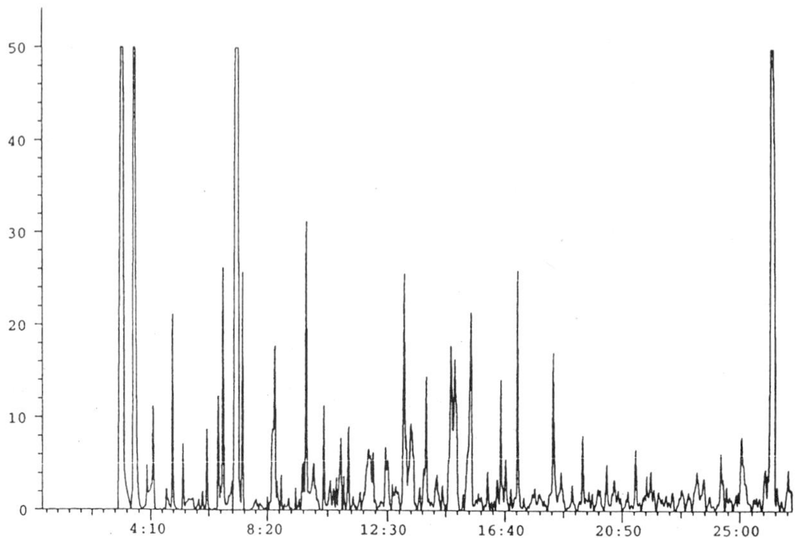

FIGURE 9 TIC of a roast and ground coffee sample moistened with water and extracted with methylene chloride.

Such materials can be a relatively rich source of aromatic compounds since aroma compounds are typically lipid soluble. A number of procedures can be used to prepare a sample. In this section we will cover three useful ones.

A. Steam Distillation

The lipid material may be steam distilled at atmospheric pressure or under vacuum, as was described in Section IV, and subsequently subjected to solvent extraction. Alternatively, a modified Likens-Nickerson extractor has been described (19), which permits the introduction of steam into the system. Recoveries of model compounds from lipid systems were not as satisfactory as for aqueous samples.

B. High Vacuum Distillation

When large amounts of lipid materials are present, the sample may be subjected to a falling film molecular still. The apparatus utilizes the principle of vaporization of the flavor from a heated thin film of the oil under high vacuum. One such apparatus is shown in Figure 10 (20). Several hundred milli-

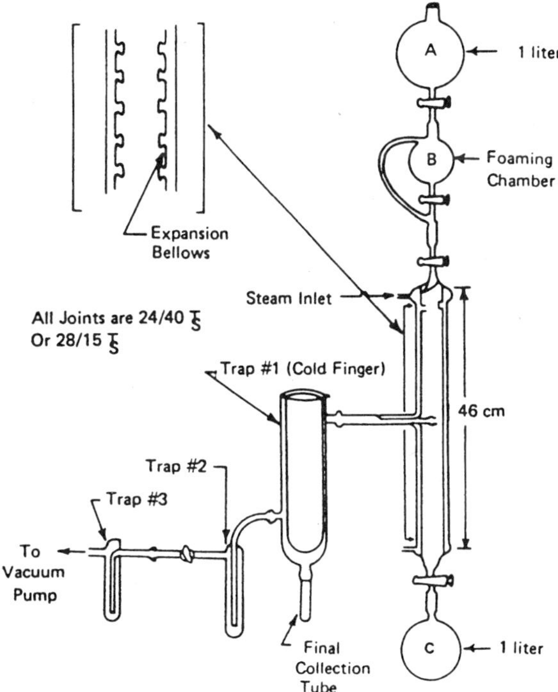

FIGURE 10 Falling film molecular still for the removal of volatiles from lipids. (From Ref. 20.)

liters of oil are placed in vessel A and slowly passed through the foaming chamber into the heated bellows chamber. The distillate is collected in a series of traps cooled with liquid nitrogen. The oil may be recycled. Another series of apparatus described by Chang et al. at Rutgers (21) has accomplished similar goals. This type of apparatus generally falls into the same category of equipment as that used to deodorize lipids.

C. Short Path Distillation

One version of the apparatus is shown in Figure 11a. The nonvolatile material is placed in the flask. The flask is heated while stirring the sample and a high vacuum is applied. The inner condenser is cooled with liquid nitrogen or dry ice-solvent (22). We have found this apparatus very useful for separating the volatile aromatics from nonvolatile residues (i.e., lipids) such as those gener-

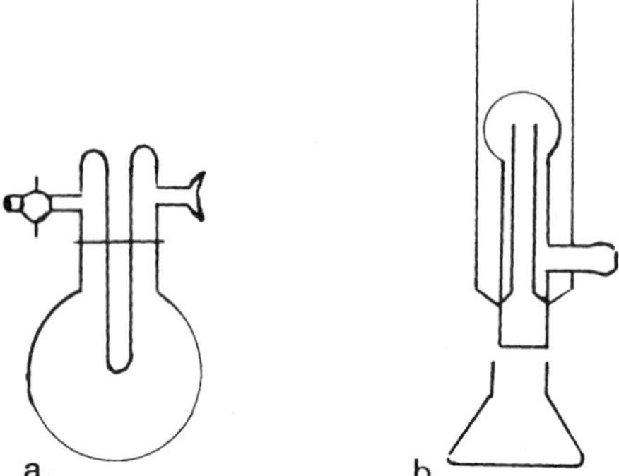

Figure 11 Apparatus for the removal of aromatics from lipids. (a from Ref. 22; b from Ref. 23.)

ated in Section VI. In that case the sample size may be only a few grams or less, and a smaller version of the short path distillation apparatus is appropriate. This apparatus can be easily fabricated by a glassblower.

An example of the application of such an apparatus is shown in Figure 12. The sample was produced by high vacuum distillation of 10 g of coffee oil ex-

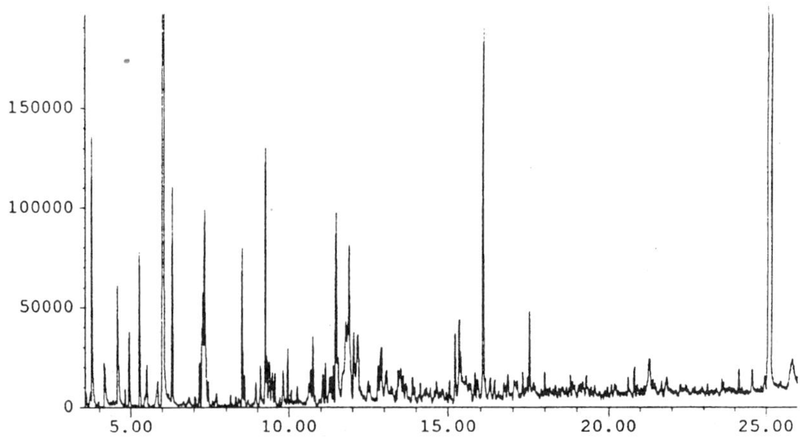

Figure 12 TIC of volatiles from roast and ground coffee oil, distilled in apparatus shown in Figure 11a.

pelled from roast and ground coffee. The volatiles were condensed with liquid nitrogen and subsequently washed off the cold finger with methylene chloride. Figure 12 shows the total ion chromatogram of the sample. The large peak eluting at 25 minutes is caffeine.

Nawar (23) has commented that the apparatus shown in Figure 11a may present problems if the sample contains water. He suggested the apparatus shown in Figure 11b. Vacuum is applied at point A, and vessel L is filled with liquid nitrogen during the 1-hour distillation period. At the end of the distillation, the cold trap is disconnected and the coolant is discarded. The condenser is inverted, the ice melted, and condensed volatiles and water extracted with a solvent. He reported greater than 80% recovery of high-boiling hydrocarbons in a model system study.

VIII. CO-DISTILLATION OF SAMPLE WITH SOLVENT

A new technique has been suggested by a group of Russian workers (24). They compared three methods of isolation, namely, distillation-extraction and two methods based on co-distillation of sample from solvent-water mixtures. In the co-distillation technique, a solvent such as diethyl ether, pentane, or methylene chloride is dispersed in the sample and the sample is distilled rapidly (at, e.g., 200°C) until all the solvent and a small amount of water have passed over. The sample is analyzed by gas chromatography. Their co-distillation technique (at atmospheric pressure) compared favorably with the Likens-Nickerson technique. They analyzed three samples: a model system, a meat sample, and a fish sample.

The chromatogram of an R&G coffee which was dispersed in water and co-distilled with solvent in our laboratory is presented in Figure 13. The curve is the total ion chromatogram of the sample, which has large caffeine peak eluting at 25 minutes.

The advantages of co-distillation are that isolates are generated without a boiled note, the process is efficient and reproducible, and it takes only 15–20 minutes for a distillation.

IX. SUMMARY

Over the years numerous procedures have been proposed for the isolation and identification of aromatic compounds. Because of the variation of sample types encountered, no single technique will always suffice. One must always be aware that none of these techniques will produce an isolate that quantitatively represents the composition of the starting material.

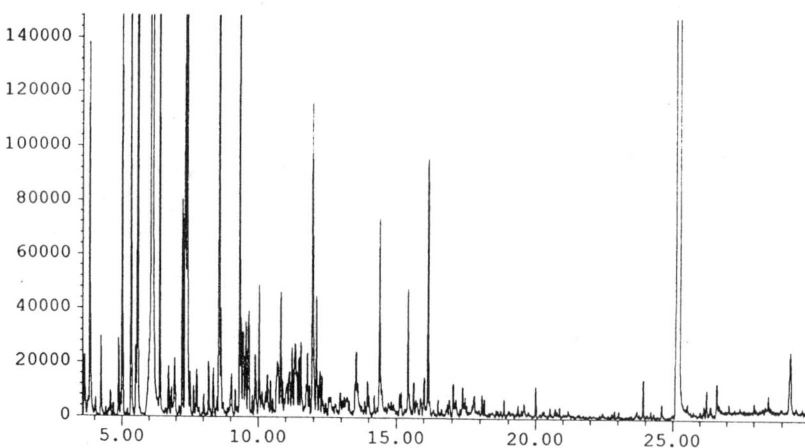

FIGURE 13 TIC of a roast and ground coffee sample co-distilled with methylene chloride

This chapter reviewed techniques that involve distillation and extraction procedures. These have the advantage of being simple and rapid, and they do not require a complex apparatus. For typical food products, some version of the Likens-Nickerson distillation apparatus is probably the technique of choice; for lipid materials, some high-vacuum distillation procedure is worth investigating initially.

REFERENCES

1. T. H. Parliment, "Sample Preparation Techniques for Gas-Liquid Chromatographic Analysis of Biologically Derived Aromas," in *Biogeneration of Aromas* (T. H. Parliment and R. Croteau, eds.), American Chemical Society, Washington, DC, 1986, p. 34.
2. G. Wasserman, H. Stahl, W. Rehman, and P. Whitman, *Kirk-Othmer Encyclopedia of Chemical Technology*, 4th ed., Vol. 6, John Wiley and Sons, New York, 1993, p. 793.
3. W. Jennings and M. Filsoof, Comparison of sample preparation techniques for gas chromatographic analysis, *J. Agric. Food Chem.* 25:440 (1977).
4. C. Weurman, Isolation and concentration of volatiles in food odor research, *J. Agric. Food Chem.* 17:370 (1969).
5. H. Sugisawa, "Sample Preparation: Isolation and Concentration," in *Flavor Re-*

search, Recent Advances, (R. Teranishi, R. Flath, and H. Sugisawa, eds.), Marcel Dekker, Inc., New York, 1971, p. 11.

6. S. Risch and G. Reineccius, "Isolation of Thermally Generated Aromas," in *Thermal Generation of Aromas* (T. H. Parliment, R. J. McGorrin, and C.-T. Ho, eds.), American Chemical Society, Washington, DC, 1989, p. 42.
7. H. Maarse and R. Belz, *Isolation, Separation, and Identification of Volatile Compounds in Aroma Research*, Akademie-Verlag, Berlin, 1981.
8. C.-T. Ho and C. H. Manley, eds., *Flavor Measurement*, Marcel Dekker, New York, 1993
9. P. Schreier, *Chromatographic Studies of Biogenesis of Plant Volatiles*, Huthig, New York, 1984.
10. *Restek Advantage 4*:7 (1993).
11. M. Leahy and G. Reineccius, "Comparison of Methods for the Isolation of Volatile Compounds from Aqueous Model Systems," in *Analysis of Volatiles. Methods. Applications* (P. Schreier, ed.), de Gruyter, New York, 1984, p. 19.
12. W. Schultz and J. Randall, Liquid carbon dioxide for selective aroma extraction, *Food Technol. 24*:1283 (1970).
13. D. A. Moyler, Carbon dioxide extracted ingredients for fragrances, *Perf. Flav.* 9:109 (1984).
14. T. H. Parliment, A new technique for GLC sample preparation using a novel extraction device, *Perf. Flav. 1*:1 (1986).
15. T. H. Parliment and H. D. Stahl, "Generation of Furfuryl Mercaptan in Cysteine-Pentose Model Systems in Relation to Roasted Coffee," in *Sulfur Compounds in Foods* (C. Mussinan and M. Keelan, eds.), American Chemical Society, Washington, DC, 1994, p. 160.
16. T. Parliment and H. Stahl, "Formation of Furfuryl Mercaptan in Coffee Model Systems," in *Developments in Food Science V37A Food Flavors: Generation, Analysis and Process Influence* (G. Charalambous, ed.), Elsevier, New York, 1995, p. 805.
17. G. B. Nickerson and S. T. Likens, Gas chromatographic evidence for the occurrence of hop oil components in beer, *J. Chromatog. 21:*1–3 (1966).
18. T. Schultz, R. Flath, R. Mon, S. Eggling, and R. Teranishi, Isolation of volatile components from a model system, *J. Agric. Food Chem. 25:*446 (1977).
19. C. Aug-Yeung and A. MacLeod, A comparison of the efficiency of the Likens and Nickerson extractor for aqueous, liquid/aqueous, and lipid samples, *J. Agric. Food Chem. 29:*502 (1981).
20. B. Johnson, G. Waller, and A. Burlingame, Volatile components of roasted peanuts: basic fraction, *J. Agric. Food Chem. 19:*1020 (1971).
21. S. Chang, F. Vallese, C. Hwang, O. Hsieh, and D. Min, Apparatus for the isolation of trace volatile constituents from foods, *J. Agric. Food Chem. 25:*450 (1977).
22. J. de Bruyn and J. Schogt, Isolation of volatile constituents from fats and oils by vacuum degassing, *J. Am. Oil Chem. Soc. 38:*40 (1961).

23. J. J. Balboni and W. W. Nawar, Apparatus for direct collection of volatiles from meat, *J. Agric. Food Chem. 18:*746 (1970).
24. T. Misharina, R. Golovnya, and I. Beletsky, "Comparison of the Efficiency of Isolation of Volatiles from Foodstuffs by Co-Distillation and Likens-Nickerson Methods," in *Developments in Food Sci. V35. Trends in Flavor Research* (H. Maarse and D. van der Heij, eds.), Elsevier, New York, 1994, p. 117.

2

Analysis of Food Volatiles Using Headspace–Gas Chromatographic Techniques

THOMAS P. WAMPLER
CDS Analytical, Inc., Oxford, Pennsylvania

I. OVERVIEW

Gas chromatography (GC) involves the analysis of volatile organic compounds, that is, materials that exist in the vapor phase, at least at the typical GC operating temperatures between 40 and 300°C. Since aroma compounds must, by their very nature, leave the food matrix and travel through the air to be perceived, they are generally excellent candidates for analysis by GC. Although many of these compounds may be solvent extracted, distilled, or otherwise isolated from the food matrix, it is frequently preferable to take advantage of their volatility and rely instead on techniques of headspace analysis.

Headspace sampling techniques are frequently divided into three broad categories: static headspace, dynamic headspace, and purge and trap. In each case, however, the fundamental principle is the same—volatile analytes from a solid or liquid material are sampled by investigation of the atmosphere adjacent to the sample, leaving the actual sample material behind. In static headspace techniques, a small sample (usually about 1 ml) of the atmosphere around the sample is injected directly onto the GC column. In dynamic techniques, the organic analytes from larger samples of the headspace are first concentrated, then transferred to the GC. Dynamic headspace techniques in their simplest form then are just ways to transfer a headspace sample which is too large to inject directly. The term "dynamic headspace" is usually used when referring to the analysis of solid materials, and the term "purge and trap" generally refers to the analysis of liquid samples by bubbling the purge gas through them.

All headspace techniques share certain advantages and considerations. Chief among these is that the analytes are removed from the sample matrix without the use of an organic solvent, so the resulting chromatogram has no solvent peak. This may be especially important when the compounds of interest are early eluters or are, in fact, solvents, and the presence of a solvent peak would both dilute and mask the analyte peaks. In addition, the effects of sample temperature, matrix solubility, and the volatility of the analyte are important considerations in optimizing a headspace assay, whether static or dynamic.

II. STATIC HEADSPACE

A. General Considerations

Even though the actual separation of the analytes in a gas chromatograph does take place in the vapor phase, most samples are injected as a solution of the analyte in some volatile solvent. The entire sample, solvent and analytes, vaporizes in the hot injection port, and the volatiles formed then proceed to the GC column. Many compounds, however, exist as gases at the temperature at which they are being sampled or have sufficiently high vapor pressure to evaporate and produce a gas phase solution. In these cases, the gas itself may be injected into the GC instead of a liquid solution, either by syringe or by transferring a known volume of vapor from a sample loop attached to a valve. The amount of gas that may be injected into a gas chromatograph is limited by the capacity of the injection port, the column, and consideration of the increase in pressure and flow in the injection port caused by a gas phase injection. In practical terms, injections are almost always in the low milliliter range, with sizes of 0.1–2.0 ml being typical. The utility of a headspace injection then depends on whether or not enough of the interesting analytes exist in a 1-ml gas sample to be detected reliably by GC. Many gas phase analyses are conducted by simple injection, including quality analysis of hydrocarbon products, natural gas, medical gases, and so on, and in general analytes present at about one part per million (ppm) may be assayed in a reproducible way using this technique.

The volatile analytes in a gas sample may have always been there, like argon in air, or they may migrate there from some other source, like air pollutants from the evaporation of spilled gasoline. The controlled analysis of vapors that have migrated into an atmosphere from some solid or liquid source forms the basis of static headspace analysis.

B. Static Headspace Sampling

If a complex material, such as a piece of food, is placed into a sealed vessel and allowed to stand, some of the more volatile compounds in the sample matrix will leave the sample and pass into the headspace around it. If the concentration of such a compound reaches about 1 ppm in the headspace, then it may be assayed by a simple injection of an aliquot of the atmosphere in the vessel. How much compound enters the headspace depends on several factors, including the amount of it in the original sample, the volatility of the compound, the solubility of that compound in the sample matrix, the temperature of the vessel, and how long the sample has been inside the vessel. The concentration of the analyte in the headspace also depends, of course, on the volume of the vessel being used. At equilibrium, the amount of compound A that has escaped from the sample matrix and exists in the surrounding atmosphere is just the total amount of A minus the amount still in the matrix:

$$A_{\text{Headspace}} = A_{\text{Total}} - A_{\text{Matrix}}$$

and the partition coefficient is just:

$$K_A = \frac{A_{\text{Headspace}}}{A_{\text{Matrix}}}$$

The amount of A that actually gets into the gas chromatograph depends on what portion of the total headspace is injected:

$$A_{\text{Injected}} = \frac{V_s}{V_T} A_H$$

where V_s is the volume of the syringe injection, V_T is the total volume of the headspace sampling vessel, and A_H is the amount of compound A in the total headspace.

Therefore, the amount of A injected is

$$A_I = (A_T - A_M)\frac{V_S}{V_T}$$

In practice, the food sample is placed into a headspace vial, sealed and warmed to enhance vaporization of the volatiles, and then allowed to stand for a period of time to establish equilibrium at that temperature. Once the volatiles have equilibriated, an aliquot of the headspace gas is withdrawn with a syringe and injected into the gas chromatograph injection port. As an alternative, the equilibrated headspace may be allowed to pass through a sample loop of known volume, which is subsequently flushed into the injection port. Static headspace analysis has been applied to a wide variety of sample types, including herbs (1) and fragrances (2).

C. Advantages of Static Headspace Sampling

Chief among the advantages of static headspace sampling is the ability to analyze a sample for low molecular weight volatiles without the presence of a solvent peak. This is especially important since many samples analyzed by static headspace are actually being assayed for residual solvent content. Packaging, pharmaceuticals, and many other processed materials incorporate the use of solvents in some step of their production, and the amount of those solvents retained in the finished product must be determined. Since the solvents are determined as analytes in a gaseous matrix, they are not diluted by a solvent that produces a response on the GC detector, so the chromatography is simplified and more sensitive.

In addition to eliminating the solvent peak, static headspace presents a technique that is easily automated (3,4), making it attractive for sample screening applications (5). Commercial instruments are available from many suppliers which automatically warm the sample vials, inject the headspace, and begin the GC run. These automated systems frequently transfer a measured sample loop full of headspace to the chromatograph instead of using a syringe. The combination of careful temperature monitoring, equilibrium time, pressure control of the sample loop, and automatic injection to the chromatograph provides increased reproducibility over manual attempts at headspace analysis, as well as freeing the analyst's time for other functions.

Additional advantages of the static headspace technique include relatively low cost per analysis, simple sample preparation, and the elimination of reagents. Since the sample analytes are not extracted from the sample material using a solvent, there is no need to deal with solvent reduction by evaporation either into the air, with its concerns about pollution, or by recondensing.

D. Disadvantages of Static Headspace Sampling

As discussed in Section II.B, any static headspace analysis can inject only a fraction of the compound of interest to the chromatograph, since the concentration in the headspace is in equilibrium with that still in the sample matrix, and only a portion of the headspace is withdrawn and transferred. Consequently, for very low levels of analyte concentration in the original sample material, static headspace techniques may lack the sensitivity required for the determination. Elevating the temperature of the sample generally increases the volatility of the analyte, but most static headspace instruments have the capability of heating samples only to about 150°C.

Analyses at fairly low temperatures also limit the usefulness of static headspace for analytes with higher boiling points. Many materials that may be extracted and solvent injected onto a GC column and that may elute well at higher column temperatures will be poorly represented in a static headspace sample produced with the sample at a cool temperature. Finally, reproducibility depends on analyzing a sample after it has reached equilibration, and the time required to achieve this point may, especially for less volatile compounds, be a drawback for some analyses.

III. DYNAMIC HEADSPACE

A. General Considerations

As the name implies, dynamic headspace involves moving the analytes away from the sample matrix in the headspace phase. Instead of allowing the sample volatiles to come to equilibrium between the sample matrix and the surrounding headspace, the atmosphere around the sample material is constantly swept away by a flow of carrier gas, taking the volatile analytes with it. This performs two functions relative to the concentration of the volatiles. First, it prevents the establishment of an equilibration state, causing more of the volatile dispersed in the sample matrix to leave the sample and pass into the headspace. Second, it increases the size of the headspace sample used beyond the limit of the actual sample vessel. It is not unusual to collect samples using a total volume of 100 ml to 1 liter of headspace, which may result in an essentially quantitative removal of the volatile analytes from the sample matrix.

To take advantage of this increased amount of volatile analyte, the entire dynamic headspace sample should be transferred to the gas chromatograph for a single analysis. This is accomplished by venting the carrier gas of the dynamic headspace through a collection trap, which retains the organic compounds while letting the carrier pass through. In this way, the analytes from a large headspace volume are concentrated in the trap, and a dynamic headspace instrument is frequently called a "sample concentrator." Since the sample is being purged with a flow of carrier and the analytes trapped for analysis, the technique is also frequently called "purge and trap." In general, the term "purge and trap" is used to refer to liquid samples analyzed by bubbling the carrier through the liquid, while "dynamic headspace" is used when the sample material is a solid. In either case, however, the principle of retaining, or concentrating, the organic analytes in a trap while venting a large headspace volume is the same. The trapping step may involve adsorption onto a high–surface area sorbent material or cold trapping by condensing or freezing the analyte in the trap.

A generalized diagram of a dynamic headspace instrument is shown in Figure 1. The valve may be a 6-port or an 8-port one, providing for directing flow from the sample to the trap in one direction and from the trap to the GC in the other. During sample collection, the headspace gas flows from the sample vessel through the valve, to the trap and out the vent, while GC carrier flow goes directly through the transfer line to the column. When the valve is rotated, the GC carrier is diverted through the trap, which is heated rapidly to revolatilize the collected organics, transferring them to the gas chromatograph for analysis.

Commercial instruments also provide for automatic drying of moisture from the trap, baking the trap at elevated temperatures between runs, and may include special options to handle water vapor from liquid samples, cryogenic

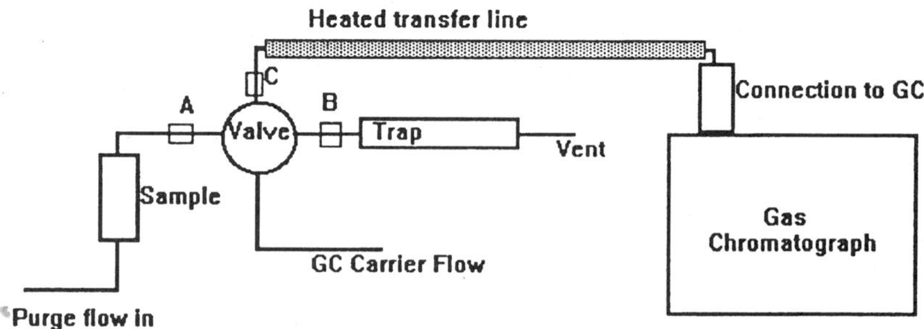

FIGURE 1 Simplified diagram of a general purge-and-trap/GC system.

ability for cold trapping, cryogenic refocusing on the GC column for sharper peaks, and automation of multiple samples.

B. Advantages of Dynamic Headspace/Purge and Trap

Dynamic headspace techniques offer many of the same advantages of static headspace (for a detailed comparison, see Ref. 6), including elimination of the solvent peak, analysis of just the volatiles, automation, and easy sample preparation. In addition, the trapping stage of the analysis offers increased sensitivity, permitting the analysis of volatiles present at the parts per billion (ppb) level routinely. With careful attention to contaminants and instrument background, it has been demonstrated that purge-and-trap techniques are capable of routine application in the parts per trillion (ppt) range (7). Further, sorbents offer some selectivity within the range of volatiles collected, so it may be possible to select a combination of sorbent and temperature which permits the collection and concentration of specific analytes while venting others, thus simplifying the analysis.

C. Disadvantages of Dynamic Headspace/Purge and Trap

Because the instrumentation requires the monitoring of several steps, valving, heating zones, and so on, purge-and-trap instrumentation is more complex, and may be more expensive to purchase, than other types of sample introduction. In addition, again because of the functioning of the instrument, there are many opportunities for malfunctions, including heater damage, valve leaking, contamination, and cold spots. The sources of error in purge-and-trap instruments have been reviewed by Washall (8), including sample storage, trap heating effects, carry-over and purging efficiency. Compared to static headspace, purge-and-trap techniques require a little more time per sample, for purging, trap drying, and trap transfer, all of which require approximately 15 minutes for a typical analysis. Some of this time is generally transparent, however, since there is no equilibration time, and much of the sample processing may be done while the gas chromatograph is still analyzing the previous sample.

D. Purging Vessels

1. Liquid Samples

Early applications of purge and trap were targeted at the environmental laboratory for the analysis of water samples. By purging the water with a flow of helium and trapping the purged organic pollutants, it was possible to assay analytes such as solvents at the low ppb and high ppt level routinely. Figure 2

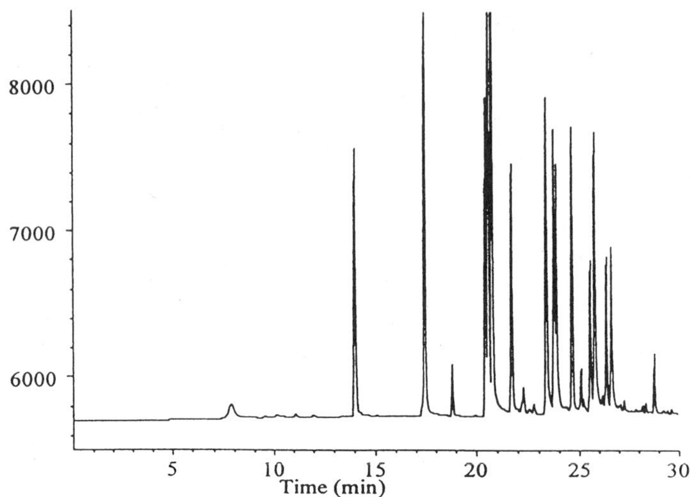

Figure 2 Purge-and-trap analysis of 5-ml water sample containing aromatics at 20 ppb each.

shows a typical analysis of water for aromatics, present at 20 ppb each. To maximize the surface area between the water and the bubbles of the purge gas, the gas was forced through a porous frit at the bottom of the vessel, making a stream of very fine bubbles, which then passed through the water, carrying away the volatile organic contaminants. These fritted vessels work well with clean samples, such as drinking water, but are not idea for all samples. If the sample contains solid particles, they may clog the frit, making it difficult to clean, creating carryover and impairing the efficiency. For samples other than clear water, a needle or impinger arrangement is used (Fig. 3). The purge gas is introduced through a needle or thin tube, which projects below the surface of the water. While the bubbles are larger, and therefore the purging is a little less efficient than with a fritted sparger, the whole system is easier to clean and permits the use of simpler, even disposable sample vessels. This type of purging vessel is especially well suited for the analysis of foods, which contain many constituents that make samples foam, and almost certainly include solids, oils, and other contaminating materials. A further advantage of the needle or impinger style vessel is that the tube is adjustable, so that the depth into the liquid sample is variable. For some samples, in fact, it may be best to have the purge gas enter just above the surface of the liquid, instead of actually bubbling through it. The purging efficiency is reduced, but if samples are

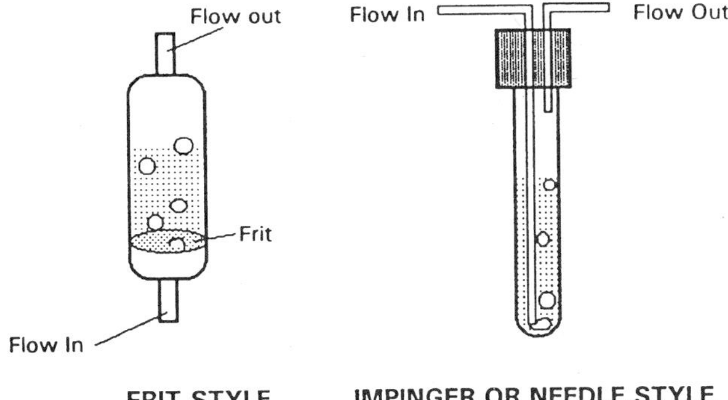

FIGURE 3 Purging vessels for liquid samples.

prone to foaming, this is an intermediate between static headspace and true purge and trap, which will provide increased sensitivity without contaminating the valving of the instrument by having the sample foam over into the pneumatics.

2. Solid Samples

Solid materials, including soils, polymers, foods, vegetation, and arson debris, just to name a few, are rarely purged in the kind of vessel used for a liquid sample, since the frit serves no purpose in these cases and would only be a point of contamination. Instead, the samples are generally placed into a heated flow-through cell (for small samples, just a tube). Flow is brought in at one end, passes through or around the sample, and exits out the other. For larger samples, including whole pieces of fruit, entire containers like cans and bottles, and so on, large "bulk" headspace samplers have been developed with internal volumes as large as 1 liter (Fig. 4). Flow is usually brought in and exits through smaller tubing, rather than making the large sampler a huge tube, because of sealing considerations.

In general, some additional sampling problems are introduced when using such large sample containers. These problems should be considered when choosing whether to analyze a portion of a sample in a small tube or the entire sample in a large vessel. Some analysts are concerned about the representative quality of a small piece taken from a large sample and therefore choose to analyze the entire thing, requiring a sample vessel with considerable volume. It must be remembered, however, that the larger the fittings used, the more difficult it is to seal them, and the more likely the sample vessel will leak. Further,

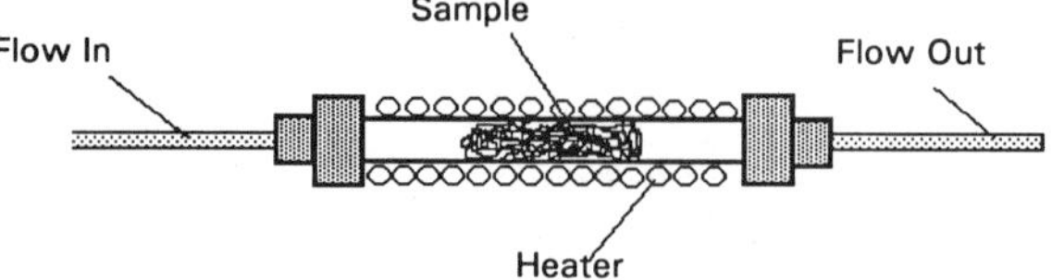

THERMAL DESORPTION TUBE

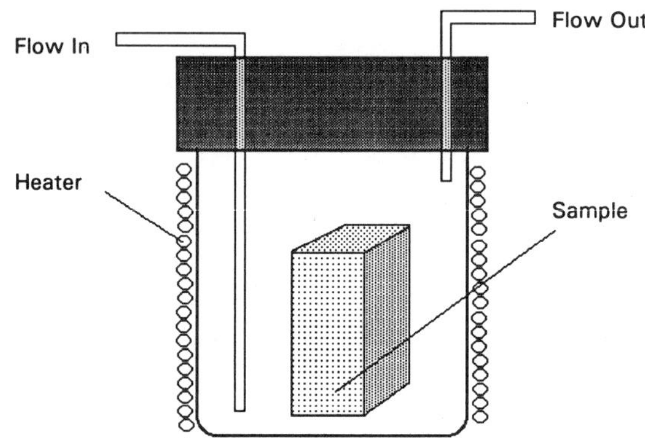

BULK HEADSPACE SAMPLER

FIGURE 4 Sample vessels for dynamic headspace analysis of solid materials.

if the sampling is to be done by introducing a flow of carrier gas into the sample chamber, the entire chamber must be pressurized enough to overcome the backpressure of the sorbent trap before any carrier will flow out of the vessel to the trap. In a small vessel this is not usually a problem, but in a larger vessel, because of the increased surface area, it becomes much more likely that the seals will leak or even that the top of the will pop off before flow is established to the trap. In addition, the time required to sample such a large volume is increased, since there is mixing and turbulence inside the headspace chamber. Finally, there are temperature considerations. The larger a sample, the less likely that all parts of it are at the same temperature and the longer it takes to establish thermal equilibrium. Since most sample vessels are heated from the outside, the larger the vessel, the larger the temperature gradient across it. It may be necessary to monitor the temperature at both the heater location and at the actual sample location, or at several sample locations, to have a clear idea of what the actual temperature is during sampling.

Some of these problems may be avoided by using a vacuum sampling approach instead of a pressurized sample purge for large vessels. In this way, the sample vessel does not have to be pressurized to overcome the backpressure of the trap, and loss of analytes due to vessel sealing is less likely. Instead, the vent of the trap is connected to a vacuum pump, and the sample is pulled from the vessel through the trap, then sent out the pump vent. An inlet tube into the sample vessel provides for replacement air or sample gas, so that the vessel stays at one atmosphere throughout the sampling.

E. Trapping

Regardless of the sample vessel type—fritted, impinger, thermal desorption tube, or bulk sampler—its function is to remove volatile organics from the sample matrix and carry them away in the purge gas flow. The carrier gas then proceeds to the trap, where the volatiles are retained and the carrier is vented. Selection of the trapping technique and medium depends on several factors, including:

Chemical nature of the analyte
Thermal stability of the analyte
Sorption and desorption characteristics of the sorbent
Breakthrough volume of the analyte on the sorbent
Availability and cost of cryogen
Presence of contaminating materials, including water vapor

1. Sorbent Trapping

Many organic compounds can be removed from a stream of gas by passing them through a tube packed with a finely divided sorbent material. Because of the high surface area of the sorbent, the organic vapor is likely to collide with it and may be adsorbed onto its surface. This is the same principle used for purifying gases and liquids by forcing them through a filter, frequently filled with activated charcoal, but in this case the fluid (carrier gas) is discarded and the trapped materials are the compounds of interest. In an ideal case, the organic volatile is held by the sorbent at room temperature while other materials pass through, and the analyte can be desorbed by heating the trap only enough to revolatilize it but not enough to cause thermal degradation. In fact, this is the case for many organic compounds, which makes the analysis of water samples for organic pollutants like solvents very straightforward by purge and trap. Other compounds are not well sorbed, or behave well only on sorbents that also collect unwanted materials. Some sorbents are quite stable thermally, whereas others produce artifacts at desorption temperatures. Some sorbents hold volatiles so efficiently that they must be heated to quite high temperatures to release them, perhaps causing thermal damage in the process. Part of the method-development stage of any dynamic headspace technique involves evaluation of the sorbent/analyte interaction and selection of the best trapping material. It is sometimes necessary to use more than one sorbent in a trap, especially if a wide range of volatiles is to be trapped, and some analysts prefer to collect the volatiles by cryogenics onto some inert surface and eliminate sorbents altogether.

Tenax®

Most sorbent materials are porous polymers similar to (or identical to) the kinds of materials used to fill packed GC columns for gas analyses. Tenax® (poly-2, 6-diphenyl-*p*-phenylene oxide) is perhaps the most widely used, general purpose sorbent for dynamic headspace techniques. It is capable of sorbing a fairly wide range of organic volatiles, is especially good with aromatics, may be heated to relatively high temperatures for desorption, and is long lasting. It is not suitable for very volatile hydrocarbons (pentane and below) or for small alcohols, which is frequently an advantage. Because it has been used for dynamic headspace–type analyses for such a long time, there is much information available in the literature regarding its suitability for particular analyses.

Other Sorbents

Although it is sometimes regarded as a "universal sorbent," Tenax® is not suitable for every application, and many analysts choose to augment or replace it with other sorbent materials (9). In an effort to extend the purge-and-trap technique, the U.S. Environmental Protection Agency (EPA) has devised additional traps, which use Tenax® as the primary sorbent backed by other, more retentive sorbents. To concentrate on a wide range of volatiles, such as in EPA method 502.2, which includes compounds as light as vinyl chloride and as heavy as trichlorobenzene, the trap specifies Tenax®, silica gel, and activated charcoal. As a general rule, the more retentive the sorbent or the smaller the molecules it is capable of retaining, the more heat is required to desorb the analytes and regenerate the trap. A particular problem with activated charcoal, and especially silica gel, is their tendency to adsorb water, which must be dealt with if it is not to be transferred to the gas chromatograph.

For the analysis of small molecules by trapping and thermal desorption, several new sorbent materials have been introduced that provide the retentive ability of activated charcoal, but collect less water. Graphitized carbon sorbents (Carbotrap, Carbopack) can collect hydrocarbons larger than propane and release then thermally. Very small molecules, such as chloromethane, may be trapped using carbon molecular sieves, which differ from standard, inorganic molecular sieves in that they are prepared by charring polymers at high temperatures. These include the various Carbosieves™, Carboxen™, and Ambersorb™ materials, with Carboxen™-569 in particular reported as having a very low water affinity, increasing the ability to collect small organics without transferring too much water to the analytical instrument. Various combinations of these sorbents, with and without Tenax®, have been demonstrated to provide both good trapping efficiency and may be desorbed at relatively high temperatures, producing a tighter analyte plug transferred to the gas chromatograph. This results in better chromatographic resolution, particularly for the early eluting peaks in the chromatogram.

Breakthrough Volume

When a volatile organic compound enters a bed of trapping material in a carrier gas stream, it may be adsorbed by the packing, but not irreversibly, since it is important to desorb it later for analysis. Some materials are quite firmly adsorbed and will remain on the surface of the sorbent for a considerable time, requiring fairly high temperatures (150–250°C) to remove them. Other compounds are not as well adsorbed, even at room temperature, and will eventually work their way through the sorbent bed, just as a retained compound works its way through a GC column. The volume of carrier gas that may be passed through a trap before a particular analyte leaves the other end of the sorbent bed is called the breakthrough volume. The breakthrough volume depends on the nature of the compound, its volatility, the interaction between the compound and the sorbent, the amount of sorbent used, and the temperature of the trap. In practice, a safe sampling volume is used to develop a sampling technique, which is a smaller volume than the actual breakthrough volume and is reported per gram of sorbent material.

2. Cryogenic Trapping

Advantages

Even well-conditioned solid sorbents exhibit out-gassing at the temperatures required for thermal desorption of adsorbed compounds. Tenax®, for example, produces aromatic volatiles at temperatures above 180°C. For many applications, the amount of organic material produced from the polymer sorbent may be negligible, but for trace-level applications the presence of background peaks from the sorbent may be a problem. This is accentuated in the analysis of heavier organics, since they require a higher desorption temperature to transfer from the trap to the gas chromatograph. Frequently the desorption parameters become a compromise between temperatures high enough to desorb the analytes efficiently but low enough to minimize artifacts. One solution is to eliminate the sorbent altogether and collect the analytes cryogenically (10).

Liquid nitrogen (boiling point –196°) and solid carbon dioxide (boiling point –79°) have both been used to chill traps for cryogenic sample concentration. Whether one uses liquid nitrogen or carbon dioxide depends on availability, cost, and the temperature range desired. Although it may seem that CO_2 would suffice for many purposes, the fact is that many analysts find they need temperatures of –100°C or colder to collect their analytes efficiently. The pneumatics involved in delivering liquid nitrogen and CO_2 as cryogens are significantly different and generally not interchangeable. Liquid nitrogen is usually used at about 20 psi, while CO_2 is supplied at about 900 psi. Further, nitrogen stays as a liquid when delivered, while CO_2 becomes a solid, so the cryogenic wells used as reservoirs to cool the trap must be designed differently.

By replacing the trap packing with glass beads, glass wool, or some other inert material, surface area is provided for the analytes to condense upon during trapping. When the collection step is complete, the trap need only be heated enough to volatilize the analyte, since it is not necessary to desorb the compounds from the surface of a sorbent. This has additional advantages for the collection of thermally unstable materials, which could decompose at temperatures required for desorption from a porous polymer or charcoal.

Perhaps the greatest advantage of cryogenic trapping is the ability to tune the trap to the analytes of interest. By chilling the trap just enough to condense a particular analyte, other, more volatile compounds may be allowed to pass through and vent from the system, simplifying the analysis. On the other hand, since traps may be cooled to temperatures below –180°C using liquid nitrogen, very volatile analytes (with the exception of methane) may be collected, which would break through ordinary sorbent traps. Some analysts use a combination of sorbent and cryogenics to extend the range of the sorbent, for example, using a cryotrap filled with Tenax®. For applications needing only sorption, the Tenax® is used at room temperature. When light hydrocarbons or small alcohols are needed, the collection temperature is dropped and the sorbent becomes a cold surface for condensation, just like glass beads in a standard cryotrap.

Disadvantages

Although in theory one can tune the trap temperature to collect only the desired compounds, in practice there may well be compounds that behave similarly to the analytes of interest and are collected anyway. In general, any compound with a boiling point higher than that for which the trap collection temperature was designed will also be trapped. Perhaps the most troublesome is water, since it is present in many samples and creates significant chromatographic problems. Since the point of using cryogenics is to collect at subambient temperatures, it should be assumed that if water is present in the sample, it will be condensed or frozen in the cryotrap.

A second drawback to cryogenic collection is the cost of the additional instrumentation needed to handle the cryogen, including solenoids capable of functioning at 180°C below zero, control electronics, and the cost of the cryogen itself. If the trap is filled with glass beads for a clean background, cryogen must be used for every run. In addition, there is a finite time—a few minutes each run—needed to bring the trap from a rest temperature to the cryogenic temperature for collection. A finial caution involves cold spots. It is important to consider the effects on the system as a whole of cooling a portion of it to −100°C. Even if the cryogenic trap has its own heater, adjacent portions of the pneumatic path, especially unheated fittings, will also be cooled, and may warm slowly if not specifically heated. The longer the trapping time, the more pronounced this effect becomes, and the more important it is to investigate portions of the flow path that may be inadvertently cooled, creating a source for subsequent poor chromatography, bleed, inefficient transfer of heavier materials, etc.

F. Water Management

Whether performing purge-and-trap analysis of a water sample, a beverage, or dynamic headspace of a food material, the sample matrix is likely to contain substantial amounts of water, much of which may be carried away from the sample and collected with the analyte compounds. Since the presence of even 1 µl of water on a capillary GC column poses a serious analytical problem, it is important to remove this water one way or another before transferring the trapped organics to the chromatograph.

There are several approaches to managing water vapor in dynamic headspace analyses, including selection of a trapping medium that is hydrophobic, trapping the water independently of the analytes (11), venting the water independently, and combinations of these.

One reason for the popularity of Tenax® as a sorbent is its low affinity for water, even if the sample being purged is aqueous, so the purge gas is essentially saturated. A trapping tube filled with 100–150 mg of Tenax® will still retain about 1 μl of water for each of 40 ml of purge gas used in the process, so a 10-minute purge cycle at 40 ml/min would deliver about 10 μl of water to the trap. Since Tenax® does not adsorb water, however, it is usually enough to pass a source of dry carrier gas through the trap for a minute or two to vent the water from the trap without disturbing the organics, which are actually adsorbed onto the surface of the Tenax®. The carbon molecular sieve Carboxen™-569 is reported also to be highly hydrophobic and useful in collection of smaller molecules or in conjunction with Tenax® for a wider-range sorbent trap.

In addition to drying the trap by purging it with a dry carrier, there are approaches used to prevent the water from reaching the trap in the first place or to eliminate it from the analytes as the trap is backflushed to the gas chromatograph. In the simplified diagram of a purge and trap shown in Figure 1, the positions marked A, B, and C are possible locations for water-removal devices. Position A is located just after the sample, before the carrier gas goes through the valve to the trap, B is located just upstream of the trap, after the valve, and C is positioned after the trap, just before the gas chromatograph itself. At location A or B, a device could be added that would remove water vapor from the purge stream but not affect the organic volatiles, which would still be collected on the trap. Since A and B are upstream from the trap, the size, volume, and so on involved here would not affect the quality of the chromatography. A device at location C, on the other hand, must be designed keeping in mind that the analytes passing through it are on their way to the GC column and additional volume here could cause peak broadening.

Two types of devices are in current use to help remove water vapor from the analytical stream of a purge-and-trap instrument, namely, condensation and permeation. The condensation units produce an intentional cold spot in the pneumatics of the system, providing an area for water to condense out of the carrier. There is always the concern that less volatile organics will drop out as well, at least partially, reducing recovery and contaminating subsequent runs. In general, most of the water present in a purge stream can be removed by passing the carrier through a zone at about 25°C, while many organics, even substituted aromatics and naphthalene, stay vaporized and pass through to the trap. Some instruments use a plain piece of stainless steel or nickel tubing at positions A or B to accomplish this, whereas some fill the tubing with glass beads to increase the surface area. These zones should have independent heaters permitting the collected water to be vaporized and vented from the water trap before the next run, or eventually the water trap will become saturated and stop functioning. Some instruments actively cool these zones, using either a cryogen or a Peltier device to increase the efficiency of the water collection. Care must be taken to control the temperature, since the colder the trap, the more likely that compounds other than water will be condensed in the zone. If the cold spot is placed between the trap and the gas chromatograph at position C, the effect of either the internal volume or the temperature on the quality of the chromatography must be taken into account. For some techniques, a fairly large volume is used, and split capillary chromatography is recommended to provide more rapid transfer of the analytes through the volume, reducing peak broadening. As an alternative, spitless chromatography may still be performed regardless of the volume of the water trap at C if cryogenic refocusing is performed at the gas chromatograph connection.

Permeation or diffusion devices eliminate water by having it pass through the wall of the drying tube while the analyte molecules stay in the carrier stream. Nafion® tubing is quite efficient in its ability to remove water vapor from a gas stream, partly becuase its polymer structure includes sulfonic acid groups. A drying tube made with Nafion® is usually a double-walled device, with the analytical stream passing through the center of the Nafion® tube in one direction and a flow of dry air passing the outside of the Nafion® in the other direction. Water is removed from the inside gas stream by the sulfonic acid groups in the polymer and transferred through the polymer tube to the dry countercurrent air flow, where it is removed from the system.

Whichever water-elimination device is used, its effect on the organic analytes in the carrier stream is increasingly pronounced the more similar the analyte is to water. Polar compounds, especially small alcohols, are likely to be affected by diffusion-type dryers, while the higher the boiling point of an organic, the more likely it is to be slowed in its transfer though a condensation trap.

G. Applications

1. Liquid Samples

Since purg and trap was originally developed for the analysis of volatile organics in water, it seems a logical extension to apply the technique to food samples that are largely aqueous. In fact, a significant amount of work has been done by purge and trap in the analysis of beverages, [an excellent early compilation is by Charalambous (12)] including wine (13,14), beer (15), milk (16), coffee (17), and fruit juices (18–20). There are several important practical consideratins when applying a process designed for the analysis of trace levels of volatiles in water to samples like fruit juices, including the fact that many of the volatile constituents are present at levels much higher than those encountered in environmental analyses. Beers and wines have levels of alcohol in the percent range, rather than the ppb range, so care must be taken to select an appropriate sample size, and dilution or carrier gas splitting may be required to prevent overloading the gas chromatograph. In addition, many beverages contain high levels of sugars, and undissolved solids, and oils, which can produce foaming in the sample vessel, contamination, and carry-over to the next run.

For many beverage samples, it is wise to start with a significant dilution for the first analysis and increase the strength of the sample after an initial evaluation of the chromatography and the behavior of the sample in the instrument. Fritted purging vessels are frequently a problem, since the bubble size is intentionally small, which accentuates foaming, and the foam can be forced out of the vessel into the pneumatics of the instrument. Better results are frequently obtained using an impinger or needle style of sparging arrangement, which results in a few larger bubbles and reduced foaming. Even here, some samples like fruit juices can produce large bubbles, which continue up the vessel and into the plumbing. There are two approaches that can help limit this effect. The incorporation of a bubble breaker into the top of the purging vessel will prick the bubbles and allow the fluid to run down the sides of the vessel. The second idea is to place the sparging gas delivery tube just above the surface of the sample liquid instead of below it. While this reduces the efficiency of the purging process, many samples are sufficiently concentrated to provide ample volatiles even if the liquid is not actively bubbled. A variation of this approach is to take a very thick liquid such as a juice concentrate and coat a small sample as a film onto the surface of the purging vessel. This increases the surface area of the sample and promotes increased recovery from the purge gas without causing foaming. In such cases, a smaller, concentrated sample may be easier to analyze than a larger, dilute one.

Figures 5 and 6 show chromatograms of two samples of diet cola. In each case, 0.5 ml of the soda was diluted to 5 ml, then purged at room temperature with an impinger to a Tenax trap. Most of the volatiles recovered are citrus oil constituents, which are used to give colas most of their flavor, with the largest peak at about 10 minutes being limonine. Considerable variation was found among various colas, including diet and regular, canned and fountain. The differences were in both the absolute amount of the oil compounds present and in the relative amounts of specific peaks, indicating that a variety of citrus oils was used in flavoring the different beverages.

Vegetable oils (21–23), fish oils (24) and other nonaqueous liquids (25), including emulsions have also been studied using purge-and-trap techniques, especially for volatile constituents that indicate the freshness, stability, oxidation, or spoiling of the oils.

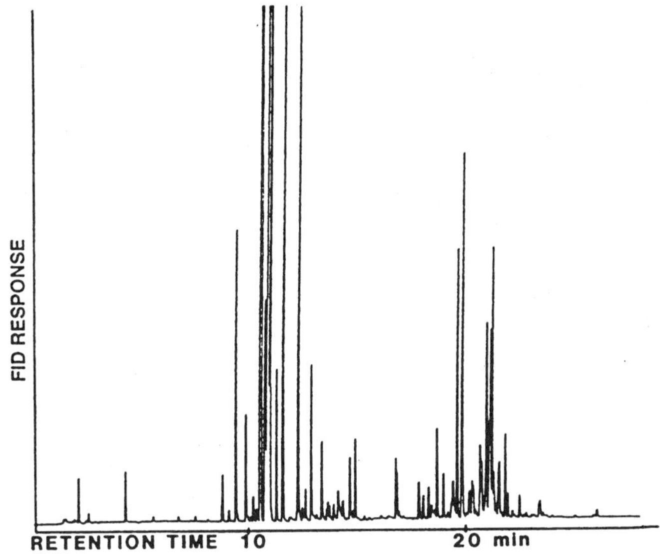

FIGURE 5 Purge and trap analysis of 5 ml of a 1/10 dilution of diet cola beverage.

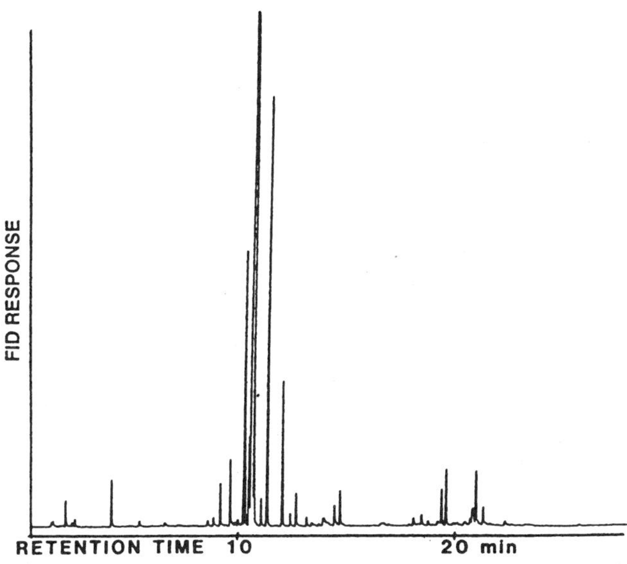

FIGURE 6 Purge and trap analysis of a 5-ml sample of a 1/10 dilution of another diet cola beverage.

2. Semisolid Samples

Some sample materials are neither free-flowing liquids nor stable solids, but blended to be pastes, gels, spreads, etc. These materials may provide a special sampling consideration. While liquids may be placed into a small bottle or vessel to purge and solids (see next section) may be warmed and purged from a tube or cartridge, semisolids may change their character while being sampled. If the sample is to be warmed to increase volatility of the analytes, the effect of increasing the temperature on the sample composition must be taken into account. A material may be fairly solid at room temperature, so thermal desorption in a tube may seem appropriate, but if it melts and flows at a warmer temperature, the sample material may run into the pneumatics of the instrument and cause considerable contamination. These samples may be diluted with water and sparged, or a small sample may be suspended in a large amount of material to provide surface area for the melted sample to spread onto. Figure 7, for example, shows a 2-mg sample of toothpaste sampled at 70°. Dilution of the toothpaste in water before running could produce a foaming problem, so the sample was placed in the center of a glass tube filled with glass wool. There was much more glass wool than toothpaste, so when the sample was warmed and began to spread, it just migrated into the glass wool. After a few minutes, the water from the sample was purged out, and a solid residue of the nonvolatile materials remained in the glass wool af-

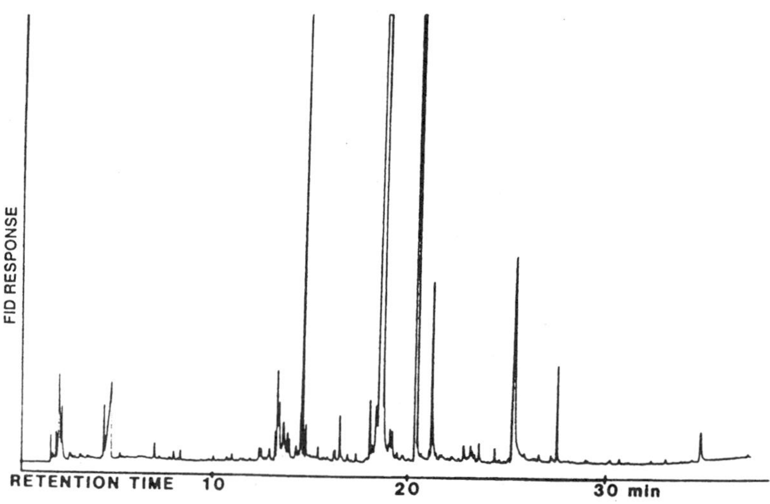

FIGURE 7 Dynamic headspace analysis of 2-mg sample of toothpaste at 70°C.

ter sampling. Other semi-solid foods such as cheeses (26) have been assayed using dynamic headspace techniques. Figure 8 shows a comparison of cheddar and American cheeses analyzed in the same manner as the toothpaste. Thirty-milligram samples were placed into glass tubes and surrounded by glass wool to prevent the oils from migrating into the sample concentrator oven.

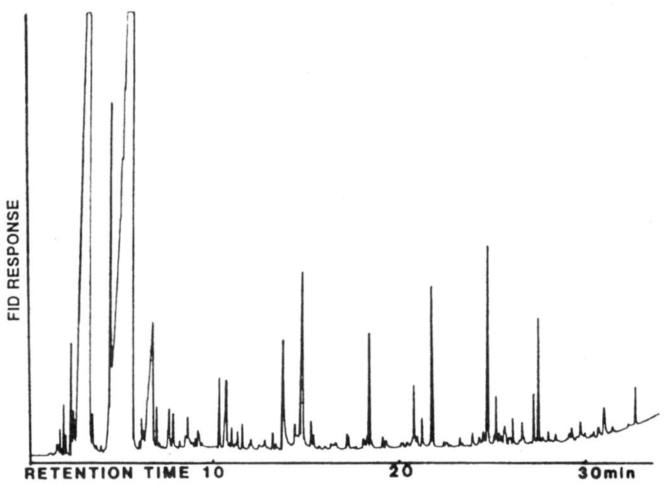

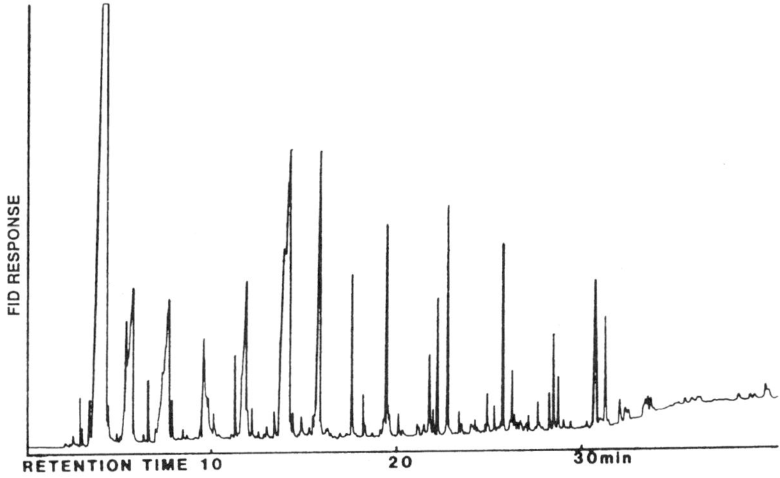

FIGURE 8 Comparison of dynamic headspace analyses of 30-mg samples of (top) American cheese and (bottom) cheddar cheese.

3. Solid Samples

In some respects, solid materials are actually easier to sample by dynamic headspace than are liquids and semisolids. If the sample material is truly solid, and not likely to melt at sampling temperatures, then a small portion of the material may be placed into a thermal desorption tube or cartridge, heated, and purged to the trap. For many foods, warming the sample to 50–100°C while purging it enhances recovery of volatiles, but some analytes are temperature unstable and are better purged at temperatures as low as possible. Dynamic headspace analysis has been applied successfully to such diverse foods as herbs and spices (27), beet sugar (28), and canned fish (29). To produce the headspace chromatogram of raw garlic shown in Figure 9, a small slice of the garlic was warmed to 70° and purged for 10 minutes to a Tenax trap. Citrus oils may be purged from the peel in the same way, as shown in Figure 10, where a small piece of grapefruit peel was purged for 10 minutes at 75°.

Having a variety of purging devices for sample manipulation makes comparisons between different sample types fairly straightforward, as shown in Figure 11. The top chromatogram shows a purge and trap (impinger vessel) of a diluted sample of orange soda. The label on the soda indicated that it was created using only natural flavors. To compare natural orange oil to the chromatogram of the orange soda volatiles, a small piece of orange peel was ther-

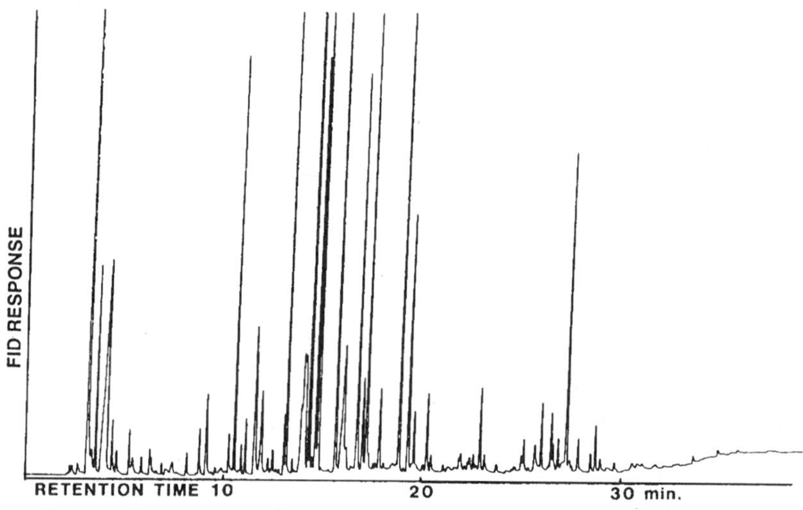

FIGURE 9 Dynamic headspace analysis of raw garlic at 70°C.

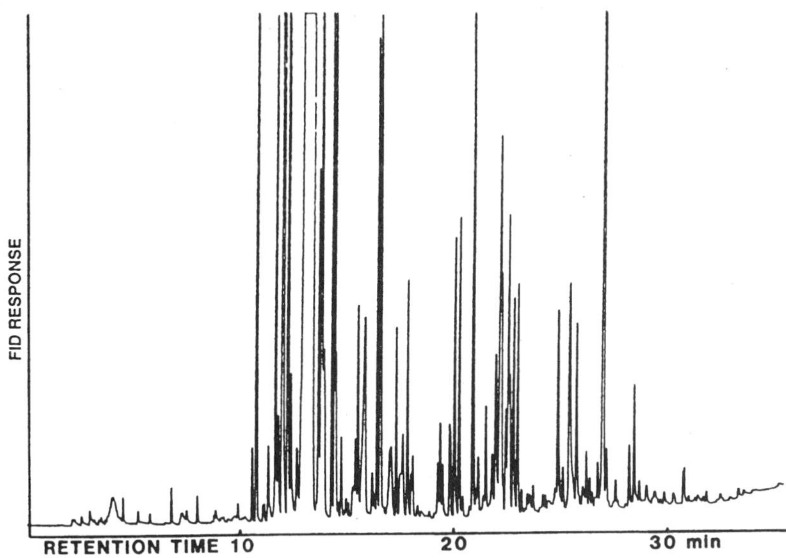

FIGURE 10 Dynamic headspace analysis of grapefruit peel at 75°C.

mally desorbed as for the grapefruit sample shown before. The resulting chromatogram is shown at the bottom of Figure 11. Only peaks 1, 2, and 3 are identified (α-pinene, β-pinene, and limonene, respectively), but the presence of many of the orange oil peaks in the soda clearly shows that the flavoring is from oranges as the manufacturer indicated.

Although small samples generally suffice for dynamic headspace of foods, it is sometimes preferable to examine a rather large amount of material. It is possible to make sampling vessels in whatever shape and size is desirable, but it is important to remember that the larger the sample vessel volume, the more purging is required to evacuate it. If the sample vessel is to be quite large, it may be a problem to have it seal properly. Since the purge gas must overcome the backpressure of the sorbent trap before it can flow through it, the sample vessel must be pressurized to some extent before the analytes will be transported to the trap. The larger the vessel—and more importantly, the larger the lid that must be sealed—the more likely it is that the vessel will leak and the sample volatiles escape to the atmosphere rather than being transferred to the trap. This may be prevented by using a vacuum pump attached to the vent of the trap to draw the sample out of the container, rather than trying to pressurize the whole sampling system. In this way, liter size or larger ves-

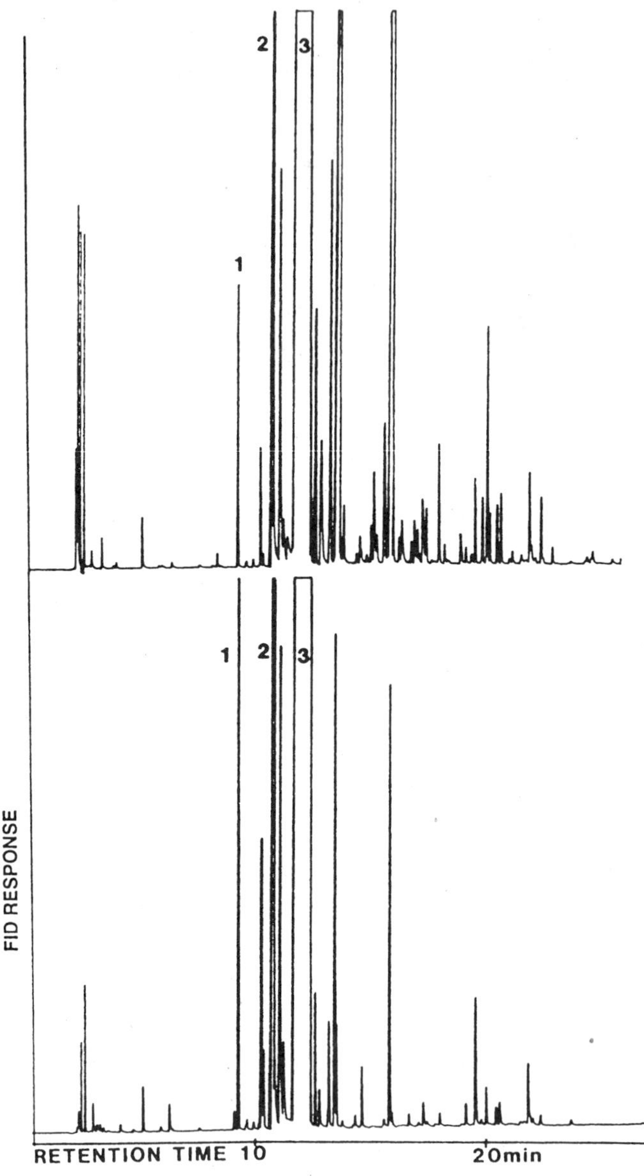

FIGURE 11 Comparison of volatiles purged from orange soda (top) with dynamic headspace of orange peel (bottom).

sels may be used, with the atmosphere inside the jar drawn directly to the trap. This approach was used to sample the atmosphere around whole fruits, producing chromatograms like those shown in Figures 12 and 13. The entire banana, kiwi, or other fruit was put into a liter jar that had a fitting connecting it directly to the inlet of the trap and another that allowed filtered air into the jar to replace that withdrawn during sampling. The fruit was allowed to stay in the jar for a period of several days, with a 500-ml sample of the headspace withdrawn once each day to evaluate the volatiles. A comparison of the chromatograms obtained over 3 days for a whole lemon is shown in Figure 14.

It is sometimes equally important to analyze the materials that come in contact with foods as well as the food itself. Packaging materials may impart odors or flavors to foods by transferring volatile or semivolatile compounds

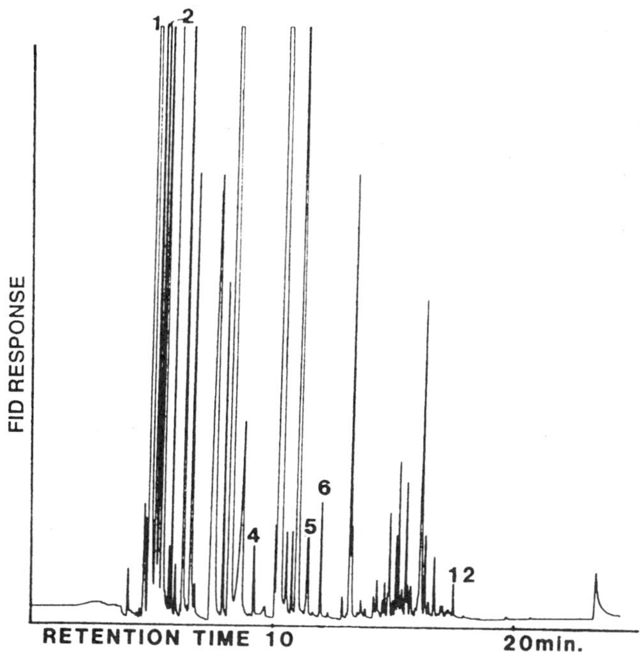

FIGURE 12 Dynamic headspace analysis of one whole banana at room temperature. Peaks are as follows: 1, butyraldehyde; 2, ethyl acetate; 3, ethyl butyrate; 4, butyl acetate; 5, heptanone; 6, amyl acetate; 7, methyl hexanoate,; 8, α-pinene; 9, β-pinene; 10, limonene; 11, octanol; 12, nonanal; 13, decanal

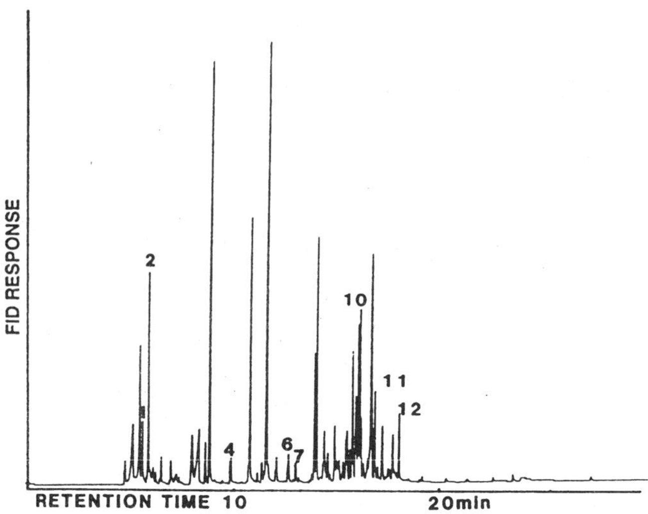

FIGURE 13 Dynamic headspace analysis of one whole kiwi; peaks as identified in Figure 12.

from the wrapping or container to the food (30–32). These compounds may have resulted from the manufacture of the packaging [e.g., solvents, residual monomers (33) and other low oligomers, plasticizers] or could themselves be contaminants not intended to be part of the formulation. Sometimes a packaging product adsorbs contaminants from the factory air, oil from processing machines, or other contaminants and then transfers them to the food, resulting in consumer complaints. Alternatively, the packing may adsorb aroma compounds from the food instead (34). The packaging materials may easily be assayed using dynamic headspace techniques, liberating the volatiles from the packaging matrix for analysis. Figure 15 shows the dynamic headspace analysis of a piece of Styrofoam from a hot beverage cup. Residual styrene monomer, as well as other organic volatiles, are clearly present in the cup. These organics may be passed into the food or beverage that is held the container. Figure 16, for example, shows the results of a purge-and-trap analysis of a microwaveable soup prepared in the Styrofoam cup in which it was sold. Here a short, wide-bore column was used, for quick analysis and sensitivity, which shows the presence of styrene monomer, passed from the cup to the soup. Similar analyses show the same effect for hot coffee and tea allowed to stand in a Styrofoam cup for 5 minutes before sampling.

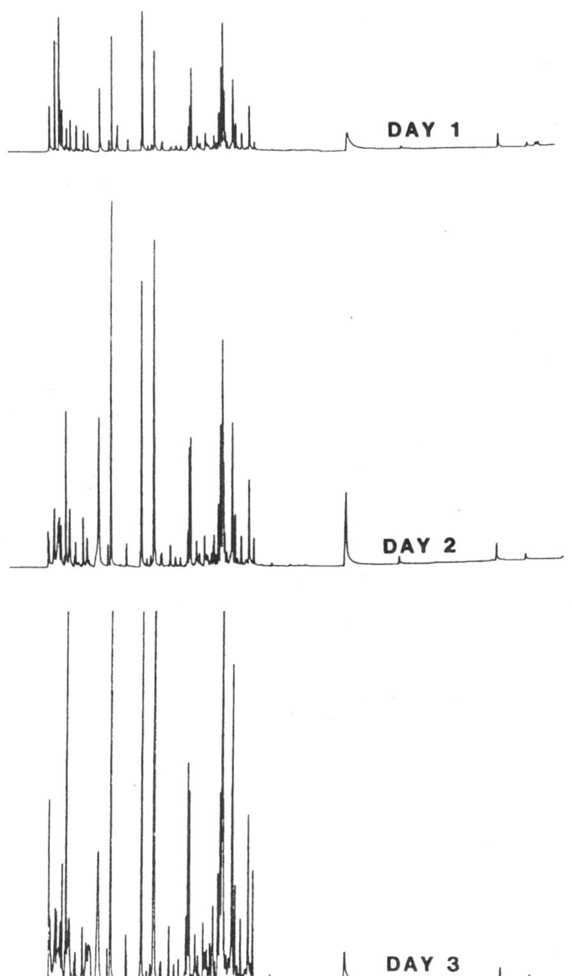

FIGURE 14 Volatiles collected from one whole lemon after 1, 2, and 3 days.

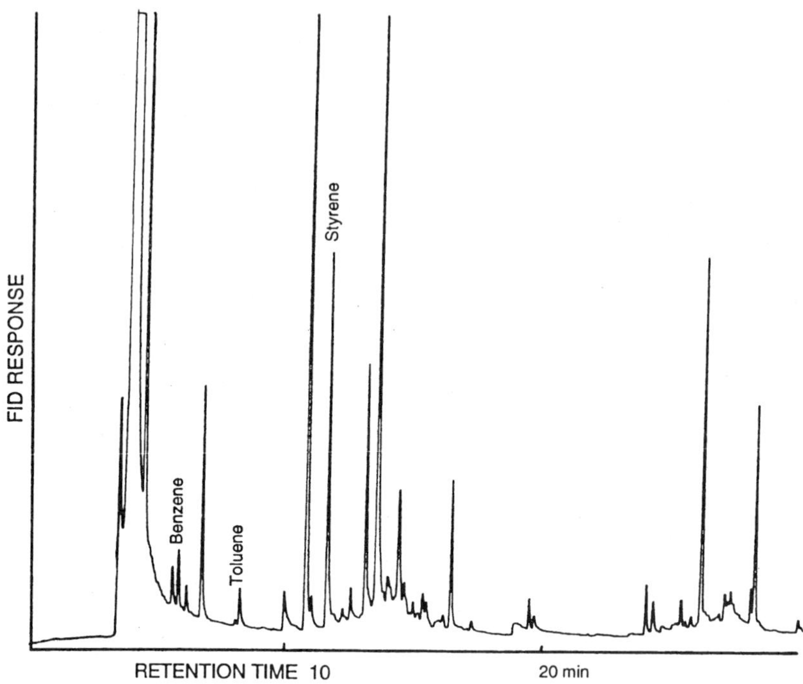

FIGURE 15 Dynamic headspace of styrene foam cup material.

H. Quantitative Analysis Using Purge and Trap

From its inception, as a way to determine the levels of organic pollutants in water, purge and trap has been applied in a quantitative approach. Typical methods developed by the EPA require rigorous standardization and calculations based on internal standards. As with similar techniques, the internal standard is added to the sample matrix just before analysis so that it is processed in the identical way that the sample volatiles are.

For nonenvironmental samples, the same approach should be used. If a quantitative determination is to be made on a liquid sample, the internal standard solution should be miscible with the sample matrix to ensure proper dispersion and, consequently, identical behavior of the analyte and internal standard volatiles. For solid materials, it is sometimes difficult to add the internal standard to the sample matrix without the possibility of the internal standard vaporizing as the sample is placed into the purging tube or vessel. Addition of the internal standard solution to the sample tube just before purg-

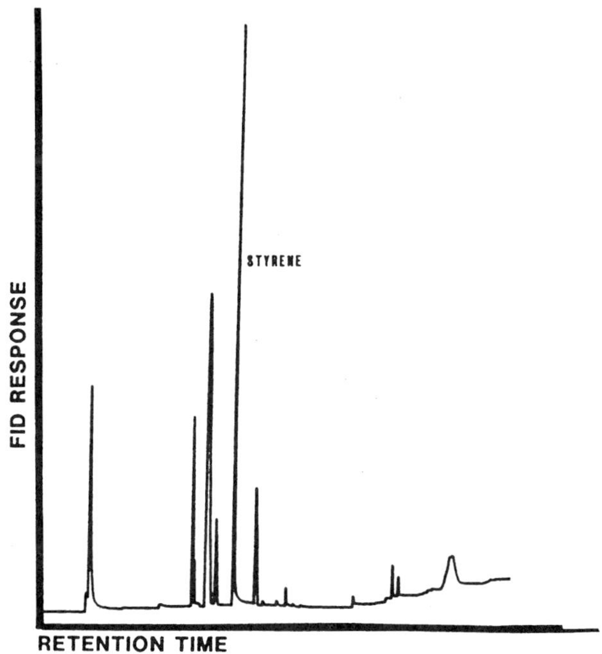

FIGURE 16 Purge-and-trap analysis of soup made in foam cup in microwave showing styrene from packaging.

ing reduced the chance that the internal standard will be preferentially volatilized, as does the selection of an internal standard of similar volatility to the analyte materials. If the solid material is a powder, the syringe may be inserted into the center of the sample plug in the tube and the solution expelled directly into the sample. This approach has been used successfully for the determination of residual solvents in pharmaceuticals (35,36) by dynamic headspace. If the sample is a solid piece, such as citrus peel or peppercorns, the sample may be placed in the tube and held in place with a generous quantity of glass wool. The internal standard may then be injected into the glass wool before thermal desorption. Quantitative procedures have been developed for a variety of food and packaging analyses, including the determination of ethylene dibromide in prepared foods (37) and the use of multiple runs to quantitate N-nitrosodimethylamine in baby bottle nipples (38).

Some purge-and-trap instruments have trap injection ports that permit the injection of the internal standard solution onto the trap directly while the sample is being purged, which ensures that the whole injection is trapped but does not compensate for any loss due to purging efficiency, vessel leaking, and so on. With attention to sampling parameters and the selection of a compatible internal standard, purge-and-trap analyses can easily provide quantitative results with relative standard deviations for replicates below 5%.

REFERENCES

1. F. Chialva, G. Gabri, P. A. P. Liddle, and F. Ulian, Qualitative evaluation of aromatic herbs by direct headspace GC analysis, *J. H.R.C. & C.C. 5*:182 (1982).
2. E. Jones, M. Davis, R. Gibson, B. Todd, and R. Wallen, Application of headspace GC to complex liquid samples, *Am. Lab. 16*:74 (1984).
3. B. Kolb, D. Boege, and L. S. Ettre, Advances in headspace gas chromatography: instrumentation and applications, *Am. Lab. 20*:33 (1988).
4. P. Wessels and G. Schwinger, Pressure-balanced headspace sampling using an electronic-pressure-controlled, on-column injector, *LC.GC 13 (6)*:480 (1995).
5. C. A. Weston, R. P. Albert, D. N. Speis, L. Williams, and W. Martin, Screening environmental samples for volatile organics utilizing a static headspace sampler, *Am. Lab. 24*:30 (1992).
6. M. E. McNally and R. L. Grob, A review: current applications of static headspace and dynamic headspace analysis, *Am. Lab. 17*:20 (1985).
7. L. Lepine and J. Archambault, Parts-per-trillion determination of trihalomethanes in water by purge and trap gas chromatography with electron capture detection, *Anal. Chem. 64*:810 (1992).
8. J. W. Washall and T. P. Wampler, Sources of error in purge and trap analysis of volatile organic compounds, *Am. Lab. 22*:38 (1990).
9. R. D. Barnes, L. M. Law, and A. J. MacLeod, Comparison of some porous polymers as adsorbents for collection of odor samples and the application of the technique to an environmental malodor, *Analyst 106*:412 (1981).
10. H. T. Badings, C. de Jong, and R. P. M. Dooper, Automatic system for rapid analysis of volatile compounds by purge and cold-trapping/capillary gas chromatography, *H.R.C & C.C. 8*:755 (1985).
11. R. Westendorf, Managing water in purge and trap GC/MS, *Environ. Lab. 24*:36 (1992).
12. *Analysis of Foods and Beverages, Headspace Techniques*, (G. Charalambous, ed.) Academic Press, New York, 1978.
13. S. Datta and S. Nakai, Computer aided optimization of wine-blending, *J. Food Sci. 57*:178 (1992).
14. H. Kallio, Method of sensitive analysis of wine headspace volatiles based on selective capillary column trapping, *J. Chromatogr. Sci. 29*:438 (1991).
15. A. Kaipainen, A study of the aroma profiles of non-alcoholic beer by thermal desorption and GC-MS, *J. High Resolut. Chromatogr. 15*:751 (1992).
16. H. T. Badings, C. De Jong, and R. P. M. Dooper, Rapid analysis of volatile com-

pounds in food products by purge and cold-trapping capillary gas chromatography, *Progress in Flavor Research* (J. Adda, ed.), Elsevier Science Publishers B.V., Amsterdam, 1984, p. 523.

17. D. Robertys and W. Bertsch, Use of computerized pattern recognition in the analysis of stress induced changes in coffee aroma, *H.R.C. & C.C. 10*:244 (1987).
18. G. Blanch, G. Reglera, M. Herriaz and J. Tabera, Comparison of different extraction methods for the volatile components of grape juice, *J. Chromatogr. Sci. 29*:11 (1991).
19. R. Marsili, Measuring volatiles and limonene-oxidation products in orange juice by capillary GC, *LC GC 4*:358.
20. R. J. Phillips, Routine analysis of volatile components in foods and beverages, *Am. Lab. 24*:110 (1992).
21. D. M. Wyatt, Dynamic headspace gas chromatography/mass spectromety technique for determining volatiles in ambient stored vegetable oils, *J. Chromatogr. Sci. 25*:257 (1987).
22. S. Raghavan, S. Reeder, and A. Khayat, Rapid analysis of vegetable oil flavor quality by dynamic headspace capillary gas chromatography, *J. Am. Oil Chem. Soc. 66*:942 (1989).
23. J. M. Snyder and T. L. Mounts, Analysis of vegetable oil volatiles by multiple headspace extraction, *J. Am. Oil Chem. Soc. 67*:800 (1990).
24. T. Hsieh, S. Williams, and W. Vejaphan, Characterization of volatile components of menhaden fish (Brevortia tyrannus) oil, *J. Am. Oil Chem. Soc. 66*:114 (1989).
25. J. Merkle and D. Larick, Conditions for extraction and concentration of beef fat volatiles with supercritical carbon dioxide, *J. Food Sci. 59*:478 (1994).
26. W. Yang and D. Min, Dynamic headspace analysis of volatile compounds of Cheddar and Swiss cheese during ripining, *J. Food Sci. 59*:1304 (1994).
27. T. Wampler, W. Bowe, and E. Levy, Spitless capillary GC analysis of herbs and spices using cryofocusing, *Am. Lab. 16*:25 (1985).
28. R. Marsili, N. Miller, G. Kilmer, and R. Simmons, Identification and quantitation of the primary chemicals responsible for the characterization malodor of beet sugar by purge and trap GC-MS-OD techniques, *J. Chromatogr. Sci. 32*:165 (1994).
29. B. Girard and S. Nakai, Grade classification of canned pink salmon with static headspace patterns, *J. Food Sci. 59*:507 (1994).
30. D. Wyatt, Analytical analysis of tastes and odors imparted to foods by packaging materials, *Plastic Film Sheeting* 2:144 (1986).
31. R. Marsili, Testing packaging materials: why and how, *Food Product Design (June)*:78 (1993).
32. T. Wampler, Automated analysis of volatiles in pharmaceutical environments and products, *Pharm. Manuf. 1*:5 (1984).
33. H. Ehret, V. Ducruet, A. Luciani, and A. Feigenbaum, Styrene and ethylbenzene migration from polystyrene into dairy products by dynamic purge and trap gas chromatography, *J. Food Sci. 59*:990 (1994).

34. J. Konczal, B. Harte, P. Hoojjat, and J. Giacin, Apple juice flavo compound sorption by sealant films, *J. Food Sci. 57*:967 (1992).
35. T. Wampler, W. Bowe, and E. Levy, Dynamic headspace analyses of residual volatiles in pharmaceuticals, *J. Chromatogr. Sci. 23*:64 (1985).
36. J. Washall and T. Wampler, A dedicated purge and trap/GC system for residual solvent analysis of pharmaceuticals, *Am. Lab. 25*:20C (1993).
37. S. Moon, T. Healy, A. Lichtman, and R. Porter, An automated method for ethylene dibromide (EDB) determination in food products, *Am. Lab. 18*:106 (1986).
38. R. Westendorf, A quantitative method for dynamic headspace analysis using multiple runs, *J. Chromatogr. Sci. 23*:521 (1985).

3

The Analysis of Food Volatiles Using Direct Thermal Desorption

Casey C. Grimm, Steven W. Lloyd,
James A. Miller, and Arthur M. Spanier
United States Department of Agriculture, New Orleans, Louisiana

I. INTRODUCTION

Volatile compounds released from foods are monitored to determine composition, quality, and safety of the product. The very nature of food, a complex mixture of proteins, carbohydrates, and fats, results in a continuous change in the formation of the volatile compounds generated by the food over time. The application of heat during the cooking process, with variable amounts of oxygen and moisture present, greatly affects the volatile composition of a food sample. The volatile composition may become more complex with time as labile compounds react to form new compounds. The presence of some compounds at concentrations as low as the parts per billion range can have a major impact on the overall flavor and acceptability of food. Geosmin and methylisoborneol can be detected in water at the parts per trillion range (1).

For these compounds, the human nose is more sensitive than current analytical instrumentation.

Volatile analysis of foods is used to determine various properties including quality, purity, origin, and composition. Due to the relatively low concentrations of volatile materials that can affect the acceptance or rejection of a food, a procedure is normally employed to extract and concentrate the sample sufficiently prior to instrumental analysis. The predominant method for analyzing volatiles is gas chromatography (GC). Typically, compounds need to be delivered to the head of the GC column in the nanogram range in order to be detected. However, specialized detectors such as ion trap mass spectrometers (ITMS) or sulfur chemiluminescence detectors (SCD) are capable of detecting compounds in the picogram range.

The analysis of volatiles is generally accomplished by an extraction step, followed by concentration, chromatographic separation, and subsequent detection. Well-established methods of analysis include solvent extraction, static and dynamic headspace sampling, steam distillation with continuous solvent extraction, and supercritical fluid extraction. An overview of sample preparation methods is provided by Teranishi (2). The chromatographic profile will vary depending upon the method of sample preparation employed, and it is not uncommon to produce artifacts during this step (3,4). Thermally labile compounds may decompose in the heated zones of instruments to produce a chromatographic profile that is not truly representative of the sample.

A chromatographic "snapshot" of a food sample's volatile composition is taken at one moment in time in order to compare one sample to the next. The fewer parameters that are varied, the more likely the analysis will be reproducible. Hence, the less sample manipulation, the fewer variables in the experiment, the more likely the results can be repeated. Sample manipulation not only includes the analytical methodology, but also how the food is cooked and stored.

Direct thermal desorption (DTD) is the technique of sparging the volatiles from a sample matrix and transferring them directly onto the head of a chromatographic column. The matrix is heated to facilitate the extraction of the volatile compounds from the sample. A cryofocusing unit, or cold trap, is often employed to focus the analytes at the head of the column for improved chromatographic peak shape. This technique allows for the qualitative analysis of volatile compounds with little or no sample preparation. Quantitation of volatiles may be possible, but is problematic. Variations in purging efficiency, loss of purged volatiles through split/splitless injectors, carryover, and the mechanics of the addition of an internal standards are some of the problems encountered in quantitative DTD. Problems with sample carryover have been minimized with the introduction of newer instrumentation that eliminates transfer lines.

II. HISTORY

In an attempt to facilitate sample preparation methods, early researchers would unscrew the top of the injection port on a gas chromatograph, remove the liner, and place a second liner filled with their sample directly into the injection port (5). The sample would be held in place with a plug of glass wool. The hot injection port, with its flow of carrier gas, would serve to thermally desorb the volatiles from the food sample onto a packed column held at room temperature. The volatiles from samples such as peanuts and vegetable oils were analyzed by this method. In addition to burned fingers, this method had a few drawbacks such as broad peak shapes. Liquid CO_2 was used to cool the column to subambient temperatures, focusing the desorbed volatiles onto the front end of the column, resulting in enhanced chromatographic separation.

An improvement was made in this approach by moving the sample outside of the injection port into its own heated block. Grob, Zlatkis, and Fisher/Legendre developed devices for stripping volatiles from samples and introducing them into the gas chromatograph (6,7). The external closed-loop inlet device (ECID) was developed and marketed by Scientific Instrumentation Services (SIS) of River Ridge, Louisiana (Fig. 1). The apparatus consisted of a heating chamber, a six-port valve, heated stainless steel tubes, and an electronics unit for controlling the source block and valve temperatures. A number of these instruments were sold to researchers primarily in the food industry and are still in use (8).

Figure 1 shows the instrument in the load position. When the valve is turned, the gas flows are diverted along the dashed lines. Approximately 2g of sample can be placed in a glass tube with the sample held in place with glass wool. Oil samples can be analyzed by putting a few drops of the oil directly onto the glass wool (9). The tube is then inserted into the sample chamber, which could be preheated over a wide range of temperatures from ambient to 300°C. After placing the sample into the sample chamber, the heated valve is rotated to allow the carrier gas to pass through the sample chamber and to sweep the desorbed volatiles through the valve and into the injection port of the gas chromatograph. Since all the purge gas goes onto the column, the carrier flow rate is equivalent to the purge flow rate. Desorption takes place over a period of 4–30 minutes. Following the purge, the valve is rotated to the run position; the carrier gas then bypasses the sample chamber and flows directly

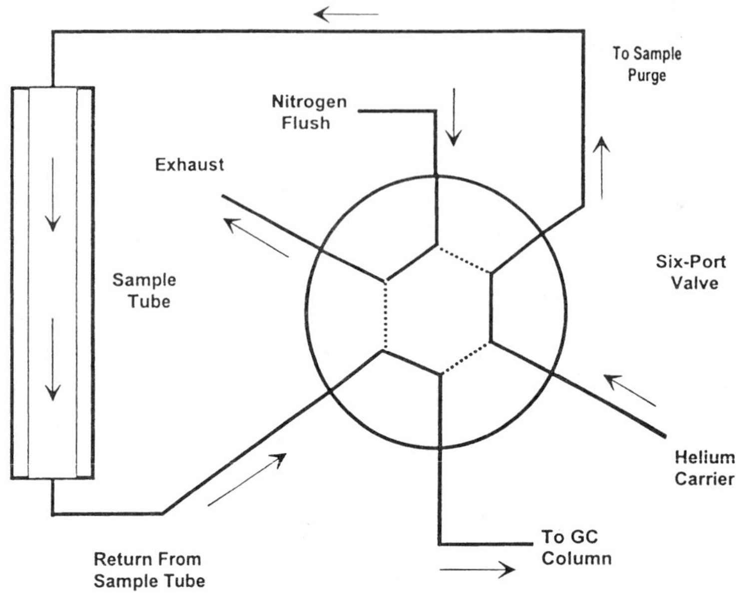

FIGURE 1 The extenal closed-loop injection device is shown in the load position. The dashed lines represent the flow of gases following sample loading.

into the GC. At this time a GC temperature ramping program is initiated. The sample tube is then removed, and a stream of nitrogen is used to sweep out any residual volatiles in the sample chamber and accompanying transfer lines. This system has been used to directly desorb the volatiles from a wide variety of food samples including peanuts, sugar, and meat.

In 1984 the ECID was adapted for use with capillary columns (10). The capillary columns required lower flow rates and had a lower sample capacity. The lower flow rates going through the transfer lines resulted in more acute problems with carryover and moisture. When purging samples with high moisture content, and using cryofocusing, the capillary columns would freeze up and block all carrier flow. Carryover from volatiles in the transfer line was observed on blanks run between samples. The application of the ECID to capillary columns was not as successful as with the more robust packed columns.

Subsequently, an alternative method of introduction was devised employing a stainless steel glass-lined tube and with a needle secured to the end

(11–13). The device would then, like a syringe, be inserted through a septum into the GC injection port, analogous to a direct injection, and the carrier gas diverted by a three-port valve to pass through the sample and purge the volatiles directly from the sample into the injection port. There they would condense at the head of a column held at subambient temperature. Originally designed for the desorption of adsorbent traps, the system was readily amenable for use as a direct thermal desorption system. These home-built systems have reduced purge/carrier flow rates, but avoided the problem of contaminated transfer lines with resultant carryover from one run to the next. As the ECID, the interface with the split/splitless injectors required that the split flow be capped off to prevent sample loss. If left open, the purged volatiles would exit the split vent in the same proportions as the carrier gas. Under normal conditions with injections by a syringe, the sample is volatilized by the injection port and the entire sample is forced onto the head of the capillary column, with only pure carrier gas exiting the split vent. However, when the carrier gas is used to first purge the sample, the analytes are mixed with the carrier gas and any split results in a loss of sample being deposited on the head of the column. With typical split ratios of 50:1 to 100:1, this limits the quantity of volatiles that can be detected to the parts per thousand range.

An automated system called the short-path thermal desorber (SPTD) (Fig. 2) was developed jointly by researchers at Rutgers University and Scientific Instrument Services of Ringoes, New Jersey (an independent company, separate from the previously mentioned SIS) (14). This instrument is placed on top of the GC injection port and can be adjusted to allow conventional injections without disconnecting the unit. The sample is placed in a glass-lined stainless steel tube and held in place with glass wool. An injection needle is affixed to one end and the other end is screwed into the SPTD. The injection is made pneumatically, and the sample is not heated prior to injection. Control of the temperature, desorption time, and equilibration are provided by an electronic controlling unit. An automated system has an inherent advantage over manual systems for improved reproducibility from one run to the next. Quantitative data with a precision of less than 5% STD has been reported (15).

III. PARAMETERS

The setting of the parameters of direct thermal desorption will directly affect the desorption efficiency, collection, and quantitative analysis of the sample. Desorption temperatures must be set high enough to facilitate the stripping of

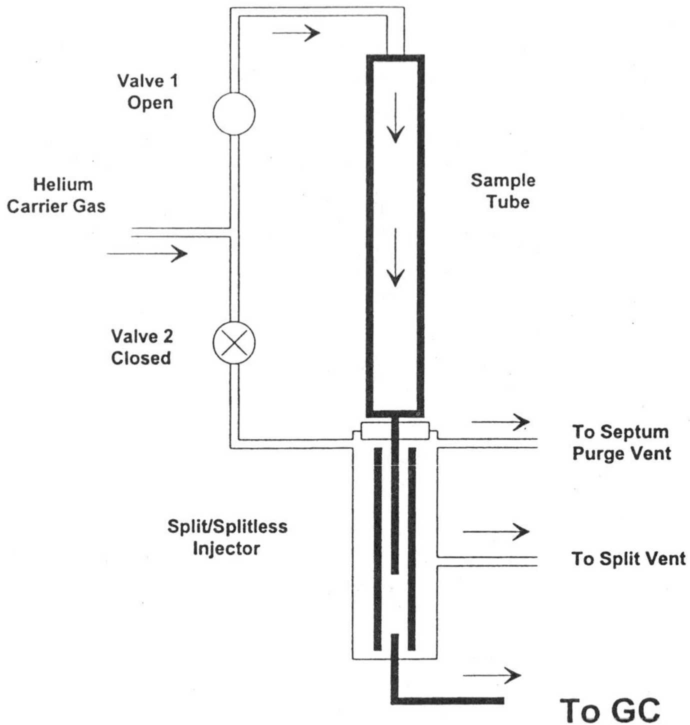

FIGURE 2 The short-path thermal desorber is here shown in the load position. Following desorption, valve 1 is closed and valve 2 is opened.

the volatile compounds, yet not alter the sample or analyte. Desorption times should be sufficient to remove the majority of the volatiles. Purge/carrier gas flow rates should be sufficient to purge the analyte from the sample but not push the desorbed volatiles through the cryofocusing zone. GC columns must allow sufficient flow for efficient desorption of the sample and must be suitable for analysis by direct thermal desorption.

A. Optimization

Sunesson et al. have performed a multivariant optimization of parameters for the thermal desorption–cold trapping of volatiles (16). Their conclusions, although based on the use of a specific instrument, are generally applicable for all direct thermal desorption devices:

1. Set the cold trap to its lowest setting.
2. The highest temperature possible that does not alter the sample should be used in the injection block.
3. The lining of the cold trap should be a thick stationary phase.
4. The heating of the temperature ramp rate should be as high as possible.
5. The flow rate should be as high as possible.

B. Sample Constraints

The two major sample limitations to DTD of volatiles are moisture content and sample size. An excess amount of water will result in a blocked capillary and/or the extinguishing of a GC detector's flame. When used with packed columns the moisture contents can be higher. For capillary columns, the upper limit is approximately 5% moisture in the sample (17). The sample size generally ranges from 1 to 1000 mg. The lower value results from the mechanical inability to handle small amounts of material and the amount of analyte being present at a concentration below the limit of detection. Since the purging efficiency is always less than 100% and is often less than 10%, a 1-mg sample containing an analyte present at 100 ppm would result in a maximum of 100 ng of analyte at the detector.

For optimum reproducibility, the more uniform the sample particles, the more consistent the packing will be. The purge/carrier gas flow through the sample will contact a similar amount of surface area if the sample particles are uniform. The ideal sample for DTD is a thermally inert low-moisture powder with the analytes present at concentrations between parts per million to parts per thousand. This description sounds like that used to describe typical adsorbent materials like Tenax, Chromosorb, and charcoal. The more the food sample resembles these adsorbent materials, the fewer problems result from the matrix.

Some samples that have been analyzed by DTD and related techniques are presented in Table 1. This list contains some liquid samples, which are sparged and passed through a drying reagent and the analytes deposited directly onto the head of the column (18,19). Although not truly direct thermal desorption, these techniques are very similar.

C. Columns

Assuming the sample is amenable to DTD, the internal diameter (I.D.) of the chromatograph column employed is the most critical factor in determining the success of a DTD method. A trade-off must be made between sample capacity,

TABLE 1 Substances Analyzed by Direct Thermal Desorption

Sample	Ref.
Ajax detergent	24
Aspirin	24
Beef	3
	23
Candy	24
Carpets	25
Cheese	26
Coffee	27
	24
Coriander fruit	17
	14
Glad Wrap	24
Marijuana	14
Onion	28
Peanuts	29
	24
Pine needles	24
Plant material	30
Plywood	24
Polypropylene films	17
Rugs	24
Soil	14
Soybean oil	6
Spices	27
Sugar	20
	21
Vanilla beans	17
	31
Vegetable oil	9
VOCs	18
Wine	19

water tolerance, and chromatographic resolution. Packed columns are superior to capillary columns for sample loading and their ability to handle moisture, but they provide poor chromatographic resolution. Their high flow rates are consistent with typical purge rates of 40 ml/min, allowing the injection ports to deliver all of the purge gas onto the head of the column. When packed columns or mega-bore glass capillary columns (0.75 mm I.D.) are employed, even samples with high moisture contents are amenable to direct thermal desorption. With capillary columns, microgram quantities of water deposited during the direct thermal desorption may result in blockage of the column during cryofocusing.

A capillary column with a 0.32 mm I.D. has an upper flow rate of approximately 2 ml/min. Sample loading can be improved and column blockage alleviated by using wide-bore and megabore capillary columns. These columns are the best for use with direct thermal desorption when analyzing samples with a high degree of moisture such as meat (3). In going to the larger-diameter capillary columns with thicker films, a subsequent loss in chromatographic resolution should be expected. A compromise is reached between the high-capacity packed columns and the low-load high-efficiency capillary columns with the 0.75-mm-wide bore and the 0.53-mm megabore open tubular columns. These columns provide satisfactory chromatography and can handle sample loads in the microgram range. The megabore columns are made of glass, and their installation and removal can be difficult.

Even with the larger-diameter columns, water may still present a problem. High amounts of water can compromise the integrity of the column's stationary phase. As the water enters into the detector, it can quench the flames on flame ionization (FID) and flame photometric detectors (FPD). The extinguishing of the detectors can be overcome by using an increased flow rate of both hydrogen and air. This results in a slight decrease in sensitivity. This also works well with the sulfur chemiluminescence detectors, which require higher flow rates and in which hydrocarbons are converted to water and carbon dioxide, while sulfur-containing compounds produce sulfur monoxide.

D. Split/Splitless Injectors

DTD devices are typically interfaced to the gas chromatograph via split/splitless injection ports. Split/splitless injectors have been developed to allow injected volatiles to be concentrated at the head of the capillary column, yet still provide sufficient gas flow to sweep out the injection port. This is accomplished by altering the flow through the injector. During the splitless mode (Fig. 3a), the carrier gas enters at the top of the injector and applies pressure on the volatiles to drive them into the top of the capillary column. The majority of the carrier gas exits through the septum purge line at the top of the injector. After sufficient time is allowed to void the injection volume, the flow is changed so that the majority of the carrier gas sweeps through the injection liner but exits the sweep vent. This method works well for normal injections using syringes.

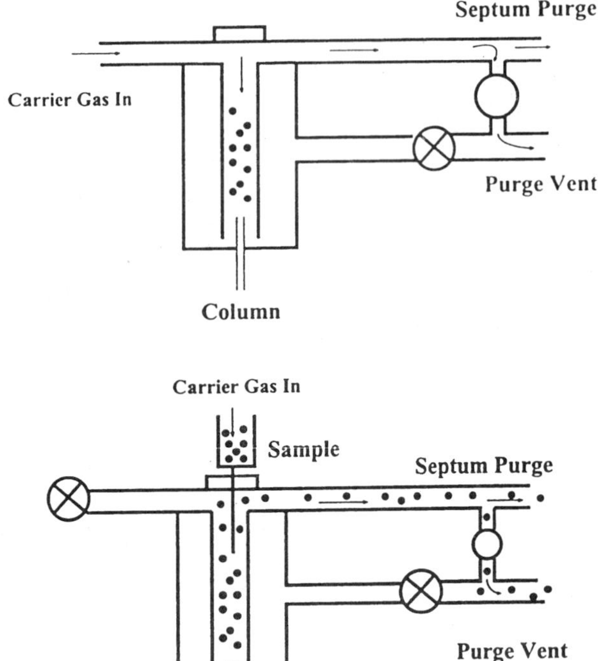

Figure 3 Diagram of gas flow of an HP split/splitless injector under normal operation (top) and under DTD operation (bottom).

Direct thermal desorption devices alter the flow through the injector. The carrier gas mixed with the analytes now enters the injection port through the sample needle (Fig. 3b). The majority of the carrier gas and volatiles exit through the septum purge, with only a fraction of the purged volatiles going onto the head of the column. For this reason, the split ratio must be decreased as much as possible, and in some cases the split vent may be capped off. However, this results in a reduced flow of carrier gas through the injection port and can lead to carryover between runs and irreproducible results. This is especially true for volatiles being desorbed from complex food samples.

IV. APPLICATIONS

A comparison of DTD was made with purge and trap (P&T) for analyzing volatiles from samples of beet sugar, roasted peanuts, and grilled ground beef. Aliquots from the same sample were used for the comparison. Method parameters were kept the same with two exceptions: the P&T method used N_2 as the purge gas, while the DTD used helium, and following P&T, the Tenax trap was thermally desorbed at 150°C. Samples were purged at temperatures determined experimentally to be optimal.

A. Experimental

A short-path thermal desorption device (SIS, Ringoes, NJ) was installed on an HP 5890 Series II gas chromatograph. The capillary column used was a DB-5, 30 m, 0.53 I.D column with a 5 μm film (J & W Sci, NJ). Following the injection port, the capillary was passed through a cryofocusing unit (SGE, Australia). A thermocouple was attached to the cryofocusing zone and the temperature held at –150°C. The gas chromatograph was held at 100°C for 10 minutes, then ramped at 3°C/min to 200°C. A second ramp of 25°C/min was used from 200 to 250°C. The temperature was then held for 5 minutes for a total run time of 50 minutes. The GC program was initiated at the beginning of the desorption so compounds not retained would be observed at the detector. The capillary flow rate was 3 ml/min with the split at 11 ml/min and the septum purge at 3 ml/min. The split/splitless injector was operated in splitless mode for 4 minutes during the desorption.

1. Purge and Trap

Sugar crystals were ground to produce free-running crystals. Frozen precooked beef patties were chopped to a fine meal. Roasted peanuts were chopped to about $^1/_8$-inch particles. Approximately 500 mg of sample was placed in a 50-ml test tube equipped with a sparge needle. The sample was purged with nitrogen for 4 minutes at a rate of 17 ml/min. An adsorbent trap consisting of 200 mg of Tenax, held in place with glass wool, was used to collect the volatiles. The sugar was held at 150°C, the beef at 70°C, and the peanuts at 120°C. These temperatures have been determined to be the highest possible without significantly altering the sample. After purging and trapping, the Tenax trap was desorbed at 150°C for 4 minutes using the SPTD under the same conditions used for DTD.

2. Direct Thermal Desorption

Aliquots of 500 mg each of the same samples used for purge and trap were taken and placed in a glass-lined stainless steel tube. Glass wool was used to hold the sample in place. The sample was purged of atmospheric oxygen for the minimal setting of 1 second prior to injection. The thermal desorption temperature was held at ambient for 1 minute following injection. This equilibration period is needed when switching the carrier gas from the normal operation to pass through the sample. Upon equilibration, the heated blocks close around the sample tube. The sample was heated to 150°C for sugar, 120°C for peanuts, and 70°C for beef. Volatiles were swept directly onto the column and cryofocused at −150°C utilizing liquid nitrogen. After a 4-minute desorption, the liquid nitrogen was cut off and the cryofocusing zone allowed to rise to the GC oven temperature of 100°C.

B. Volatiles from Beet Sugar

Beet sugars are prone to adsorb off-odors as a result of contact of sugar beets with soil microorganisms that produce potent off-flavors. Odor is a major factor in quality control of the acceptability of the sugar. The volatile compounds previously reported in beet sugar are primarily mixtures of short-chain fatty acids, furanones, aldehydes, and alcohols (20,21). The sample chosen possessed an exceptionally offensive odor and does not represent a typical chromatographic profile of beet sugars. The volatile composition of the sample is dominated by short-chain fatty acids and straight-chain aldehyes. Figure 4 shows a comparison of the beet sugar analyzed by the purge-and-trap method and by direct thermal desorption. The total amount of volatiles loaded onto the column is greater when using the purge-and-trap method. A likely explanation is that the dense packing of the sugar in the tube for DTD does not allow the purge/carrier gas to efficiently desorb the volatiles from the sugar.

Acetic acid is one of the first components to elute (Fig. 4, compound #1) with a retention time of 6.37 minutes. Propionic, butyric, isovaleric, and hexanoic acids (compounds 2,3,4, and 5) are observed in both methods. These short-chain fatty acids are the primary causes of the offensive odor of this sugar. The concentrations of these compounds are much greater using the P&T method relative to DTD. In the P&T trace (Fig. 4, top), the straight-chain aldehydes heptanal, octanal, and nonanal are also observed, while only trace levels are observed in the DTD chromatogram.

C. Volatiles from Peanuts

Figure 5 shows the chromatographic traces of a crushed peanut sample analyzed by the two different techniques. The upper chromatogram was obtained using the P&T method, while the bottom chromatogram was run using the

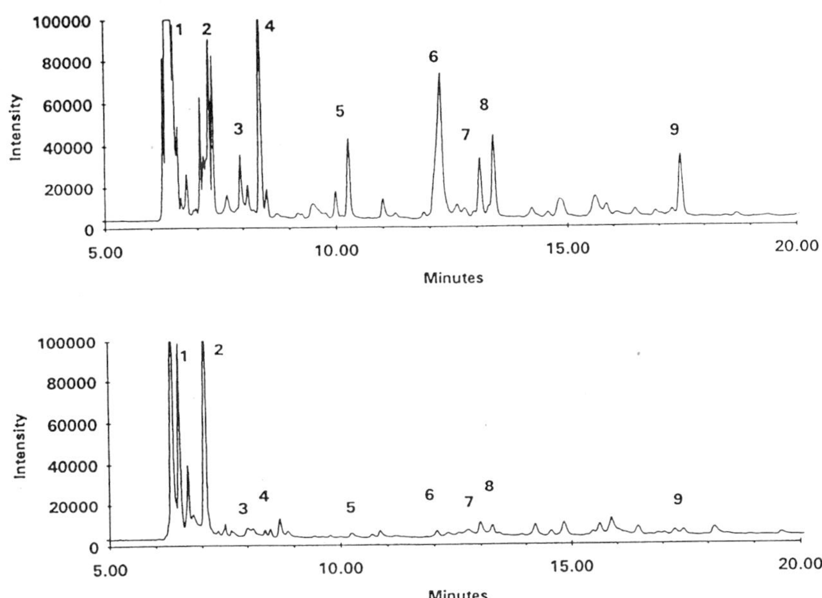

FIGURE 4 GC-FID trace of beet sugar. (Top) Volatiles desorbed by purge and trap: 1, acetic acid; 2, propionic acid; 3, butyric acid; 4, hexanal; 5, heptanal; 6, methylbutyric acid; 7, 2-octenal; 8, octanal; 9, nonanal. (Bottom) Volatiles directly desorbed onto the column.

DTD method. Again, the conditions were optimized for DTD and not for P&T.

The volatile composition of roasted peanuts consists of aldehydes, alkylpyrazines, furanones, and alcohols (22). Compounds identified by standards and retention times are shown in Figure 5. For the peanuts, the total volatile concentration is greater for the DTD method than for the P&T method. The relatively larger chunks of the peanut sample prevent close packing and result in enhanced desorption efficiency from the sample in the DTD method.

Both methods produced large amounts of acetone, pentane, and acetaldehyde, which are unresolved at the front end. The straight-chain hydrocarbons and aldehydes—pentane, hexane, heptane, heptenal, octenal, and nonanal—are observed in both chromatograms, with concentrations slightly greater in the DTD method. The pyrazines are observed in greater concentration in the DTD relative to the P&T chromatogram.

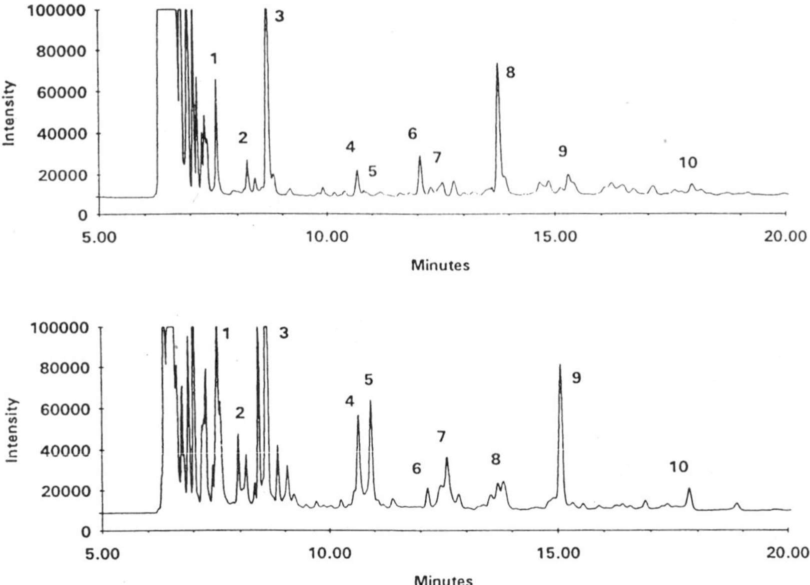

FIGURE 5 GC-FID trace of roasted peanuts. (Top) Volatiles desorbed by purge and trap: 1, pentanal; 2, N-methylpyrrole; 3, hexanal; 4, heptanal; 5, 2,5 and 2,6-dimentylpyrazine; 6, 1-octen-3-ol; 7, methylethylpyrazine; 8; 2-pentylfuran; 9, phenylacetaldehyde; 10, vinylphenol. (Bottom) Volatiles directly desorbed onto the column.

D. Volatiles from Grilled Beef

Figure 6 shows the chromatographic traces of the volatiles from grilled ground beef. The volatile profile has been shown to vary with purge temperature (23). A purge temperature of 70°C was selected because protein denaturation has been shown to occur at higher temperatures (3). The sample was taken from a 4-day-old refrigerated sample and is typical of samples having undergone meat flavor deterioration. The large peak at 8.5 minutes is hexanal, which overloads the capillary column in both the P&T trace and the DTD trace. As observed with the sugar sample, the total volatile concentration is greater in the P&T method.

Pentanal and hexanal (Fig. 6, compounds 2 and 3, respectively) are observed in higher concentrations using the DTD method, while heptanal, 2-octenal, and nonanal are present in relatively greater concentrations in the P&T method.

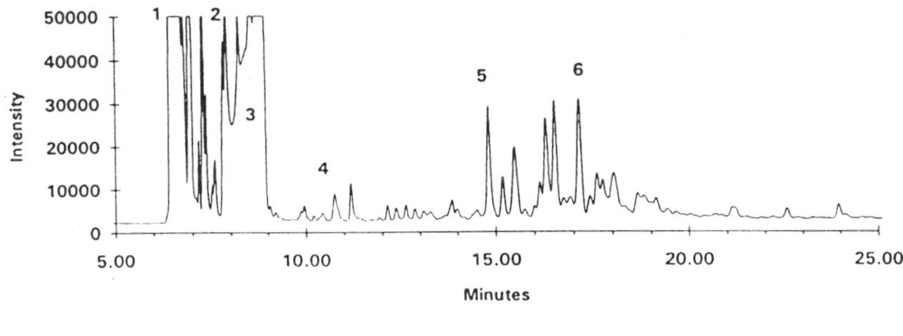

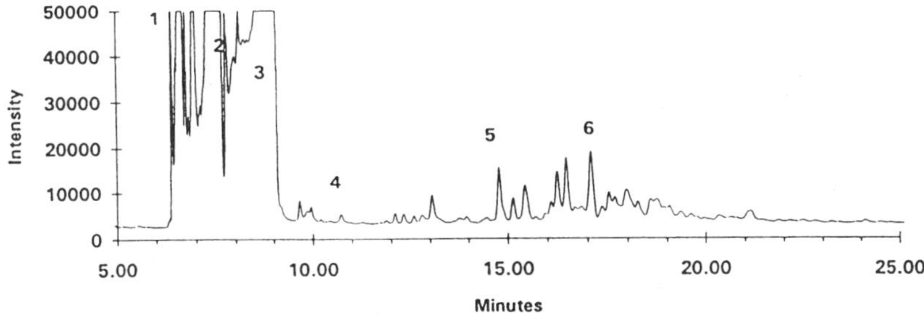

FIGURE 6 GC-FID trace of grilled beef. (Top) Volatiles desorbed by purge and trap: 1, acetaldehyde; 2, pentanal; 3, hexanal; 4, heptanal; 5, 2-octenal; 6, nonanal. (Bottom) Volatiles directly desorbed onto the column.

These three examples show that for low-boiling compounds, DTD can be more efficient for desorbing samples, but that the concentrating power of P&T is needed for higher-boiling compounds. The relative purging efficiency of P&T versus the desorbing efficiency of DTD is sample dependent.

E. Quantitative Analysis

One of the challenges encountered with direct thermal desorption is in quantitation. With automated instruments, it is fairly easy to reproduce temperatures, flow rates, and purge times. However, variability can occur as a result of sample preparation, i.e., granulation, shredding, and chopping, and as a result of sample packing in the desorption tube. The variation in gas flow through the sample affects the total amount of material desorbed. The efficiency of the purge/carrier gas to strip volatiles is directly related to the amount of the sample's surface area with which it comes into contact. The addition of a standard is often employed to calibrate the purge efficiency and the instrumental response.

There are two types of standards: a surrogate standard and an internal standard. The surrogate standard is added to the sample prior to any sample manipulation and is used to gauge purge efficiency. These types of standards work well with liquid matrices where the standard is readily incorporated into the sample matrix. An internal standard is added to the sample tube prior to DTD and is used to gauge instrument performance. With little or no sample preparation steps, the distinction between the two types becomes blurred. The standard itself should be thermally inert and nonindigenous to the sample. If gas chromatography–mass sepectroscopy (GC-MS) is being used, a stable isotope-enriched derivative of the compound being analyzed is the best standard.

Mechanical problems associated with tube seals and needle blockage may also cause difficulty with reproducibility. Since the needle remains in the injection port for several minutes (the injection period plus the desorption period), septa need to be replaced more frequently than for normal injections. A leak around the needle will result in a decrease in the sample amount loaded onto the column.

With the SPTD, fast heating of the sample can result in breakthrough at the cryotrap. A large burst of volatile compounds is blown through the cryotrap as soon as the heating units are closed. A signal prior to the end of the desorption period is an indication of the volatiles breaking through the cryotrap. Breakthrough is more severe in the case of P&T relative to DTD. A possible explanation is that as the matrix is subjected to heat, the volatiles are more readily desorbed off the Tenax, resulting in a plug of carrier gas containing an increased concentration of volatiles. A temperature ramp on the heating blocks and/or a more efficient cold trap could eliminate this problem.

Table 2 shows the averages, standard deviation, and the relative percent error for a mixture of pentanal, hexanal, heptanal, octanal, nonanal, and decanal run three times each by DTD. The mixture was desorbed at 150°C for 4 minutes and cryofocused at –150°C. Peak areas were measured using an HP 3390 integrator. The relative percent error for pentanal is 5.6% but decreases to 2.5% for nonanal.

The chromtographic traces from the DTD-GC-MS of three aliquiots of a commercial aromatic brown rice are shown in Figure 7. Three samples consisting of 0.50 g each of cracked rice were thermally desorbed at 70°C. The entire column was held at 0°C during the desorption (4 min) and then ramped at 5°C/min to 200°C. No breakthrough was observed, and the first 5 minutes

TABLE 2 Repeatability of Three Runs of a 100 ppm Mixture of Hydrocarbons by DTD

	Direct Thermal Desorption		
	Average	Std. Dev.	%
Pentanal	32923	1831	5.6
Hexanal	41436	2145	5.2
Heptanal	33072	1395	4.2
Octanal	62003	1507	2.4
Nonanal	59425	1513	2.5

of the chormatograms have been cut off. The broad peaks at the front end result from the poor cryofocusing of the low-boiling compounds. The straight-chain aldehydes resulting from lipid oxidation dominate the chromatogram. Some variability is observed between runs in the relative concentrations of the aldehydes. The amounts of acetic acid (2), 2-pentylfuran (5), and nonanal (6) remain constant between runs. However, the amounts of pentanal (3) and hexanal (4) show a slight increase between runs. These runs demonstrate the variability of the desorbing efficiency from a sample as a result of packing efficiency.

V. SUMMARY

Direct thermal desorption provides a rapid technique for the qualitative analysis of solid samples with little or no sample preparation. Volatiles are thermally desorbed from the sample and concentrated directly onto the head of a GC column. Similar chromatographic profiles may be obtained using DTD relative to P&T. Since the purge and desorption times are concurrent in the DTD method, analysis times are shorter. The relative purge efficiencies are compound and matrix dependent. DTD in some cases may provide a greater amount of material for detection. This is especially true for low-boiling compounds with higher vapor pressures.

Food samples that have moderate moisture content can be analyzed, but these ultimately require additional steps, which may affect the analysis greatly.

Quantitative analysis is possible but is dependent on the specific analyte and the matrix. The composition of the sample particles must be uni-

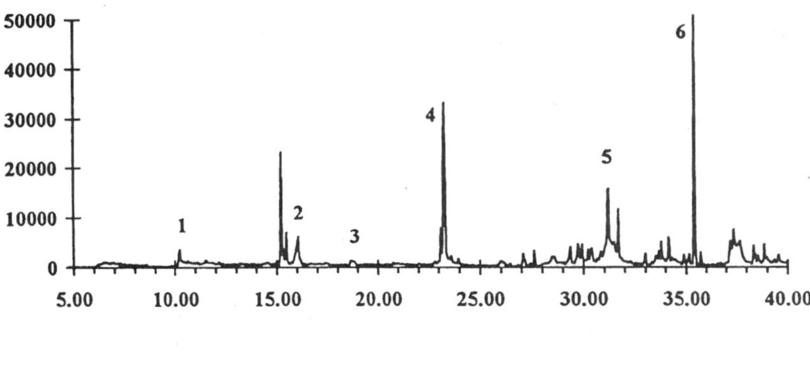

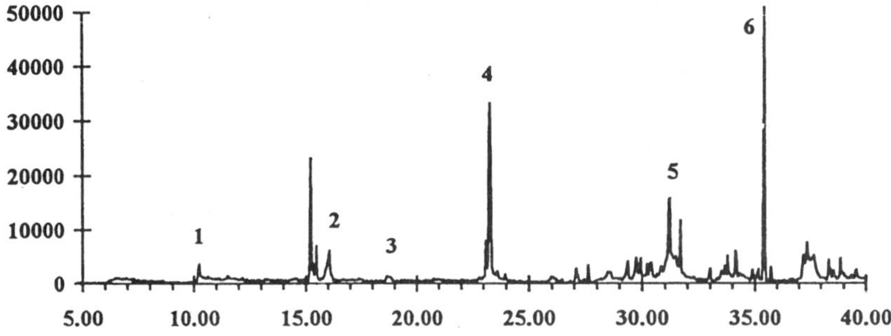

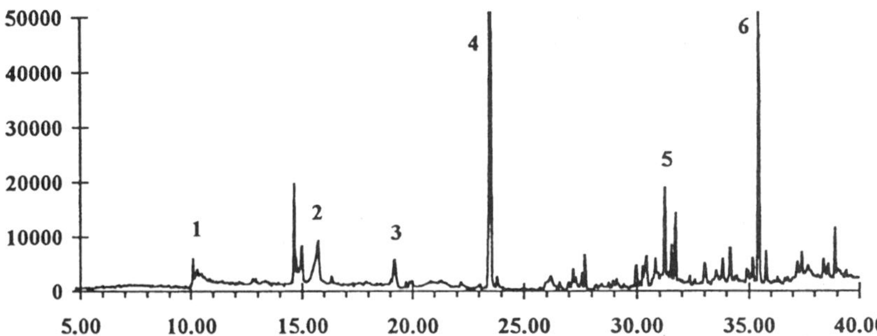

FIGURE 7 GC/MS traces of aromatic rice from three consecutive runs of (top) 875, (middle) 790, and (bottom) 750-mg samples. 1, Pentane/Acetone; 2, acetic Acid; 3, pentanal; 4, hexanal; 5, 2-pentalfuran; 6, nonanal.

form, enabling equivalent packing between runs. Septa need to be examined and replaced more frequently, and methodology for incorporating an internal standard must be developed.

ACKNOWLEDGMENTS

The authors would like to thank Mary An Godshall and J. V. Verecellotti for their editorial assistance in the preparation of this manuscript.

REFERENCES

1. P. E. Persson, Sensory properties and analysis of two muddy odour compounds, geosmin and 2-methylisoborneol, in water and fish, *Water Res. 14*:1113 (1980).
2. R. Teranishi and S. Kint, Sample preparation, *Flavor Science, Sensible Principles and Techniques* (T. E Acree and R. Teranishi eds.), American Chemical Society, Washington, DC, 1993.
3. A. M. Spanier, C. C. Grimm, and J. A. Miller, Sulfur-containing flavor compounds in beef: Are they really present or are they artifacts? *Sulfur Compounds in Foods* (C. J. Mussinan and Mary E. Keelan, eds.) ACS Symposium Series 564, Washington, DC, 1994, p. 49.
4. E. J. Block, Flavor artifacts, *J. Agric. Food Chem. 41*:692 (1993).
5. S. P. Fore, H. P. Dupuy, J. I. Wadsworth, and L. A. Glodblatt, A simplified technique used to study the shelf life of peanut butter, *J. Am. Peanut Res. Educ. Assoc. 5*:59 (1973).
6. M. G. Legendre, G. S. Fisher, W. H. Schuller, H. P. Dupuy, and E. T. Rayner, Novel technique for the analysis of volatiles in aqueous and nonaqueous systems, *J. Am. Oil Chem. Soc. 56*:552 (1979).
7. M. G. Legendre, H. P. Dupuy, R. L. Ory, and W. O. McIlrath, Inlet system for direct gas chromatographic and combined gas chromatographic/mass spectometric analysis of food volatiles, U.S. Patent 4,245,494 (1981).
8. J. R. Vercellotti, O. E. Mills, K. L. Bett, and D. L. Sullen, Gas chromatographic analyses of lipid oxidation volatiles in foods, *Lipid Oxidation in Food* (A. J. St. Angelo, ed.), American Chemical Society, Washington, DC, 1992, p. 232.
9. H. P. Dupuy, Analysis of vegetable oils, *J. Am. Oil Chem Soc. 54*:10 (19xx).
10. H. P. Dupuy, G. J. Flick Jr., M. E. Bailey, A. J. St. Angelo, M. G. Legendre, and G. Sumrell, Direct sampling capillary gas chromatography of volatiles in vegetable oils, *J. Am. Oil Chem. Soc. 62*:1690 (1985).
11. Y. Chen, Z. Li, D. Xue, and L. Qi, Determination of volatile constituents of chinese medicinal herbs by direct vaporization capillary gas chromatography/mass spectrometry, *Anal. Chem. 59*(5):744 (1987).
12. P. Werkhoff and W. Bretschneider, Dynamic headspace gas chromatography: concentration of volatile components after thermal desorption by intermediate

cryofocusing in a cold trap. I. Principle and applications, *J. Chromatogr. 483*:43 (1987).

13. G. Reglero, M. Herraiz, T. Herraiz and J. Sanz, Capillary gas chromatographic determination of volatiles in solid matrices by direct introduction using a programmable-temperature vaporizor, *J. Chromatogr. 483*:43 (1989).
14. J. J. Manura and T. G. Hartman, Applications of a short-path thermal desorption GC accessory, *Am. Lab. 24*(8):46 (1992).
15. P. Werkhoff and W. Bretschneider, Dynamic headspace gas chromatography: concentration of volatile components after thermal desorption by intermediate cryofocusing in a cold trap. II. Effect of sampling and desorption parameters on recovery, *J. Chromatogr. 488*: (1987).
16. A. L. Sunesson, C. A. Nilsson, B. Andersson, and R. Carlson, Thermal Desorption Cold Trap-Injection in High-Resolution Gas Chromatography: Multivariate Optimization of Experimental Conditions. *J. Chromatogr. 623*(1):93 (1992).
17. T. G. Hartman, J. Lech, K. Karmas, J. Salinas, R. T. Rosen, and C. T. Ho, Flavor characterization using adsorbent trapping-thermal desorption or direct thermal desorption-gas chromatography and gas chromatograph-mass spectrometry, *Flavor Measurement* (C. T. Ho and Manley, eds.) 1993.
18. D. Djozan and Y. Assadi, Optimization of the gas stripping and cryogenic trapping method for capillary gas chromatographic analysis of traces of volatile halogenated compounds in drinking water, *J. Chromatogr. A 697*:525 (1995).
19. C. Garcia-Jares, S. Garcia-Martin, and R. Cele-Torrijos, Analysis of some highly volatile compounds of wine by means of purge and cold trapping injector capillary gas chromatography. Application to the differentiation of Rias Baixas Spanish white wines, *J. Agric. Food Chem. 43*:764 (1995).
20. R. T. Marsili, N. Miller, G. J. Kilmer, and R. E. Simmons, Identification and quantitation of the primary chemicals responsible for the characteristic malodor of beet sugar by purge and trap GC-MS-OD techniques, *J. Chromatogr. Sci. 32*(5):165 (1994).
21. M. A. Godshall, C. C. Grimm, and M. A. Clarke, Sensory properties of white beet sugars, Proceedings of the 1994 Sugar Processing Conferences, Helsinki, Finland, 1994, p. 312.
22. J. R. Vercellotti, K. L. Krippen, N. V. Lovegreen, and T. H. Sanders, Defining roasted peanut flavor quality. Part 1. Correlation of GC volatiles with roast color as an estimate of quality, *Food Science and Human Nutrition* (G. Charalambous ed.), Elsevier Science Publishers, 1992, p. 183.
23. A. M. Spanier, A. J. St. Angelo, C. C. Grimm, and J. A. Miller, The relationsh of temperature to the production of lipid volatiles from beef, *Lipids in Food Flavors* (C. T. Ho and T. G. Hartman, eds.), ACS Symposium Series 558, American Chemical Society, Washington, DC, 1994, p. 78.
24. J. J. Manura, Direct thermal analysis using the short path thermal desorption system, *Short Path Thermal Desorption Note*, No. 5 (1991).
25. M. E. Lee, N. E. Takenaka, F. A. Beland, and D. W. Miller, Using direct thermal

desorption to access the potential pool of styrene and 4-phenylcylohexene in latex-backed carpets, *Short Path Thermal Desorption Note*, No. 20 (1994).
26. M. C. Vidal-Aragon, E. Sabio, J. Gonzalesz, and M. Mas, Analysis of some highly volatile compounds of wine by means of purge and cold trapping injector capillary gas chromatography. Application to the differentiation of Rias Baixas Spanish white wines. *Alimentaria 31*(258):25 (1994).
27. J. J. Manura, Direct analysis of spices and coffee, *Short Path Thermal Desorption Note*, No. 4 (1990).
28. T. Yuiko and A. Kobayashi, Isolation of volatile components of fresh onion by thermal desorption cold trap capillary gas chromatography, *Biosci. Biotech. Biochem. 56*(11):1865 (1992).
29. J. V. Vercellotti, K. L. Crippen, N. V. Lovegreen, and T. H. Sanders, Defining roasted peanut flavor quality. Part 1. Correlation of GC volatiles with roast color as an estimate of quality, *Food Science and Human Nutrition* (G. Charalambous, ed.) Elsevier, 1992, p. 183.
30. J. L. Esteban, I. Martinez-Castro, and J. Sanz, Evaluation and optimization of the automatic thermal desorption method in the gas chromatographic determination of plant volatile compounds, *J. Chromatogr. A* 657:155 (1993).
31. J. J. Manura, Methodologies for the quantification of purge and trap thermal desorption and direct thermal desorption analyses, *Short Path Thermal Desorption Note*, No. 9 (1991).
32. T. G. Hartman, S. V. Overton, J. J. Manura, C. W. Baker, and J. N. Manoa, Short path thermal desorption: food science applications, *Food Technol. 45*(6):104 (1991).

4

Solid-Phase Microextraction for the Analysis of Flavors

ALAN D. HARMON
McCormick & Co., Inc., Hunt Valley, Maryland

I. INTRODUCTION

Every flavor and aroma analysis problem begins with the same question. How does one select a technique from the myriad of well-known isolation methods that will be best suited to the solution of the current problem? The analytical flavor chemist is faced daily with the separation and identification of complex mixtures. These mixtures comprise a wide range of organic chemicals that possess varying polarities and reactivities, usually occur in trace concentrations, and are likely included in other complex organic matrices. Fortunately, most aroma chemicals are volatile, and procedures for their isolation from foods and flavors have been established that take advantage of this volatility. Not so advantageous is the length of time usually required to obtain an isolate that is representative of the original aroma or flavor of the sample. The selection of steam distillation, solvent extraction, trapping of the volatiles on adsorbents, or combinations of these methods with other techniques might require several hours before the chemist can begin his chromatographic separation. The simple act of isolation may itself introduce artifacts from impurities in the solvents or through decomposition of the matrix or of the flavor chemicals themselves. An ideal approach to flavor isolation and analysis would provide an analytical sample whose composition is identical to the chemical mixture within the matrix, which is free of solvents and other impurities, and which could be completed within a few minutes with no intermediate processing of the sample. Solid-phase microextraction approaches this ideal.

II. WHAT IS SOLID-PHASE MICROEXTRACTION?

Solid-phase microextraction (SPME) is a relatively new technique for the rapid, solventless extraction or preconcentration of volatile and semi-volatile organic compounds. It utilizes the partitioning of organic components between a bulk aqueous or vapor phase and the thin polymeric films coated onto fused silica fibers in the SPME apparatus. The technique was first described by Berlardi and Pawliszyn for the analysis of environmental chemicals in water (1). Since that time, environmental studies (2–23) and theoretical treatments and practical applications (24–29) have continued to account for most of the publications. The areas of food, beverage, and related analyses have generated only a few references (30–34).

Solid-phase microextraction techniques are independent of the form of the matrix; liquids, solids, and gases all can be sampled readily. SPME is an equilibrium technique, and accurate quantitation requires that the extractions be carefully controlled. Each component will behave differently depending on its polarity, volatility, organic/water partition coefficient, the volume of the sample or the volume of the headspace, the rate of agitation, the pH of the solution, and the temperature. The incorporation of an internal standard into the matrix and adherence to specific sampling times will usually result in excellent quantitative correlations. Since the SPME technique requires no solvents and can be performed without heating the sample, the formation of chemical artifacts is greatly reduced, if not completely eliminated.

III. THE SPME DEVICE

Figure 1 describes the apparatus introduced by Supelco (Bellefonte, PA) for manual operation. A similar device has been designed for automated techniques and is available for use with Varian 8100 and 8200 CX series GC autosamplers (Varian Chromotography Systems, Walnut Creek, CA). The manual device is essentially a modified syringe having a spring-loaded plunger and a barrel with a detent to al-

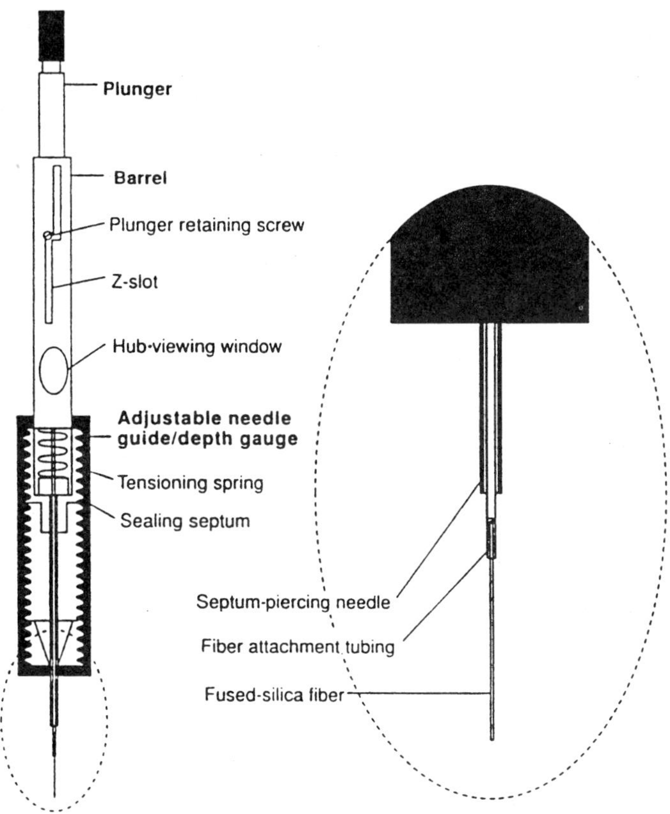

FIGURE 1 Graphical representation of a solid-phase microextraction (SPME) device. (Reprinted with permission from Ref. 29. Copyright 1994, American Chemical Society.)

low the plunger to be held in an extended position during the extraction phase and during the injection/desorption period. Also contained within the barrel is a modified 24 gauge stainless steel needle, which encloses another length of stainless steel tubing fitted tightly to a short piece of solid-core fused silica fiber. The bottom centimeter of the fused silica fiber is coated with a relatively thin film of any of several stationary phases. This film serves as the organic "solvent" during the absorption of the volatile compounds from the analytical matrix. The needle functions to puncture the septa sealing both the sample container and the GC injection port and to protect the fragile fused silica fiber during storage and use.

Fibers coated with nonpolar polydimethylsiloxane (similar to SE-30 or

OV-101) and the more polar polyacrylate are commercially available at the present time. The development of several other fiber types is actively underway, including Carbowax, Carboxen (a porous activated carbon support), and divinylbenzene copolymers. For most analyses, especially of volatile flavor compounds, a fiber having a 100-μm coating of polydimethylsiloxane is preferred. If a more rapid equilibration is needed, a fiber with a 30-μm coating of polydimethylsiloxane might be more appropriate. Fibers with a 7-μm thickness of polydimethylsiloxane will work well with samples having high boiling components, e.g., polyaromatic hydrocarbons, or where higher temperatures might be required to desorb them in the injection port of the gas chromatograph. In general, the fibers coated with thicker films will require a somewhat longer time to achieve equilibrium but might provide higher sensitivity due to the greater mass of the analytes that can be absorbed. A fiber coated with an 85-μm film of polyacrylate is available for the extraction of more polar compounds, especially those possessing phenolic structures.

IV. THE MECHANICS OF THE SPME PROCESS

The process of solid-phase microextraction is illustrated in Figure 2. A sample is placed into a vial or other suitable container, which is sealed with a septum-type cap. The fiber should be cleaned before analyzing any sample because the polymer phase can absorb aroma chemicals from the air and produce a high background in the chromatogram. Cleaning can be done in a few minutes by inserting the fiber into an auxiliary injection port or using a syringe cleaner. For liquid sampling the SPME needle pierces the septum and the fiber is extended through the needle and into the solution. During headspace sampling the fiber is extended into the vapor phase above a liquid or solid sample. The SPME apparatus and sample vial can be supported during the equilibration period by placing them inside a test tube (18 × 150 mm or larger). Both direct liquid sampling and headspace techniques often benefit from the addition of sodium chloride to the solution, which enhances the equilibrium toward the organic phase of the SPME fiber. Some care must be exercised when penetrating the septa because the needle point on the SPME device is flat. It might be appropriate to use prepunched septa both for sealing the sample vials and in the injection port of the gas chromatograph. Simply inserting a clean needle from a microliter syringe through the septum to provide a small hole before inserting the SPME fiber can prevent bending the needle.

A small stirring bar often is used to agitate the solution, which greatly increases the rate of equilibration (2). After a suitable sampling time (1–20 minutes) the fiber is withdrawn into the needle; the needle is removed from the septum and is then inserted directly into the injection port of a gas chro-

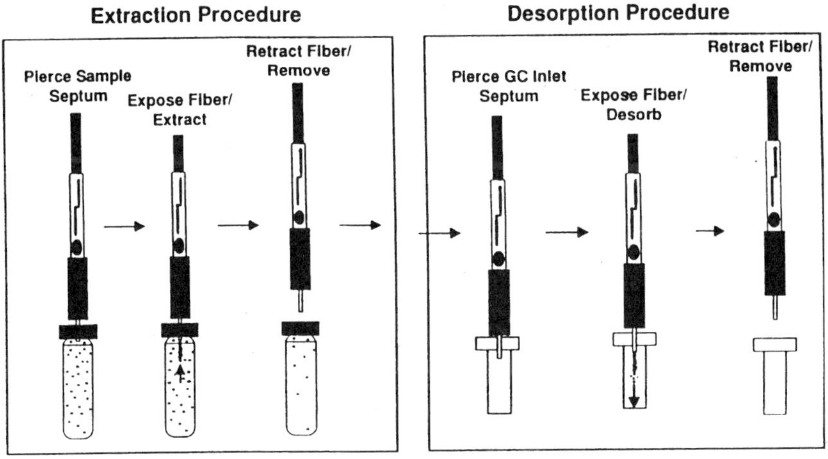

FIGURE 2 Sequence of events showing extraction steps and desorption (injection) steps followed to perform an analysis using SPME. The fiber is inserted directly into a liquid sample with the subsequent absorption of most of the analyte molecules (small circles) from the solution. (From Supelco, with permission.)

matograph for 1–2 minutes. The absorbed chemicals are thermally desorbed by the heat of the injection port and are transferred directly to the column for analysis.

Any manner of injection is suitable for SPME as long as the needle can be introduced through the septum nut and can be extended into the heated zone of any injection system. Since this technique often involves the preconcentration of very dilute substances, the split ratio of a split/splitless capillary injection port should be set to a low value (around 10:1) so that the benefit of the preconcentration step is not wasted. For some applications where the components are not at trace levels, higher split flows will work as well. The use of an injection port liner with an internal diameter of 1 mm or less usually provides somewhat sharper peaks for highly volatile compounds, although completely satisfactory chromatographic separations and peak shapes can be achieved using a standard split liner packed with glass wool. Cryogenic cooling of the column is not necessary for most applications, although some sharpening of early eluting peaks will result if that capability is available. Care should be taken to ensure that the upper surface of the glass wool or other packing material used in the injection liner is below the level of the tip of the SPME fiber when it is inserted into the injection port. The penalty for extending the fiber into glass wool is often a broken or damaged fiber.

As mentioned previously, several types of fibers are currently available that exhibit a certain degree of selectivity. For general usage the nonpolar thick film fibers will provide high sensitivity with most compounds. Polyacrylate fibers are not strictly limited to the absorption of polar molecules, but they do afford greater sensitivity for the analysis of alcohols, phenols, and certain aldehydes when compared to esters and hydrocarbons. Table 1 compares the relative amounts of a mixture of flavor chemicals extracted from the headspace above an aqueous solution containing 10 ppm of each compound. For this example, 0.5 ml of the solution was contained in a 4-ml vial maintained at 55°C without stirring and without the addition of salt. After allowing enough time for equilibration of the headspace, the mixture was analyzed by suspending the fiber above the surface of the solution for 10 minutes before gas chromatographic analysis using a flame ionization detector. The peak areas were normalized to the response for *n*-butanol after extraction with the polydimethylsiloxane fiber. For this group of flavor chemicals, the polyacrylate fiber was more effective for extraction of the alcohols

TABLE 1 Relative Effectiveness of 100-μm Polydimethylsiloxane and 85-μm Polyacrylate Fibers for the Headspace SPME Extraction of a 10 ppm Mixture of Selected Flavor Chemicals in Water

	Relative extraction efficiency calculated from raw area (%) and normalized to the *n*-butanol peak from polydimethylsiloxane	
Flavor compound	Polydimethylsiloxane	Polyacrylate
Ethyl acetate	4	3.1
n-Butanol	1	3.3
Hexanal	54	48.1
cis-3-Hexenol	6	19.5
Benzaldehyde	22	59
Ethyl caproate	320	170
Limonene	1410	590
Linalool	117	174
Eugenol	32	110
β-Ionone	530	505
Dimethyl sulfide	7	6.3
Pyrrolidine	7	7
Pyridine	11	3.7

(butanol, *cis*-3-hexenol, and linalool), benzaldehyde, and the phenolic compound eugenol. Also evident are the somewhat lower responses for esters (ethyl acetate and ethyl caproate), hydrocarbons (limonene), and pyridine. All of the components were effectively extracted using both fibers, however. In a similar study Yang and Peppard (32) compared the effectiveness of SPME extractions to the

TABLE 2 Relative GC Peak Areas of a Flavor Mixture Obtained by Direct Split Injection and by Different SPME Sampling Methods

	Relative peak area (%)		
Compound	Direct injection	SPME liquid sampling	SPME headspace sampling
Ethyl acetate	4.4	0.2	1.2
Ethyl butyrate	5.0	2.6	11.5
Limonene	6.4	1.2	2.6
Ethyl caproate	4.3	6.9	8.4
3-Hexenyl acetate	4.3	7.8	12.0
cis-3-Hexenol	4.9	0.3	2.1
Benzaldehyde	5.5	1.1	6.0
Linalool	4.5	1.1	6.0
Diethyl succinate	3.4	<0.1	<0.1
Neral	2.9	7.0	5.9
2-Methylbutyric acid	2.6	0.1	<0.1
γ-Hexalactone	3.4	0.1	0.3
1-Carvone	4.7	9.6	7.9
Geranial	5.0	13.6	9.7
Anethole	4.8	14.1	5.0
Caproic acid	3.2	0.1	<0.1
Phenylethanol	4.9	0.2	0.4
β-Ionone	4.3	14.9	8.9
Cinnamic aldehyde	4.6	2.5	0.2
Triacetin	2.1	0.2	0.2
γ-Decalactone	3.7	8.0	1.5
Heliotropin	2.4	0.5	0.2
Triethyl citrate	2.2	0.1	<0.1
Ethyl vanillin	3.3	<0.1	<0.1
Vanillin	3.0	<0.1	<0.1

Source: Adapted with permission from Ref. 32. Copyright 1994, American Chemical Society.

direct injection of a flavor mixture (Table 2). They observed similar selectivities among the sampling methods and estimated detection limits for the compounds of 0.1 ppb to >1 ppm, depending upon the extraction efficiencies and detector responses of the individual flavor components. Their data show essentially no response for diethyl succinate, caproic acid, triethyl citrate, vanillin, and ethyl vanillin using either method of SPME extraction.

Low molecular weight carboxylic acids are difficult to extract from aqueous solutions using SPME techniques. The formic through butyric acids are miscible in water, and even caprylic acid (C_8) is soluble to the extent of 68 mg/100 g (35). The low capacity factors of carboxylic acids associated with the nonpolar phases used for capillary GC columns lead to severe "fronting" of acid peaks, which often can be used to identify their presence in mixtures with other flavor compounds. The same phenomenon also has an effect on the absorption of acids by SPME phases. It is possible to enhance their extraction with SPME techniques, however. Figure 3 shows the relative extraction efficiencies for several carboxylic acids, each at a concentration of 10 ppm in water. The results show the effectiveness of headspace extractions for both the 85-μm polyacrylate and 100-μm polydimethylsiloxane fibers and of the addition of 25% NaCl to the solutions. With the exception of caprylic acid, the polyacrylate fiber is more efficient for headspace extractions. The salting out effect is dramatic for carboxylic acids more than four carbons in length.

Differences between headspace sampling and direct immersion sampling are illustrated in Figure 4. For this example, the polyacrylate fiber was used to extract aqueous solutions of the carboxylic acids both before and after the addition of 25% NaCl. During the direct immersion sampling, a 2-ml portion of each solution was maintained at 55°C without stirring, and the fiber was inserted into the solution for 5 minutes. Headspace sampling was continued for 5 minutes at 55°C with the fiber held above the surface of a 1-ml sample contained in a 3-ml vial. This experiment shows that both headspace and direct immersion sampling are effective for the extraction of carboxylic acids with more than three carbons, but that the higher the carbon number, the better they can be isolated from the solution. Irrespective of these apparently successful extractions, however, carboxylic acids remain extremely difficult to isolate from a mixture of flavor compounds in dilute aqueous solution. It has been suggested that doping the fiber with an esterifying reagent prior to SPME extraction greatly enhances the recovery and chromatography of carboxylic acids (J. Pawliszyn, personal communication). The details of this technique should be published in the near future.

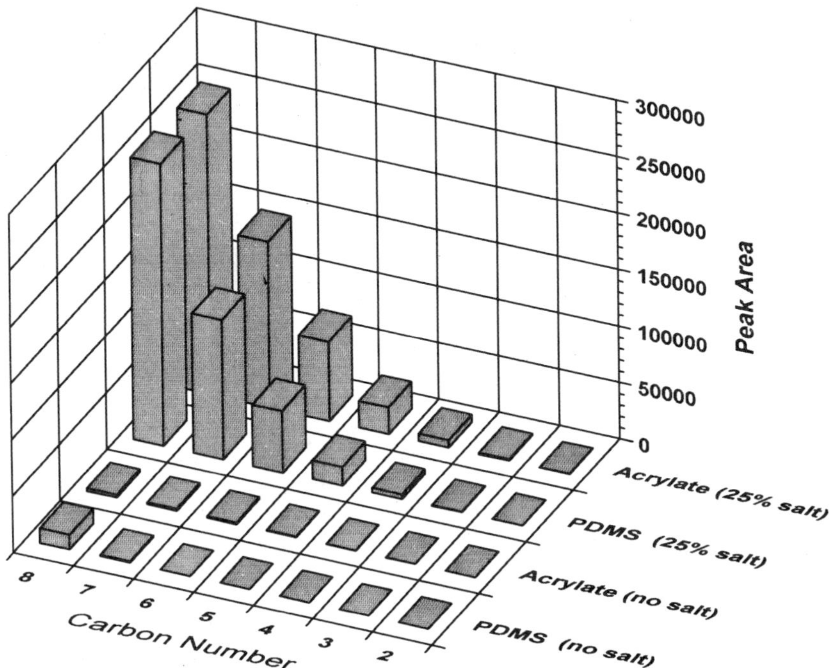

FIGURE 3 Graphical representation of the relative extraction effectiveness of a series of carboxylic acids using 100-μm polydimethylsiloxane (PDMS) and 85-μm polyacrylate (Acrylate) SPME fibers. The acids were dissolved in water at a concentration of 10 ppm each and the solutions were sampled using the headspace technique. The effect of dissolving 25% NaCl in the solutions is also represented. A 3-ml vial containing 1 ml of solution was used for the experiment, and the acids were monitored by capillary GC (30 × 0.25 mm DB-1, 1 μm film, flame ionization detection, injector temperature 235°C, split flow 8 ml/min, fiber desorb time 1.0 min).

V. THEORETICAL CONSIDERATIONS

The theoretical aspects of solid-phase microextraction have been well documented (see, e.g., Refs. 6,9,29, and 32), and the reader should refer to these references for a complete discussion. Essentially, the principles affecting extraction of organic compounds from solutions using SPME are the same ones that control

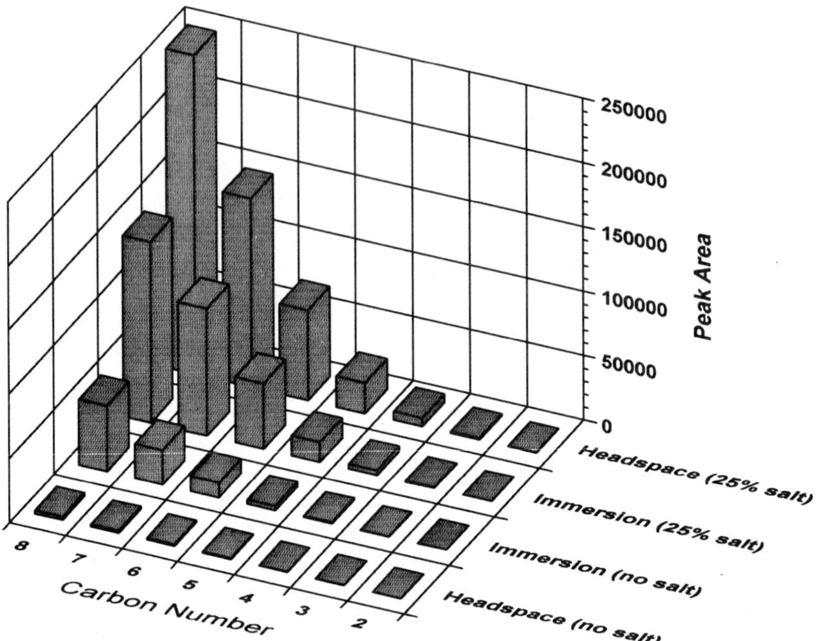

FIGURE 4 Graph showing the relative extraction differences for carboxylic acids between headspace and direct immersion SPME techniques. The acids were dissolved in water at a concentration of 10 ppm each and the solutions were extracted for 5 minutes at 40°C, without stirring, using a 85-μm polyacrylate fiber. Both aqueous and 25% NaCl solutions were examined, and the extractions were monitored by capillary GC as in Figure 3.

their partitioning between phases of immiscible liquids in a separatory funnel, a countercurrent extraction system, a Likens-Nickerson distillation head, or any other liquid-liquid extraction device. Therefore, the factors affecting efficient extraction by these methods (contact time, efficiency of mixing, pH, salt concentration, temperature, phase ratios, etc.) also affect the partitioning in SPME extractions. This is not an unreasonable concept if the SPME fiber is regarded simply as an immobilized liquid phase in contact with an aqueous solution.

The volume of the fiber coating is small relative to the bulk of the aqueous phase being extracted, and the mass of analyte absorbed by the coating at equilibrium is directly related to its initial concentration in the solution and the distribution coefficients controlling the equilibria. The principle behind the partitioning process is the equilibrium established for the analyte(s) between the fiber organic phase and the solution phase. If you consider the equilibrium expression in effect for the placement of the fiber in the solution

$$[X]_l \Leftrightarrow [X]_f$$

then

$$K_{lf} = \frac{[X]_f}{[X]_l}$$

where [X] is the concentration of the flavor chemical in solution (l) and in the organic phase of the SPME fiber (f). K_{lf} is the distribution coefficient for X between the liquid phase and the fiber. The amount of material absorbed from the solution by the fiber can be described by the relationship (9,32)

$$n = \frac{C_0 V_l V_f K_{lf}}{K_{lf} V_f + V_l}$$

where n is the amount of compound X absorbed by the fiber, C_0 is the initial concentration of X in the solution, and V_l and V_f are the respective volumes of the solution and the organic phase of the fiber. In order to obtain a quantitative extraction (>90% of the analyte absorbed by the fiber), the distribution coefficient of X needs to be about an order of magnitude greater than the volume ratio V_l/V_f of the system (6). Complete extractions are usually not necessary to obtain quantitative information, since the amounts of the analytes in the SPME phase are controlled by the various distribution constants in effect under the experimental conditions. As long as the conditions are carefully repeated from run to run, the equilibrium concentrations in the phases also will remain constant.

In the case of headspace SPME extraction, the equilibrium partitioning occurs between the liquid organic phase of the fiber and the vapor phase above a liquid or solid sample. The diffusion of analytes to the fiber in the vapor phase is about four orders of magnitude greater than in solution (9). The speed of analysis by headspace sampling should reflect this greater diffusion. In fact, headspace SPME can reduce the extraction time from 5 minutes to 1 minute or less and still maintain high sensitivities for most analytes. Heating the sample greatly increases the diffusion of analytes into the vapor phase. Zhang and Pawliszyn have taken advantage of this to effect quantitative recoveries of BTEX compounds from difficult matrices by simultaneously heating the sample and cooling the fiber (26).

Headspace SPME techniques are capable of extracting components having boiling points much higher than the sampling temperature. The chromatographic detection of a series of paraffin hydrocarbons following headspace SPME extraction at different temperatures is shown in Figure 5. Considering the mild temperatures utilized, the recovery of *n*-heptadecane (boiling point 302°C) is remarkable. In fact, a room temperature extraction also provided a significant peak for each of the nine components. It is not surprising, then, that headspace extractions of food samples can provide considerable detail about the composition of spices, herbs, and flavors. According to Zhang and Pawliszyn, compounds with Henry's constants greater than 90 atm·cm^3·mol^{-1} can be isolated using headspace SPME at ambient temperature (9). This would

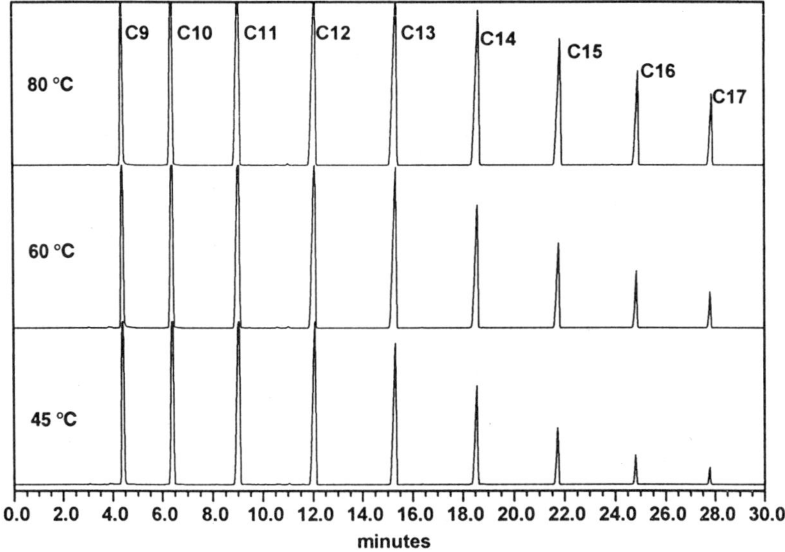

FIGURE 5 Stacked chromatograms showing the gas chromatographic analysis of a series of *n*-hydrocarbons isolated by headspace SPME at various temperatures. The sample was prepared by transferring 1 µl of individual hydrocarbon standards into a 4-ml vial and sealing with a Teflon-coated septum. After 10 minutes equilibration at the indicated temperature, the headspace vapor was extracted using a 100-µm polydimethylsiloxane fiber and was analyzed by GC with flame ionization detection. The injector temperature for this sample was set at 300°C, and the fiber was desorbed for 1 minute.

include three-ring polyaromatic hydrocarbons with boiling points around 340°C, for example.

For compounds that have appreciable water solubility, both the transfer to the vapor phase and the corresponding decrease in the magnitude of K_{lf} can prevent observing them in chromatograms obtained by SPME extraction. This is not necessarily a problem during flavor analysis because it becomes possible to analyze very low concentrations of volatile flavor compounds in the presence of high concentrations of polar solvents and other less volatile compounds using SPME extraction techniques. On the other hand, a complete analysis of every volatile and semi-volatile compound contained within a flavor mixture might not be possible when using SPME as the only isolation technique.

VI. PRACTICAL APPLICATIONS OF SPME FOR FLAVOR ANALYSIS

A. Quantitative Analysis

1. The Analysis of Ethanol

When new techniques are introduced, most analytical chemists want to know whether they are appropriate for quantitative analysis. The SPME process can be readily adapted for the rapid quantitative analysis of volatile compounds. Ethanol is a common solvent used in flavors and fragrances. It is miscible with water, has a high vapor pressure, and also has solubility in organic solvents. There are several official methods for the quantitative measurement of ethanol in flavors, extracts, and beverages. Some of these include distillation followed by specific gravity determination of the distillate (37) (method 28.1.04), direct gas chromatographic analysis after incorporation of a standard and, perhaps, a carrier solvent such as tetrahydrofuran (36) (method 36.1.01), and dichromate oxidation (36) (method 28.1.07). All of these methods are accurate, but they can be time consuming, utilize hazardous chemicals, or perhaps contaminate the gas chromatographic system with nonvolatile substances. Headspace SPME extraction is another alternative that can be used for the rapid quantitative determination of ethanol in liquids or aqueous solutions of solids. Since only volatile materials are isolated from the sample, there can be no contamination of the chromatographic system with nonvolatile contaminants.

Figure 6 shows the relative FID responses obtained for an aqueous solution of ethanol and *n*-propanol following headspace SPME with 100-µm polydimethylsiloxane and 85-µm polyacrylate fibers. A calibration curve for ethanol concentrations from 0.1 to 20% by volume is indicated in Figure 7.

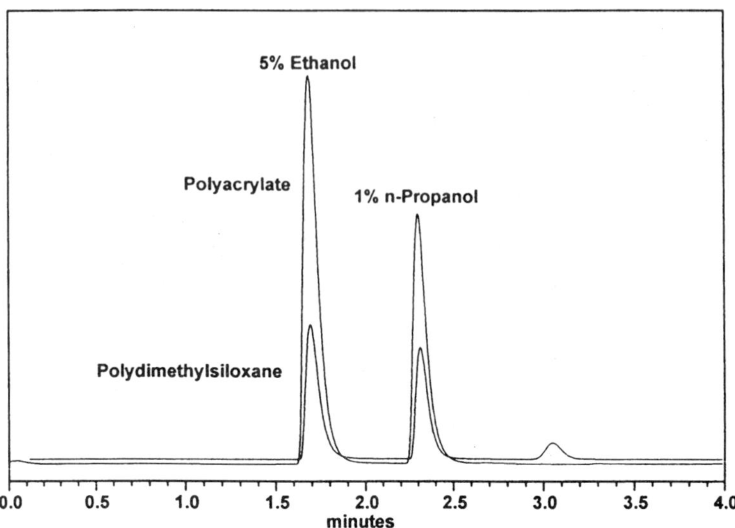

FIGURE 6 Overlaid capillary gas chromatograms showing the response differences of ethanol and n-propanol toward 100 μm polydimethylsiloxane and 85 μm polyacrylate SPME phases. The solution was analyzed by headspace SPME over 1.0 ml of solution contained in a 4 ml Teflon sealed vial. An extraction time of 5 minutes at 40°C was used for the experiment.

Both alcohols have a greater affinity for the more polar polyacrylate fiber, but the correlation coefficients for both systems show nearly ideal behavior over the concentration range. These data were collected manually by transferring 1.0 ml of solution to 4-ml vials and then extracting the headspace for 5 minutes at a temperature of 40°C. Injection into the gas chromatograph was completed by desorption for 1 minute with an injection port temperature of 235°C and a split ratio of about 10:1. Samples may be evaluated simply by introducing an appropriate amount of the internal standard into the sample, mixing, transferring a suitable amount to another vial, and repeating the headspace absorption using the same parameters that were used for calibration. The ratio of the area of the ethanol peak to the area of the *n*-propanol peak remains consistent from run to run. Linearity is maintained at concentrations above 20% for ethanol, but when analyzing other chemical classes that have a higher affinity for the fiber phase, concentrations in this range might saturate the small volume of the fiber and lead to nonlinear behavior. This would be more likely to

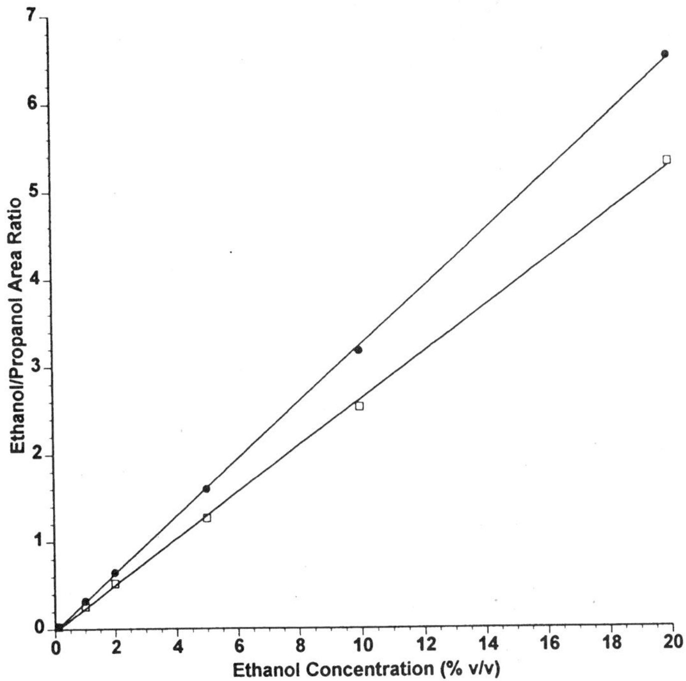

FIGURE 7 A calibration curve for ethanol prepared using *n*-propanol as an internal standard at 1.0% and gas chromatographic analysis following headspace SPME extraction. The upper curve (solid circles) was obtained with an 85-μm polyacrylate fiber and the lower curve (open squares) was obtained using a 100-μm polydimethylsiloxane fiber. The linear correlation coefficients for ethanol concentrations from 0.1 to 20.0% using both fibers is in excess of 0.999.

occur when using fibers with thin polymeric films, for example, the 7-μm polydimethylsiloxane fiber.

It is important to maintain control of extraction times and temperatures for quantitative analyses, but the incorporation of an internal standard that has characteristics similar to the analyte removes some of the error that would be associated with an externally calibrated method. More effective control of the analysis can be assured using automated sampling (24,28). The software associated with the automated version of SPME allows precise control of the absorption and desorption times, a preabsorption delay, and multiple samplings from each vial using either headspace or direct liquid immersion. It also allows the absorption phase of an extraction to begin during the chromatographic run of a preceding sample, which can greatly increase the throughput for busy laboratories.

2. Relative Quantitation of Isothiocyanates in a Seafood Cocktail Sauce

Horseradish volatiles consist primarily of allyl and phenylethyl isothiocyanates (37). These compounds provide the characteristic pungency and flavor of horseradish and impart that character to the products into which horseradish is formulated. Seafood cocktail sauces often use varying amounts of horseradish for these flavor notes. Methods are often needed to measure volatiles in finished products to determine how much flavor is being lost through evaporation, chemical conversion, absorption by packaging materials, or other effects of aging. Accelerated storage conditions can provide excellent information if the resources are available to observe and measure the chemical changes that occur. Headspace SPME was used to determine the changes in concentration of the horseradish volatiles in a control sample of cocktail sauce stored at 4°C and in a subsample of the sauce stored at 30°C for 5 days. Figure 8 shows the chromatographic differences observed using GC/mass spectrometry (MS) to detect and quantify the isothiocyanate components. For this analysis phenyl isothiocyanate was added to the cocktail sauce samples as an internal standard at a concentration of 10 ppm (1 mg/100 g). The phenyl isothiocyanate standard was prepared and used as a dilute solution in triacetin. Each sample was thoroughly mixed with the standard in sealed blender jars, and 5-g portions were transferred to 15-ml headspace vials for SPME extraction GC/MS analysis. Selected ion chromatograms were collected for integration based on the individual molecular weights of the compounds. These were m/z 99 for allyl isothiocyanate, m/z 135 for phenyl isothiocyanate, and m/z 163 for phenylethyl isothiocyanate. The chromatogram in Figure 8a was obtained for the control sample and the one in Figure 8b was obtained for the sample subjected to elevated temperature. Phenyl isothiocyanate (peak 3) produced very stable peak areas for the two analyses, whereas the areas for allyl isothiocyanate (peak 2) and phenylethyl isothiocyanate (peak 4) decreased significantly in the heated sample. A simple calculation showed that allyl isothiocyanate decreased by approximately 71% during the 5-day test, while the less volatile and less reactive phenylethyl isothiocyanate decreased by only 29%. It would be possible to determine the kinetics associated with these declines by monitoring the concentrations at specific intervals during the storage cycle.

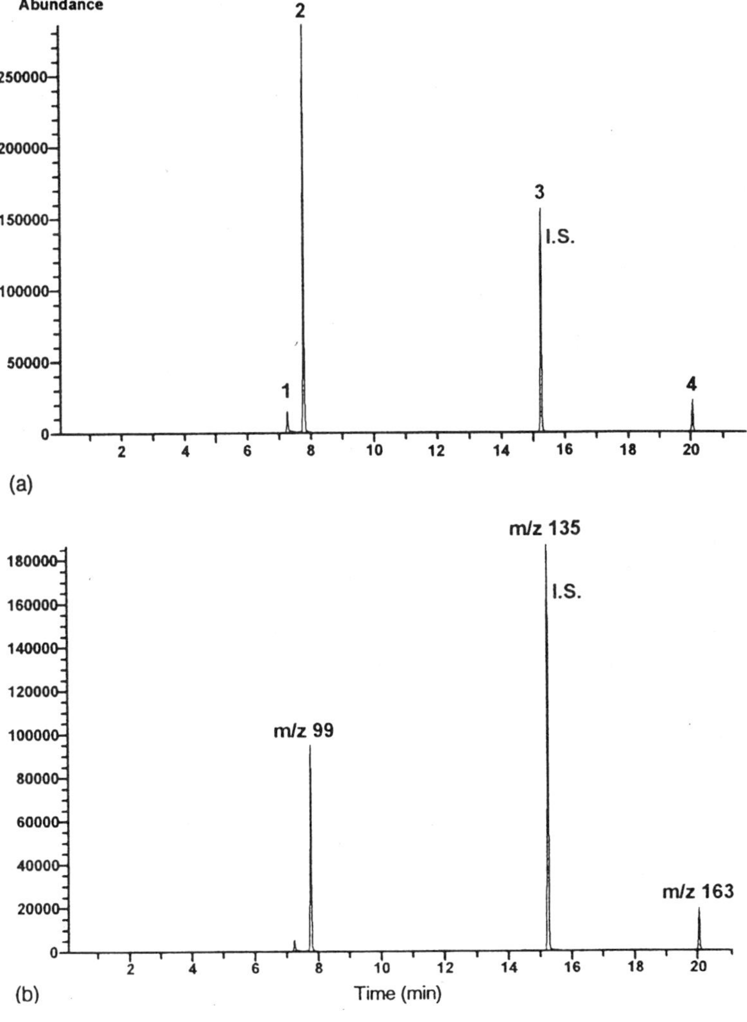

FIGURE 8 A comparison of the changes observed for the volatile isothiocyanates of horseradish isolated from (a) a sample of cocktail sauce maintained at 4°C and (b) a subsample of the same cocktail sauce held at 30°C for 5 days. The volatiles were isolated from the cocktail sauce samples by headspace SPME extraction using a 100-μm polydimethylsiloxane fiber after spiking the samples with phenyl isothiocyanate (peak 3, internal standard) at a concentration of 10 ppm. Analysis of the components was by GC/MS, and quantitation was performed using selected ion extraction chromatograms of the respective molecular ions of the isothiocyanates. The other numbered peaks are allyl thiocyanate (1), allyl isothiocyanate (2), and phenylethyl isothiocyanate (4).

The quantitation of flavor chemicals using SPME can be rapid, precise, and accurate if one takes the time to define an appropriate methodology. It is easy to detect a multitude of volatile chemicals of widely varying classes during a single analysis, but the incorporation of a single internal standard is not normally sufficient to quantify every observable component in a mixture. Because SPME is such a rapid extraction technique, however, it is possible to evaluate the effectiveness of a large number of standards in a relatively short time. Other techniques suitable for quantification by SPME are standard addition and isotope dilution analysis (30,32), but external standard calibrations may not generally be successful due to the significant matrix effects that are usually encountered.

B. Qualitative Analysis

Solid-phase microextraction is ideally suited to the characterization of unknown mixtures of volatile organic compounds. As indicated earlier, the different affinities of certain chemical classes to the various polymer films can be used to advantage when applying SPME techniques for their isolation and injection into a gas chromatograph or GC/MS system. The ability to sample solutions both by immersion and by headspace methods adds another dimension to the isolation technique. Immersion sampling may provide more sensitivity overall, but headspace extraction might separate the more volatile materials for increased selectivity. The remaining examples will illustrate these concepts more clearly.

1. A Comparison of Direct Split Injection and Headspace SPME Injection of a Punch Flavor

Liquid flavors are not always simple mixtures of flavor chemicals dissolved in single, "analytically well-behaved" solvents. Flavorists often combine diluted forms of chemicals to reach their final goal. Generally ethanol is the solvent of choice for most applications, but propylene glycol, glycerin, triacetin, benzyl alcohol, triethyl citrate, fruit juices, sugar syrups, water, and other liquids and solids often find their way into flavor mixtures. A particularly difficult flavor problem in this respect is shown in Figure 9, which shows a capillary gas chromatogram of the result of a direct split injection of a fruit punch flavor using flame ionization detection. Three solvents were used in the flavor, all in large proportion, along with a lesser amount of a fruit juice. Only ethyl caproate could be identified by GC/MS as a primary flavor chemical among the ethanol, propylene glycol, and glycerin components. The other, smaller peaks in the chromatogram were

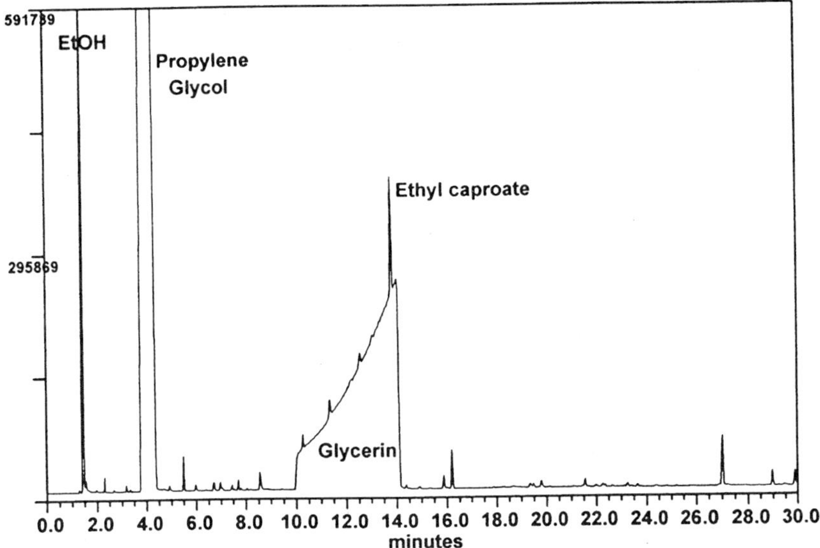

FIGURE 9 Chromatogram showing the flame ionization detector response after a direct split injection of a punch flavor onto a capillary GC column. Analytical conditions: column (30 meter DB-1, 0.25 mm, 1 μ film); injector temp. 235°C, split flow 100 ml/min; detector temp (FID) 250°C; oven temperature 60 (1 min) to 230 (6.5 min) at 4°C/min, 0.5 μl injected.

primarily associated with dimeric and polymeric ethers arising from the solvents. In addition, several artifacts associated with sugar decomposition were observed.

The same flavor evaluated using the headspace SPME technique is illustrated in Figure 10. Clearly, the two methods provide different results! One should first compare the contributions of the various solvents to the chromatograms. Headspace SPME sampling has completely eliminated the glycerin peak, which revealed 13 additional flavor components that had coeluted with that solvent as a result of direct split injection. Glycerin could not be detected even with a selected ion chromatogram. The propylene glycol peak has been reduced to a well-resolved minor component by the headspace extraction, but ethanol remains as a major solvent peak. These differences are due both to the lower volatilities of propylene glycol and glycerin and to their hydrophilic nature. The affinity of the hydroxylic sol-

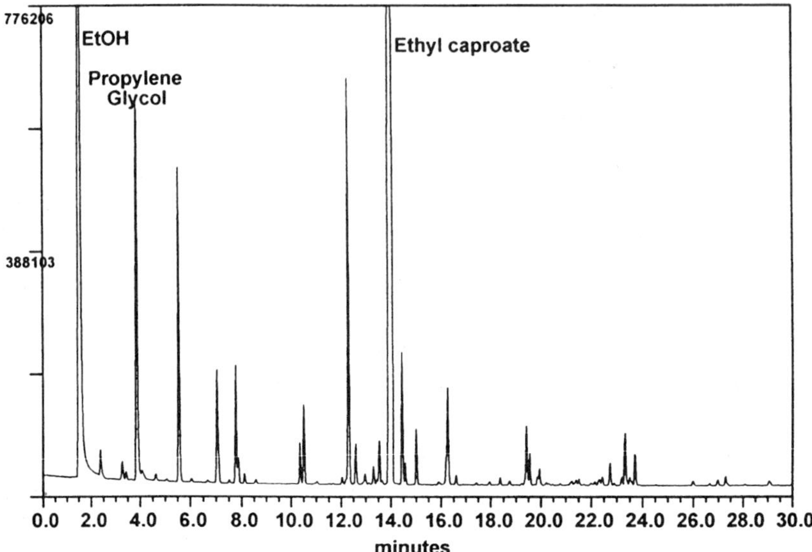

FIGURE 10 Chromatogram showing the flame ionization detector response to the headspace SPME extract obtained from six drops of a punch flavor using a 100-μm polydimethylsiloxane fiber for 10 minutes at 45°C. The chromatographic conditions were the same as for Figure 9 except that the split flow was decreased to 8 ml/min and the fiber was desorbed for 1.0 minute.

vents for the polydimethylsiloxane fiber used in this analysis is much less than the affinities of the less polar, more hydrophobic flavor chemicals. Although a chromatogram has not been included to show it, a Likens-Nickerson extraction of this flavor also did not provide a satisfactory analysis due to the formation of numerous artifacts from the thermal decomposition of sugars during the steam distillation.

2. Isolation of Aroma Volatiles from Fresh Fruits

The natural chemicals comprising the aroma of fresh fruits are usually complex mixtures of alcohols, aldehydes, esters, and terpenoids that may transform markedly during the ripening cycle. These chemicals are generally recovered from the fruit pulp or their juices by vacuum or steam distillation before separation and analysis using capillary GC or GC/MS. Such isolation techniques require relatively large amounts of fruit, sometimes on the order of several kilograms, to obtain a suitable analytical sample, which then is diluted and contaminated with the organic solvents used during the isolation. Additionally, traditional isolation methods require from 4 to 24 hours before the identification phase can begin. Purge-and-trap techniques will reduce both the amount of sample required and the time needed to prepare a suitable isolate, but the equipment is expensive and requires time to establish the operating interface to a GC or a GC/MS system. Headspace SPME can be utilized with small samples of fruit, the extract can be prepared in a few minutes with little sample preparation, and it is readily transported to any number of gas chromatographic systems.

Yang and Peppard have shown that direct liquid immersion SPME of a sample of fruit juice beverage was comparable or higher in sensitivity to a conventional solvent extraction using dichloromethane for most of the recovered flavor chemicals (32). Although they did not compare the sensitivity of headspace SPME extraction in the same study, it would have provided a similar result. For studies in our laboratories, fresh fruits have been sampled by simply removing three or four small "cores" of fruit pulp using the blunt end of a disposable Pasteur pipet and depositing the pieces into a 15-ml headspace vial. After fitting the vial with a Teflon-lined seal, the fruit is immediately extracted using headspace SPME at room temperature for 10 minutes before injection and analysis by GC/MS. The results of several of these analyses are shown in Figures 11–13.

Cantaloupe is the orange, delicately flavored fruit of *Cucumis melo* L., which becomes progressively stronger in flavor and aroma with increasing ripeness. Figure 11 shows the results of a GC/MS analysis from a 1.5-g sample of ripe cantaloupe prepared as described above. The primary aroma compounds have been identified in the figure. These compounds were not determined in a quantitative experiment, but it has been reported that isobutyl acetate, butyl acetate, and ethyl butyrate are present in cantaloupe at a level of 0.1 ppm and that hexyl acetate is present at 0.04 ppm (38). Obviously these amounts will vary from sample to sample, but if these levels are indicative of the concentrations in this melon, the headspace SPME technique is able to detect very low levels of nonpolar volatile chemicals.

A ripe banana (*Musa sapientum* L.) was also examined in the same manner. After transferring about 2 g of banana "cores" to a vial, the headspace SPME extract provided the GC/MS chromatogram shown in Figure 12. This chromatogram is considerably more complex than a "typical" banana flavor, which usually is highly concentrated in isoamyl acetate. Quantitative values have been reported (38) for several of the compounds from banana extracts, among them isoamyl alcohol (2–12 ppm), isobutyl acetate (47 ppm), isoamyl

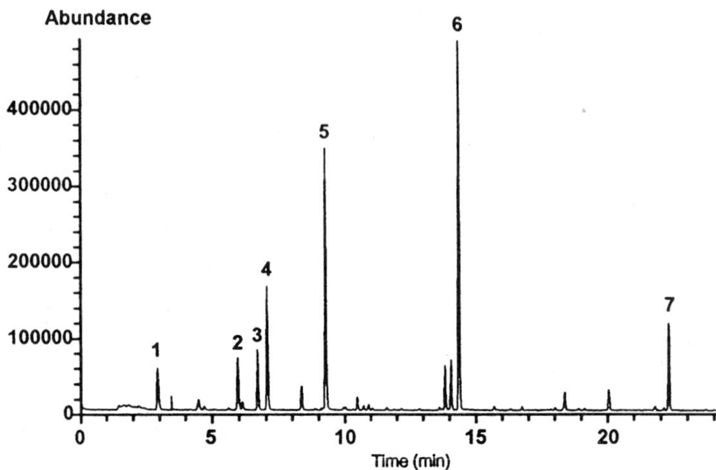

FIGURE 11 Total ion chromatogram of a portion of the volatile components obtained from a sample of ripe cantaloupe by headspace SPME using a 100-μm polydimethylsiloxane fiber. The fruit was placed into a 15-ml headspace vial by removing small "plugs" of the pulp with the blunt end of a disposable pipet. The SPME extraction was carried out at room temperature for 10 minutes before analysis by GC/MS using the same chromatographic conditions specified for Figure 10 and a Hewlett-Packard 5989 GC/MS system. The numbered components are ethyl acetate (1), isobutyl acetate (2), ethyl butyrate (3), butyl acetate (4), 2-methylbutyl acetate (5), hexyl acetate (6), and 2-ethylhexyl acetate (7).

acetate (12–75 ppm), isoamyl isobutyrate (0.7 ppm), isoamyl butyrate (6 ppm), isoamyl caproate (0.07 ppm), eugenol (1.2 ppm), and elemicin (7.5 ppm). The relative peak areas shown in this chromatogram suggest a different quantitative profile, but this might have been affected by the different ripeness of the samples and the relative extraction efficiency of the SPME fiber. 3-Hexenyl caproate was found in the SPME extract but was not listed among the banana flavor compounds in that reference.

A final example from the analysis of fruits is shown in Figure 13. Figure 13a represents the volatiles obtained from the flesh of a ripe Bartlett pear (*Pyrus communis* L.) prepared in the manner described above. Figure 13b was obtained by forcing a single pear-flavored jelly bean into a 4-ml vial and acquiring a headspace SPME sample for 10 minutes at room temperature. The transfer of the jelly bean into the vial resulted in the crushing of its outer

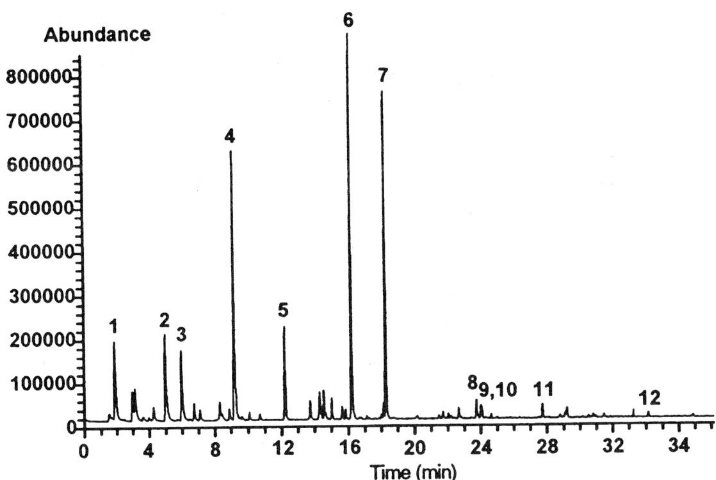

FIGURE 12 Total ion chromatogram showing the volatile components obtained from a ripe banana by headspace SPME using a 100-μm polydimethylsiloxane fiber. Small plugs removed from the banana using the blunt end of a disposable pipet were placed into a 15-ml headspace vial for the extraction. The SPME equilibration time was 10 minutes at room temperature, and the same chromatographic conditions as listed in Figure 11 were used. The numbered components are ethanol (1), isoamyl alcohol (2), isobutyl acetate (3), isoamyl acetate (4), isobutyl butyrate (5), isoamyl isobutyrate (6), isoamyl butyrate (7), isoamyl isovalerate (8), isoamyl caproate (9), 3-hexenyl caproate (10), eugenol (11), and elemicin (12).

sugar shell, which allowed the flavor compounds to escape into the surrounding headspace. With samples of this type, it is sometimes necessary to introduce water to dissolve the matrix or the flavor-encapsulating agents before the chemicals are released. It is evident by comparing the two chromatograms that the aroma chemicals obtained from the fresh Bartlett pear are different from those observed in the jelly bean flavor. This is not unusual because "nature's biochemists" are usually allowed more freedom when compounding a flavor than are flavor chemists trying to recreate what nature has provided.

According to the TNO compilation (38), Bartlett pear aroma contains very low levels of butyl acetate (0.16 ppm), hexyl acetate (0.09 ppm), methyl *trans*-2-*cis*-4-decadienoate (0.05 ppm), ethyl *trans*-2-*cis*-4-decadienoate (0.04

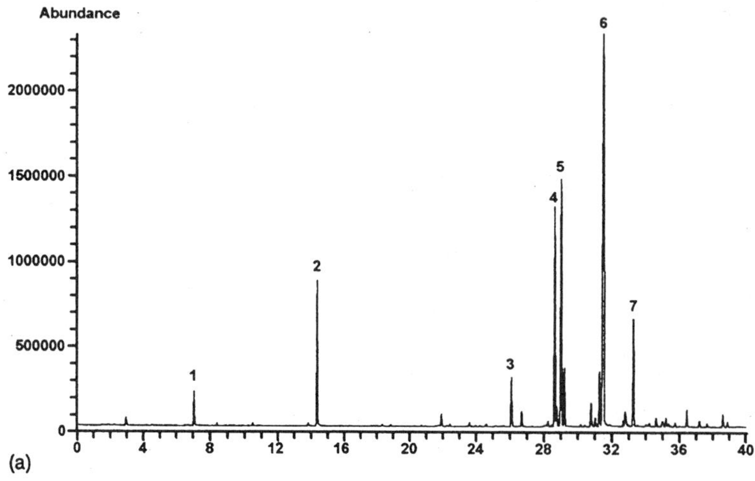

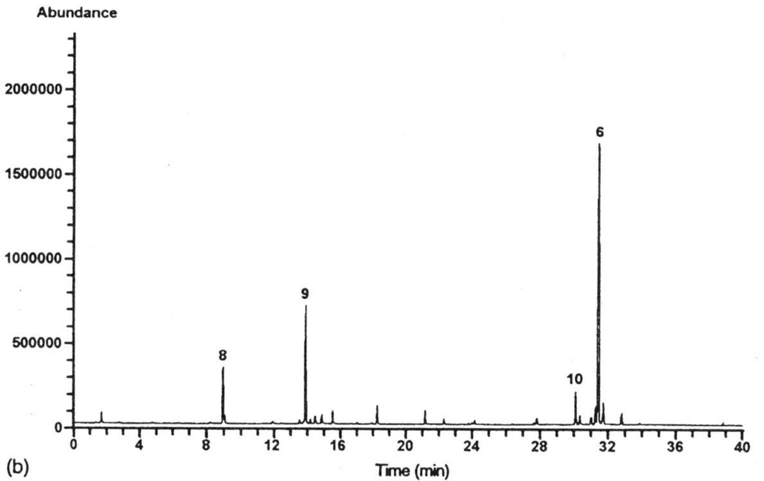

Figure 13 A comparison of the total ion chromatograms of the volatile aroma components of a ripe Bartlett pear (a) and a pear-flavored jelly bean (b) isolated by headspace SPME. Small plugs of the pear were removed with the blunt end of a disposable pipet and placed into a 15-ml headspace vial for extraction. The jelly bean was forced into a smaller 4-ml vial. Headspace extraction was performed on each sample for 10 minutes at room temperature using a 100-μm polydimethylsiloxane fiber. Peak identities are as follows: (1) butyl acetate, (2) hexyl acetate, (3) methyl *cis*-4-decenoate, (4) ethyl *cis*-4-decenoate, (5) methyl *trans*-2-*cis*-4-decadienoate, (6) ethyl *trans*-2-*cis*-4-decadienoate, (7) α-farnesene, (8) isoamyl acetate, (9) *cis*-3-hexenyl acetate, and (10) carveol propionate.

ppm), and α-farnesene (0.04 ppm). The concentrations of the other compounds identified in Figure 13 were not reported in the reference.

It is apparent from these few examples that SPME can be a powerful tool for the rapid isolation of volatile chemicals from fresh fruit and fruit juice products. It should be possible to establish a method to determine the degree of ripeness of different fruits by matching the chemical profiles with sensory or other established parameters. The changes occurring during ripening can be observed within a few minutes, and the analysis can be repeated using the same piece of fruit if shallow core samples are taken and proper storage conditions are maintained between analyses. A different treatment of the samples using buffers, salt solutions, homogenization, different SPME fiber types, separation with chiral capillary columns, etc. might provide a completely different insight into the chemical profile and biochemistry of these plants. SPME will not provide a complete chemical profile for every sample, but as a rapid isolation technique it can alert the chemist to the types of compounds occurring in the sample during the time it takes to prepare an extract using a more typical isolation scheme.

3. More Useful Examples of the Headspace SPME of Food and Beverage Products

For many spices and herbs the aroma and flavor will vary depending upon its country of origin, processing conditions, the age of the sample, the type of packaging, the ratio of essential oil volatiles to heat-producing principles, and many other factors. Black pepper is one of the most widely consumed spices in the world. It might be of benefit to be able to evaluate the chemical composition of the volatile oil of single peppercorns to correlate with sensory attributes. An example of such an analysis is shown in Figure 14. This chromatogram was the result of a 5-minute room temperature headspace SPME extraction of a single black peppercorn (42 mg) that had been crushed with pliers and rapidly transferred to a 4-ml vial. The chromatogram has been expanded along the vertical axis to show the smaller components in the mixture. The composition is somewhat atypical of a "normal" chromatogram obtained by steam distillation, but the general appearance is readily identified. Considering that the whole sample could have provided no more than 1.5 mg of volatile oil, the sensitivity of the extraction is remarkable.

Figure 15 represents the analysis of a sample of curry powder that was thought to be lacking one of its spice components. Since the spice was known to contain a unique aroma chemical, it was an easy matter to transfer a small amount of the curry to a vial, perform a headspace extraction, and determine

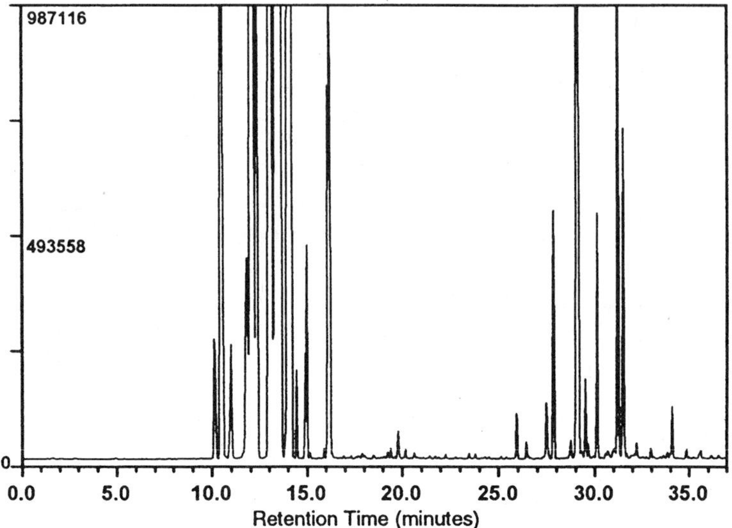

FIGURE 14 Chromatogram showing the volatile compounds isolated from a single black peppercorn using headspace SPME. Sample preparation included crushing the peppercorn with pliers and quickly placing it into a 4-ml vial. The volatiles were collected using a 100-μm polydimethylsiloxane fiber for 5 minutes at room temperature. Chromatographic conditions were the same as those listed in Figure 10. The peak heights have been increased by a factor of 5 to show the minor oxygenated terpene components around 20 minutes in the chromatogram.

whether the spice had been added. The complete analysis required less than one hour from the time the sample was received. As a quality control measure, SPME can have a significant impact on the analysis of raw materials and finished products.

Beverage manufacturers often compete with one another for customer approval of their flavors. Typical among these were the "cola wars" conducted a few years ago. SPME would have provided a rapid technique to compare various brands of cola volatiles to determine whether they really were different. The chromatograms shown in Figure 16 offer a comparison between two cola products. Obviously these two products are very similar in their aroma profiles, and they have probably been formulated using similar ingredients. Unfortunately, nothing can be determined regarding the more subtle volatile

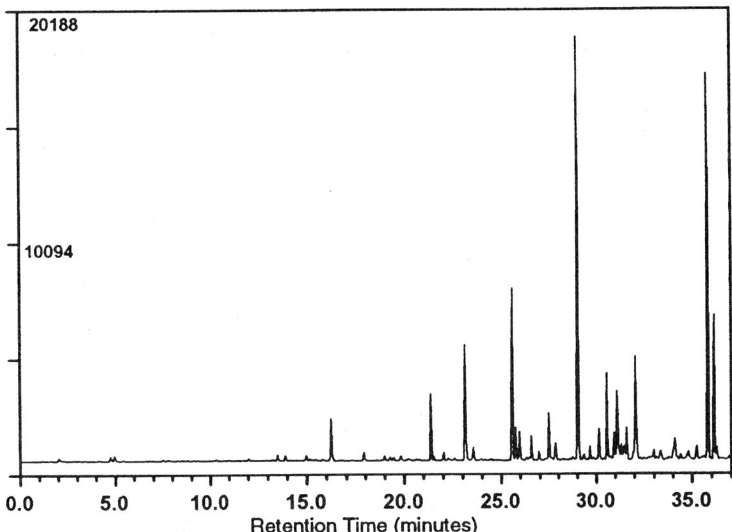

FIGURE 15 Chromatogram of a portion of the volatile components obtained by headspace SPME of a sample of curry powder. For this analysis a 100-mg sample of the dry curry powder was equilibrated in a 4-ml vial at 55°C for 10 minutes and then extracted for 5 minutes using a 100-μm polydimethylsiloxane fiber.

compounds or the nonvolatile and more polar portions of the beverages using headspace SPME. A chromatogram of a much less complex beverage flavor is shown in Figure 17. Few people would confuse the flavor of root beer with a typical cola. Even fewer would find it difficult to discriminate between their chromatograms.

VII. SUMMARY

Solid-phase microextraction is still in its infancy. As research continues toward the development of different fiber materials and techniques, the resulting greater specificity and enhanced performance can only benefit the analytical flavor chemist. Even now the applications for SPME in flavor analysis appear to be limited only by the imagination. Automation will move the techniques into quality control applications and will greatly improve the quantitative aspects of our analyses. SPME will result in a need for smaller samples and will decrease the likelihood of the identification of artifacts as flavor components.

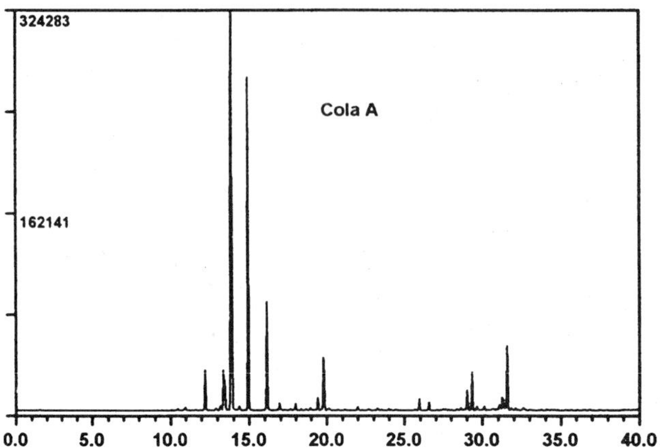

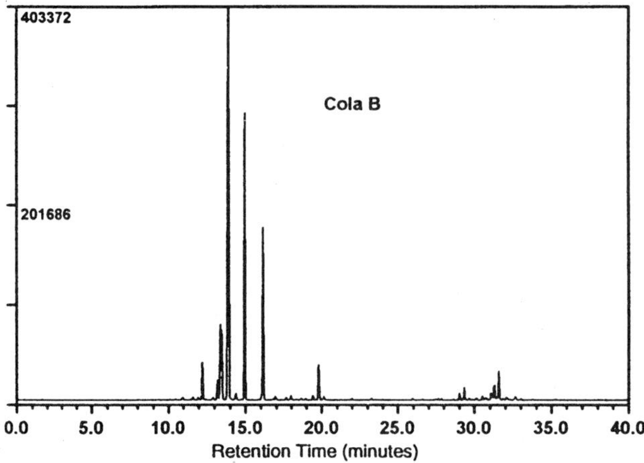

FIGURE 16 Chromatograms showing the similarities between two popular brands of cola beverages. The volatile compounds were isolated from 1-ml samples of the beverages using headspace SPME extraction at 55°C for 5 minutes with a 100-μm polydimethylsiloxane fiber.

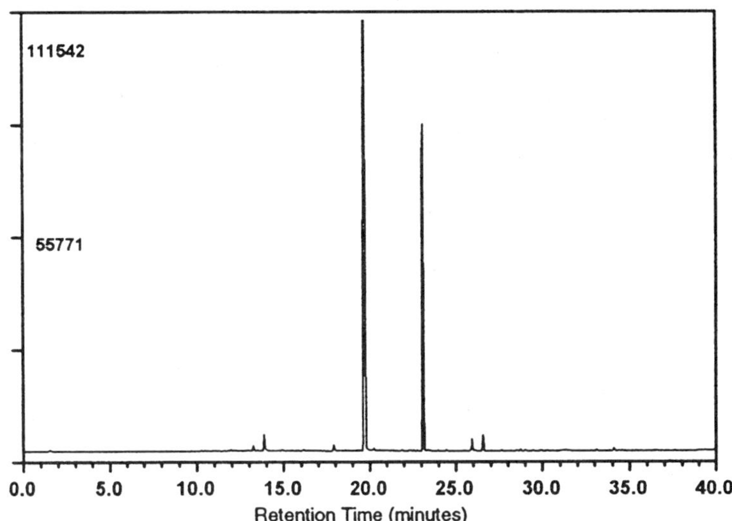

FIGURE 17 Chromatogram showing the volatile compounds isolated from a sample of root beer–flavored beverage. The extraction conditions were the same as those described in Figure 16.

We will begin to examine the differences between fresh aroma volatiles and those obtained through more harsh isolation techniques. SPME has become the method of choice for the initial isolation and analysis of aroma chemicals in our laboratory. For many applications it is the only technique required to solve the problem.

REFERENCES

1. R. Berlardi and J. Pawliszyn, The application of chemically modified fused silica fibers in the extraction of organics from water matrix samples and their rapid transfer to capillary columns, *Water Pollution Res. J. Canada 24*:179 (1989).
2. C. L. Arthur and J. Pawliszyn, Solid phase microextraction with thermal desorption using fused silica optical fibers, *Anal. Chem. 62*:2145 (1990).
3. C. L. Arthur, D. W. Potter, K. D. Buchholz, S. Motlagh, and J. Pawliszyn, Solid phase microextraction for the direct analysis of water: theory and practice, *LC-GC 10*:656 (1992).
4. C. L. Arthur, L. M. Killam, K. D. Buchholz, D. W. Potter, M. Chai, Z. Zhang, and J. Pawliszyn, Solid phase microextraction: an attractive alternative, *Environ. Lab 11*:10 (1992).

5. C. L. Arthur, L. M. Killam, S. Motlagh, M. Lim, D. W. Potter, and J. Pawliszyn, Analysis of substituted benzene compounds in groundwater using solid-phase microextraction, *Environ. Sci. Technol. 26*:979 (1992).
6. D. Louch, S. Motlagh, and J. Pawliszyn, Dynamics of organic compound extraction from water using liquid-coated fused silica fibers, *Anal. Chem. 64*:1187 (1992).
7. D. W. Potter and J. Pawliszyn, Detection of substituted benzenes in water at the pg/ml level using solid-phase microextraction and gas chromatography-ion trap mass spectrometry, *J. Chromatogr. 625*:247 (1992).
8. C. L. Arthur, R. P. Belardi, K. F. Pratt, S. Motlagh, and J. Pawliszyn, Environmental analysis of organic compounds in water using solid phase microextraction, *J. High Res. Chromat. 15*:741 (1992).
9. Z. Zhang and J. Pawliszyn, Headspace solid-phase microextraction, *Anal. Chem. 65*:1843 (1993).
10. K. D. Buchholz and J. Pawliszyn, Determination of phenols by solid-phase microextraction and gas chromatographic analysis, *Environ. Sci. Technol. 27*:2844 (1993).
11. E. Otu and J. Pawliszyn, Solid phase micro-extraction of metal ions, *Mikrochim. Acta 112*:41 (1993).
12. M. Chai, C. L. Arthur, J. Pawliszyn, R. P. Belardi and K. F. Pratt, Determination of volatile chlorinated hydrocarbons in air and water with solid-phase microextraction, *Analyst 118*:1501 (1993).
13. Z. Zhang and J. Pawliszyn, Analysis of organic compounds in environmental samples by headspace solid phase microextraction, *J. High Res. Chromatogr. 16*:689 (1993).
14. D. W. Potter and J. Pawliszyn, Rapid determination of polyaromatic hydrocarbons and polychlorinated biphenyls in water using solid-phase microextraction and GC/MS, *Environ. Sci. Technol. 28*:298 (1994).
15. K. D. Buchholz and J. Pawliszyn, Optimization of solid-phase microextraction conditions for determination of phenols, *Anal. Chem. 66*:160 (1994).
16. R. Eisert, K. Levsen and G. Wunsch, Element-selective detection of pesticides by gas chromatography-atomic emission detection and solid-phase microextraction, *J. Chromatogr. A 683*:175 (1994).
17. L. P. Sarna, G. R. B. Webster, M. R. Friesen-Fischer, and R. Sri Rajan, Analysis of the petroleum components benzene, toluene, ethyl benzene and the xylenes in water by commercially available solid-phase microextraction and carbon-layer open tubular capillary column gas chromatography, *J. Chromatogr. A 677*:201 (1994).
18. H. B. Wan, H. Chi, M. K. Wong, and C. Y. Mok, Solid-phase microextraction using pencil lead as sorbent for analysis of organic pollutants in water, *Anal. Chim. Acta 298*:219 (1994).
19. J.-Y. Horng and S.-D. Huang, Determination of the semi-volatile compounds nitrobenzene, isophorone, 2,4-dintrotoluene and 2,6-dinitrotoluene in water using

solid-phase microextraction with a polydimethylsiloxane-coated fiber, *J. Chromatogr. A 678*:313 (1994).
20. B. MacGillivray, J. Pawliszyn, P. Fowlie, and C. Sagara, Headspace solid-phase microextraction versus purge and trap for the determination of substituted benzene compounds in water, *J. Chromatogr. Science 32*:317 (1994).
21. B. Wittkamp and D. C. Tilotta, Determination of BTEX compounds in water by solid-phase microextraction and raman spectroscopy, *Anal. Chem. 67*:600 (1995).
22. R. Eisert and K. Levsen, Determination of organophosphorus, triazine and 2,6-dinitroaniline pesticides in aqueous samples via solid-phase microextraction (SPME) and gas chromatography with nitrogen-phosphorus detection, *Fresenius J. Anal. Chem. 351*:555 (1995).
23. M. Chai and J. Pawliszyn, Analysis of environmental air samples by solid-phase microextraction and gas chromatography/ion trap mass spectrometry, *Environ. Sci. Technol. 29*:693 (1995).
24. C. L. Arthur, L. M. Killam, K. D. Buchholz, J. Pawliszyn, and J. R. Berg, Automation and optimization of solid-phase microextraction, *Anal. Chem. 64*:1960 (1992).
25. C. L. Arthur, M. Chai, and J. Pawliszyn, Solventless injection technique for microcolumn separations, *J. Microcol. Sep. 5*:51 (1993).
26. Z. Zhang and J. Pawliszyn, Quantitative extraction using an internally cooled solid phase microextraction device, *Anal. Chem. 67*:34 (1995).
27. S. Motlagh and J. Pawliszyn, On-line monitoring of flowing samples using solid phase microextraction-gas chromatography, *Analytica Chim. Acta 284*:265 (1993).
28. J. R. Berg, Practical use of automated solid phase microextraction, *Am. Lab.* (Nov.):18 (1993).
29. Z. Zhang, M. J. Yang, and J. Pawliszyn, Solid-phase microextraction: a solvent-free alternative for sample preparation, *Anal. Chem. 66*:844A (1994).
30. S. B. Hawthorne, D. J. Miller, J. Pawliszyn, and C. L. Arthur, Solventless determination of caffeine in beverages using solid-phase microextraction with fused-silica fibers, *J. Chromatogr. 603*:185 (1992).
31. B. D. Page and G. Lacroix, Application of solid-phase microextraction to the headspace gas chromatographic analysis of halogenated volatiles in selected foods, *J. Chromatogr. 648*:199 (1993).
32. X. Yang and T. Peppard, Solid-phase microextraction for flavor analysis, *J. Agric. Food Chem. 42*:1925 (1994).
33. Measure flavors using solid phase microextraction, *Food Qual.* (Jan./Feb.):40 (1995).
34. A. P. Jayatilaka, S. K. Poole and C. F. Poole, Solid phase microextraction of flavor compounds from cinnamon and their separation by series coupled-column GC for the identification of botanical origin of cinnamon of commerce, Abstr. of the 1995 Pittsburgh Conf., #472P, New Orleans, March 5–10, 1995.

35. *The Merck Index*, 11th ed. (S. Budavari, ed.), Merck & Co., Inc., Rahway, NJ, 1989.
36. *Official Methods of Analysis of AOAC International*, 16th ed., Vol. II, *Food Composition; Additives; Natural Contaminants* (P. Cunniff, ed.), AOAC International, Arlington, VA, 1995.
37. G. Mazza, Volatiles in distillates of fresh, dehydrated and freeze dried horseradish, *Can. Inst. Food. Sci. Technol. J. 17*:18 (1984).
38. *Volatile Compounds in Food. Qualitative and Quantitative Data, Supplement 3* (H. Maarse and C. A. Visscher, eds.), TNO Biotechnology & Chemistry Institute, Zeist, The Netherlands, 1992.

5

Application of Multidimensional Gas Chromatography Techniques to Aroma Analysis

DONALD W. WRIGHT
Microanalytics Instrumentation Corporation, Round Rock, Texas

I. INTRODUCTION

Since its original introduction in the 1950s gas chromatography has emerged as the cornerstone analytical technique in the field of general volatile analysis. Given this importance, it is not surprising that gas chromatography is of particular importance to the specialized field of aroma investigation. By definition aroma questions involve the range of chemical compounds that are of sufficient volatility to reside in the vapor space surrounding a particular matrix. In even its most elemental form, gas chromatography is capable of revealing several pieces of key information regarding the volatile composition of a fragrant sample. This basic process, involving the single column separation of a volatile mixture followed by detection at a single universal detector, can be referred to as single dimension gas chromatography (SDGC) for the sake of reference. Among the key pieces of information that can be extracted from basic SDGC separations are the following:

Absolute retention times for a set of compounds on a particular column operating under a specific set of operating parameters
General indications of the relative concentrations of the various components in the mixture
General indications of the relative volatilities of the various components in the mixture

Conspicuously absent from this list is the capability of assigning definitive identification, structural, or functional group information to the peaks in a chromatogram. Therein lies one of the major limitations of SDGC—its limited usefulness in providing definitive qualitative information regarding the analyzed sample. This factor is especially important in the specialized field of aroma or odor analysis, since within this field the single most important characteristic of interest is qualitative in nature, namely, the relationship between a chromatographic peak and the olfactory response. As a result of this limitation, various techniques have been employed in an attempt to extract increased qualitative information from the SDGC process. These include the use of retention indices or sample spiking and absolute retention time matching. At best, however, these techniques can only serve to narrow the field of possible matches to what, on a completely unknown sample, is still a very large group of possible "hits."

Another major limitation of SDGC relates to its limited usefulness as even an absolute volatile separation technique. This limitation is understandable considering the tremendous number of volatile components potentially present in the headspace surrounding natural products. It has been proposed (1,2), for example, that for an analysis at a target concentration level of 10 parts per trillion (ppt) there is the theoretical possibility of a total component population ranging between 10^6 and 10^9. This possibility must then be considered in relation to the fact that there are at best several hundred theoretical resolution "windows" available for the complete separation of such a complex mixture under SDGC limitations. The actual number of these windows available from any chromatographic system depends on a number of factors, including column efficiency, system performance, column temperature limits, and system operating parameters. However, these limits can be assumed to typically number considerably less than 1000. In addition, since this number assumes perfect spacing of theoretical peaks, it is obvious that this level of optimal resolution will never exist for a real-world sample representing random peak distribution. The added separation challenge presented by the random peak distribution factor was recently proposed (3) and shown to be formidable. It was proposed, by way of example, that although only approximately 40,000 plates are required for the separation of 100 ordered (i.e., perfectly spaced) components, a 100-fold plate count increase (i.e., approximately 4 million plates) is required for the separation of only 82 of 100 peaks representing random distribution. Unfortunately, as this relates to aroma volatiles analysis, all of these factors are brought to bear in the extreme—component concentration levels of significance to low ppt coupled with highly disordered peak distribution. An excellent example of this limitation was shown in one study (4), which revealed in excess of 1500 resolved or partially resolved peaks from tobacco essential oil extracts. In this case, multidimensional gas chromatographic techniques were utilized to enhance these complex separations, making possible the mass spectral identification of 80 compounds not previously reported for these extracts.

II. MULTIDIMENSIONAL GAS CHROMATOGRAPHY: DEFINITIONS

A number of different techniques have been developed and utilized to offset the limitations of SDGC and increase both the quality and quantity of information that can be extracted from gas chromatographic separations. These techniques represent a number of hardware configurations and are loosely bound under the broad definitions that have become known as multidimensional gas chromatography (MDGC). W. Bertsch in his 1978 review (1) of multidimensional techniques stated that, in the strictest sense, for a technique to qualify for inclusion into the MDGC field it must meet one of two principles:

1. Two columns of different selectivity in combination with a system [integration, mass spectroscopy (MS) identification, etc.] which will permit assignment of retention indexes

or

2. Two columns of different selectivity and a device (prep scale collection tube, valve, etc.) to selectively transfer a portion of a chromatographic run from one into another column

In practice such restrictive definitions leave out a number of techniques and concepts that are very useful in overcoming the previously stated limitations of SDGC. As a result, this author prefers to include many techniques under the general heading of MDGC that do not meet the strictest limits of the

Bertsch definitions. In these cases, the overriding consideration is whether a concept, when added onto the basic SDGC technique, serves to overcome the limitations of SDGC. In other words, to qualify under the somewhat broader definition of MDGC, the concept or technique under consideration should accomplish one of the following:

1. Provide increased qualitative information regarding peak identification, functionality, or other characteristics (e.g., sensory) than could otherwise be provided by SDGC alone

or

2. Increase peak resolution beyond that which would be achievable through simple column efficiency increases on a single column type

III. MDGC TECHNIQUES FOR QUALITATIVE ANALYSIS

A. Hyphenated Detector Strategies for Chemical Characterization

There are several important analytical techniques that meet the above broadened definitions of multidimensional gas chromatography. Among these are included several hyphenated GC techniques which link a single GC column effluent with primary chemical structure characterization devices. Among the most important of these configurations are GC-MS (4–7), GC–Fourier transform infrared spectroscopy (GC-FTIR) (4), GC–atomic emission detector (GC-AED), and GC–inductively coupled plasma (GC-ICP). Coupling these detectors with even single-dimension chromatographic separations permits detailed chemical structure data to be assigned to eluting peaks. This information ranges from actual peak identification or confirmation in the case of GC-MS and GC-FTIR to functional group identification or elemental analysis in the case of GC-FTIR, GC-AED, and GC-ICP.

B. Selective Detectors Operating in Parallel

Another detector strategy that can be used to expand the qualitative information provided by a single GC column separation is the use of multiple selective detectors operated in parallel. In this process the effluent from a single chromatographic column is split between two or more detectors representing different selectivities. The simplest hardware devices used to effect this effluent splitting are very simple fixed splitters, which are based on fixed restrictor transfer lines and low dead volume connectors (8). Alternately, somewhat greater flexibility is provided by variable splitter control devices, which are based on a combination of fixed restrictor transfer lines and needle valve control. Regardless of the mechanism used to effect the effluent splitting, this process makes it possible to utilize detector response ratios from the two detectors to confirm peak identification or possibly assign chemical functionality or sensory characteristics. Detector combinations that have found particularly wide spread usage in the environmental field are photoionization detector/flame ionization detector (PID/FID) (9), PID/electron capture detector (ECD), and PID/Hall electrolytic conductivity detector (ELCD). Configurations that are particularly important to the field of aroma profiling are PID/flame photometric detector (FPD), PID/nitrogen phosphorus detector (NPD) (8,10) and PID/olfactory detector (11). Utilizing the latter, for example, it is possible to determine the aroma characteristics of a peak eluting at the olfactory detector and match that to an electronic signal that is simultaneously generated at the PID operating in parallel.

C. Selective Detectors Operating in Series

One of the most useful detector strategies for the specialized field of aroma and odor profiling is the series coupling of detectors representing different selectivities. These techniques are a logical outgrowth of the previous category and are made possible if one of the two detectors is nondestructive in principle. Thermal conductivity (TCD) (12) and photoionization (13) detectors both meet this criteria and have often been used as the first detector in a variety of series coupled detector configurations. In this author's experience, however, TCD has limited usefulness in the field of aroma and odor investigations due to both its limited sensitivity and its limited selectivity. In contrast, these same factors make the photoionization detector the single most generally useful to this field. In practice it is found that the PID exhibits excellent sensitivity toward most compounds and classes of compounds that are also important to the human olfactory response (14). Correspondingly, the PID exhibits relatively poor response to lower molecular weight saturated hydrocarbons, thereby eliminating a relatively large pool of potential interference peaks which might otherwise obscure the critical early regions of aroma profile chromatograms. The end result of these factors is that the PID represents the best overall match to the human olfactory response in both detection thresholds and detector selectivity.

Several configurations that incorporate the PID as part of a series coupled detector system have applications to the field of aroma profiling. These include PID–flame photometric, PID–nitrogen-phosphorus, and PID-chemlumin-scence. In each of these, the PID serves as a high-sensitivity general detector, which responds to most of the classes of compounds that are important to olfactory response. The PID can be coupled to a high-sensitivity and highly selective detector, which responds to a much narrower range of compounds that have been shown to be strong responders to the human olfactory senses: the FPD (8) and chemluminescence detectors (15,16) selectively responding to sulfur species and the NPD (8,10) selectively responding to nitrogen containing species. In this author's experience, however, the single most useful detector system in the aroma-profiling application is the series coupling of the PID and the olfactory detector (i.e., sniffport) (11). In this case the effluent from the PID is swept immediately through a heated interface link to a heated and air-swept external vent port. This port is configured such that an investigator can conveniently sniff the effluent and assign aroma or odor descriptors (17,18) to the peaks as they elute from the PID. If the PID-olfactory coupling is properly designed, the end result is the virtually simultaneous generation of an electronic signal at the PID and a corresponding sensory response at the sniff port for the effluent of the chromatographic column. This process permits the assignment of aroma characteristics to at least a retention region of a chromatographic profile and in some cases the isolated peak that is responsible for the aroma characteristic.

IV. MDGC TECHNIQUES FOR VOLATILES SEPARATIONS

As shown in the previous section creative detector strategies can be used to overcome the limitations of SDGC as a qualitative analytical technique. Without question these detector strategies can be extremely useful when applied to the special challenges of aroma profiling. However, in and of themselves, creative detector strategies can do very little toward offsetting the limitations of SDGC as an absolute separations technique. The focus of this current work is to explore the application of those forms of MDGC that do address the limitations of SDGC as a separations tool. In doing so, an attempt is made to illustrate how MDGC-based detector strategies can be coupled do MDGC-based separations strategies to develop integrated aroma profiling systems.

There are few, if any, specialized fields of chemical analysis that have a greater requirement for complex volatile separations than does the field of aroma and odor investigation. This results from a combination of the extremes in both sensitivity and selectivity that are characteristic of the human olfactory response. It is not surprising that the importance of these factors is magnified severalfold if the area of interest is extended to other members of the animal kingdom. There are many examples in the literature in which key aroma or off-odor (19) components from both natural and synthetic samples are detectable down to low ppt levels by the human olfactory response (11,20–24). An excellent example is 2-acetyl-l-pyrroline (2-AP), which, at the ppb level, is responsible for the characteristic "popcorn" (25) aroma of the aromatic Basmati rice varieties. When these particular varieties of rice are cooked, trace amounts of 2-AP are either released from some bound precursor form or possibly chemically generated and released to the vapor space surrounding the rice. The result is a very pungent and characteristic aroma, which is also very desirable from culinary and marketing standpoints. The chromatographic separation challenge presented for the isolation of 2-AP from rice and other food products results from the fact that the detection threshold for 2-AP has been estimated to be approximately 100 ppt (25) for the human olfactory response. The analytical challenge results not so much from these extremely low concentration levels of significance, but rather from the fact that, as we are forced to examine such low levels, the "forest grows." When concentrating the volatile organic compounds from the headspace surrounding any natural product, large amounts of potential interference compounds are inevitably collected and introduced into the GC system. As a result, we find that it is the rule rather than the exception that under SDGC conditions the most significant aroma peaks will be covered up by the surrounding mass of peaks, which may have little or no significance from an aroma standpoint. To address this limitation of SDGC it is necessary to explore the family of techniques which relate to the second of the previously stated MDGC definitions—to increase peak resolution beyond that which would be achievable through simple column efficiency increases on a single column type.

A simplified overview of a system that can be used to achieve this goal is illustrated in the schematic diagram shown in Figure 1. The major elements of this basic two-dimensional GC system are the injection device, a first column for preliminary separation, a flow switch device at the juncture of the first column and second column, a first detector for profiling the first column separation, and a second detector for profiling the second column separation. The first column and detector are commonly referred to as the precolumn and monitor detector, while the second column and detector are commonly referred to as the analytical column and analytical detector. Of the six basic elements shown, five elements can be viewed as being common to both MDGC and SDGC systems. If, for example, the switching device is replaced by a splitter tee, the effluent from the precolumn is simply split in its entirety between the monitor detector and the analytical column. The end result is then two SDGC chromatograms generated on two different detectors but with no additional qualitative information developed regarding the volatiles composi-

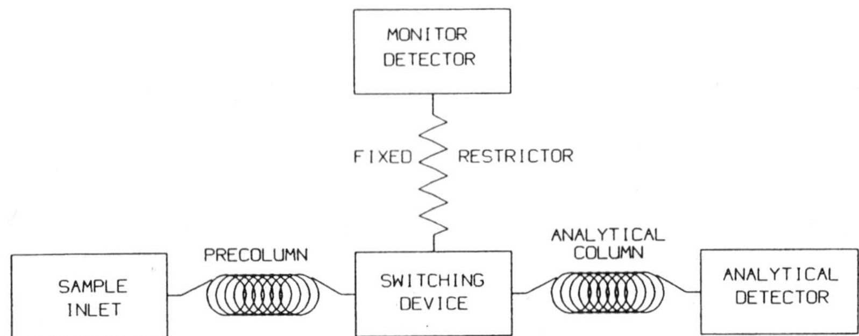

FIGURE 1 Basic MDGC components. Schematic diagram illustrating the key elements of a general MDGC separation system. This illustration is general in that it is equally representative of both rotary valve and Deans switch–based systems.

tion. Obviously, the critical difference between such a configuration and a true MDGC configuration is the presence of the flow switching device, which is located at the juncture of the precolumn, analytical column, and monitor detector transfer line. It is the presence of this device that enables the tremendous increase in separation power that is made possible through the MDGC techniques. Utilizing this critical device, the MDGC technique can be viewed as involving the following basic steps:

1. Injection of sample onto a precolumn for preliminary separation
2. Transferring those portions of the precolumn effluent that are adequately separated or are of no particular interest directly to the monitor detector
3. Shunting those portions of the precolumn effluent that are incompletely resolved or are of particular interest onto the analytical column for additional separation

The last of these steps is generally referred to as heartcutting and is called on to address a number of chromatographic separation problems. These problems may arise as the result of matrix complexity (4,26,27) due to the large number of peaks present or in some cases may be the result of gross difference in concentration between the components of interest and other matrix components (28,29). In either case these configurations permit the precolumn to serve, in essence, as an extension of the sample preparation or sample clean-up steps

(30), thereby affording the option of injecting much larger sample volumes than would be permitted under a conventional SDGC configuration. This is only possible since, under MDGC operation, the appearance of the precolumn separation at the monitor detector can be largely ignored. Mechanically transferring a small selected fraction of the resulting grossly overloaded peaks or peak groups usually results in the desired separation at the analytical column/analytical detector. Obviously, the most dramatic separation enhancements result when the heartcut transfers are carried out between columns of considerable polarity or selectivity (31) difference (e.g., a non–polar-bonded polydimethylsiloxane precolumn to a polar-bonded Carbowax 20 M analytical column). In many cases these types of MDGC operations enable a particular separation to be pushed to lower detection limits, and in most cases these improvements can be achieved while at the same time increasing the speed of analysis. Among modern separation techniques in the field of analytical chemistry, few have enjoyed more success in enabling "needle-in-the-haystack" separations.

Given the importance of these techniques, it is not surprising that several different mechanical approaches have been developed for performing the critical stream selection flow switch. This operation is carried out, either through the use of one of the new-generation low dead volume rotary switching valves (5) or, alternately, by one of the variations on the pressure balancing concept first proposed by D. R. Deans (32). Each of these approaches carries with it certain advantages and disadvantages; the rotary valve is a simpler mechanical approach, which is somewhat limited in flexibility, while the various pneumatic balance–based systems are considerably more flexible but are based on somewhat less intuitive concepts. Additional differences of note between these two approaches are the typical lower thermal mass and greater inertness possible for the pressure balance flow path connections compared to those of the rotary valve equivalents. The inertness is particularly important to aroma studies considering the extremely low levels of interest and the adsorption sensitivity of the functional groups typically present. The thermal mass is important in that it off sets the requirement for placing the Deans switch hardware components in a separate valve oven maintained at elevated temperatures. The separate valve oven is definitely a requirement for larger thermal mass rotary valves, which perform poorly when installed directly into a column oven operated under temperature-programmed conditions. These two mechanical approaches were evaluated in detail in a comparison study (5) and shown to be equally effective in performing straightforward MDGC heartcutting applications. However, considering the various comparison factors relating to these two approaches and the unique requirements of aroma profiling, it is this author's personal bias to apply the Deans pressure balance–based approach to this specialized application area. Given this personal bias, it should not be surprising that the Deans switch principle is the focus for the information presented in this current work. It is understood, however, that there are valid alternatives to this approach, which in some instances may offer simpler and less costly solutions.

V. DESIGN CONSIDERATIONS FOR A DEANS SWITCH AROMA-PROFILING SYSTEM

As stated previously, the flow switch mechanism for the Deans switch principle is less intuitive than that of the rotary switching valve. Switching a flow path with a rotary valve simply involves the mechanical shifting of a flow channel between one of two positions. In contrast, under the Deans switch principle, there are no moving parts present at the point of flow switch but rather a simple four-way tee (Fig. 2). Flow switching in this case is fluid

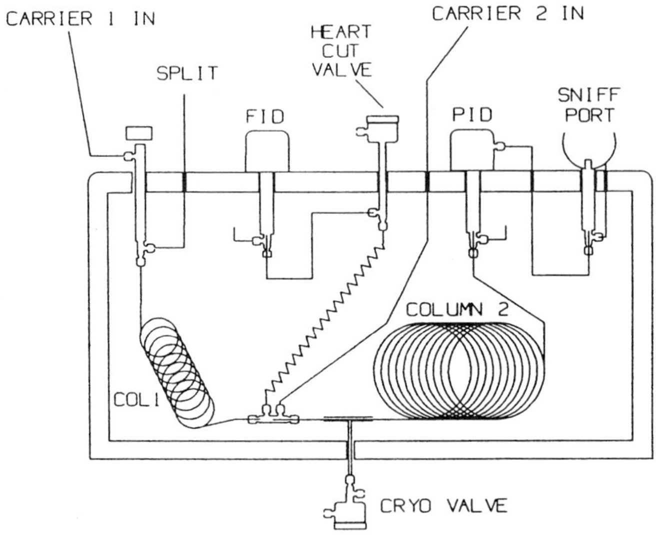

FIGURE 2 Basic MDGC system for aroma separations. Schematic diagram illustrating the key elements of a basic, single oven, Deans switch-based MDGC system. This configuration is illustrative of a relatively simple MDGC system which is optimized for the aroma-profiling application.

rather than mechanical in principle and is enabled by the addition of a second, independently regulated carrier gas supply to the juncture between the two columns. Under this configuration it is possible to tune the two carrier gas pressure inputs to the system to a state referred to as pressure balanced. This condition in essence involves supplying a balancing carrier gas pressure to the juncture between the two columns; a pressure slightly higher than that which would exist at that point if the precolumn and analytical column were simply joined together with a low dead volume union. Once this pressure-balanced condition is reached, three very useful flow switch options are made available:

1. If the system is balanced and the precolumn vent line is open, the precolumn effluent takes the path of least resistance and flows directly to the monitor detector. This flow path option is normally referred to as bypass mode.
2. If the system is balanced and the precolumn vent line is closed, the precolumn effluent is shunted across the midpoint restrictor to the second column. This flow path option is normally referred to as heartcut mode.
3. The third flow switch option is referred to as backflush and is enabled when the carrier gas pressure supply to the injector is shut off and the inlet split vent is opened. Under these conditions the balancing carrier gas supply to the midpoint restrictor takes over and reverses the direction of carrier gas flow through the precolumn. Any chromatographing component that has not reached the flow switch juncture is simply carried back to the injector and passed out the split vent line. During this time the carrier gas supply to the analytical column continues uninterrupted, with the result that any component that has been transferred past the flow switch juncture onto the analytical column continues to chromatograph in the normal manner. This function permits those heavy components of no interest to the analysis at hand to be removed from the system prior to the analytical column.

Two basic elements must be present for the Deans switch system to make possible the toggling between heartcut and bypass modes of operation. The first of these is the presence of the balancing carrier gas feed to the midpoint restrictor, while the second is a device to open and close the precolumn vent line. The second of these two requirements can be met using a pneumatically actuated high temperature on/off valve in the transfer line linking the midpoint restrictor and the monitor detector (33,34). Activation of this valve permits the instantaneous toggling of the precolumn flow between the heartcut and bypass flow paths. This device, referred to as the heartcut valve, is equipped with a make-up gas provision to ensure a rapid and complete transfer of the precolumn effluent to the monitor detector. The precolumn vent transfer line is another key element of the Deans switch system that requires special consideration. This line is, in reality, a fixed restrictor tube whose length and internal diameter are selected such that it matches the restriction of the analytical column. Relatively small ID fused silica capillary tubing is utilized to ensure that a desired level of restriction can be achieved in a short, inert, low-volume transfer line. If the restrictor is precisely matched and balancing carrier gas is fed into the midpoint restrictor at a constant pressure, equal flow rates are established through the fixed restrictor tube and the analytical column. In practice, the fixed restrictor tube is matched to the analytical column such that there is an approximate 10% bias of gas flow to the fixed restrictor/monitor detector pathway.

The last key hardware component required for the basic Deans switch system is the cryogenic trap (35). In a variety of forms and designs, these devices represent a very important element of state-of-the-art Deans switch–based MDGC systems. The cryotrap capability is useful in a number of situations, not the least of which is the refocusing of groups of unresolved heartcut components at the head of the analytical column prior to their release from the cryotrap for a separate run on a column of different polarity. A second application for the cryotrap in these configurations is the sharpening of chromatographic peaks, which may have broadened in the precolumn pathway for one of a number of reasons (30). These factors can range from injector-induced effects (e.g., adsorption, dead volumes, or large volume injections) to column-induced effects (e.g., adsorption, dead volumes, column flooding, or reverse solvent effects). In any case, if the cryotrap is properly designed and if the chromatographing components fall within the trapping range of the coolant selected, the end result is the injection of the heart cut components from the sharpest possible injection band.

Moving down from the system level to the component level, we find that design considerations are common to both MDGC and SDGC systems. If these systems are to deliver chromatographic separations which are quantitative, reproducible, and of highest possible efficiency, a number of fundamental performance requirements must be met. To meet these requirements, hardware components must be designed such that they maximize inertness while minimizing both thermal mass and flow path dead volumes. It should not be surprising that, given the low concentration levels of interest and the adsorption sensitivity of many key aroma components, these design requirements are extremely critical when the application area is aroma profiling.

VI. APPLICATION OF MDGC TECHNIQUES TO AROMA VOLATILE SEPARATIONS

When examining the range of options made possible by the basic Deans switch principle, it is easy to understand the separation power of these systems. Instead of the single opportunity for resolving any particular group of components, as is the case with SDGC configurations, the basic MDGC configuration described above offers three:

1. There is a possibility of separating the components of interest on the precolumn by itself.
2. Through the use of the heartcut option and without cryotrapping, there is the possibility of separating the components of interest based on the combined selectivity of the precolumn and analytical column.
3. Through the use of the heartcut and cryotrap options, there is the possibility of separating the components of interest on the analytical column by itself.

After the desired chromatographic separation has been achieved through the use of one of these options, the backflush function can then be called on to quickly remove uninteresting higher boilers from the precolumn. Doing so often results in the reduction in turnaround time between chromatographic runs and eliminates the requirement for a high-temperature bake-out of the columns between runs. The following series of chromatograms illustrates how these processes can be used to advantage for difficult chromatographic separations. This example is taken from an actual method development project and presents an excellent demonstration of the evolution of a Deans switch–based MDGC procedure, which in this case was developed for an aroma critical component.

A. Example Application: 2-Acetyl-l-Pyrroline from Rice Extracts

The thrust of this project was the development of a method for the separation and quantification of 2-acetyl-l-pyrroline (2-AP) from crude rice extracts. In this project the previously described MDGC techniques were used to develop an analytical procedure for this analysis, which met some very stringent requirements. The challenge, in this case, was to develop a chromatographic procedure which could be used for the rapid quality control screening of rice cultivars from a cross-breeding program. The goals for the project were not unlike those usually encountered in the development of GC methodologies. Simply stated, these goals were "rapid but complete resolution of a sub ppb level component from a complex matrix which was obtained directly from a natural product and doing so without the necessity for pre GC sample clean up or column oven temperature programming." Although these goals can be stated simply enough, actually achieving them in the laboratory is quite another matter. Several of these goals clearly run counter to each other and when limited to an SDGC approach, meeting such a challenge would not be possible. However, through the application of the MDGC techniques of heartcutting, cryotrapping, and backflushing, these goals are shifted within range. In this particular case only a few grains of rice are available from each cultivar for analysis, resulting in a sample size limitation of 0.3 g. The small, ground rice sample is cooked directly in a small amount of methylene chloride solvent to promote the release and extraction of the 2-AP. This is followed by the direct injection of up to 8 μl of the methylene chloride extract without additional clean-up, followed by the MDGC-based chromatographic separation at 110°C isothermal.

B. MDGC-Based Aroma Method Development Narrative

1. Precolumn Separation

All MDGC method development processes begin with the injection of the sample, chromatographic separation on the precolumn, and the diverting of all

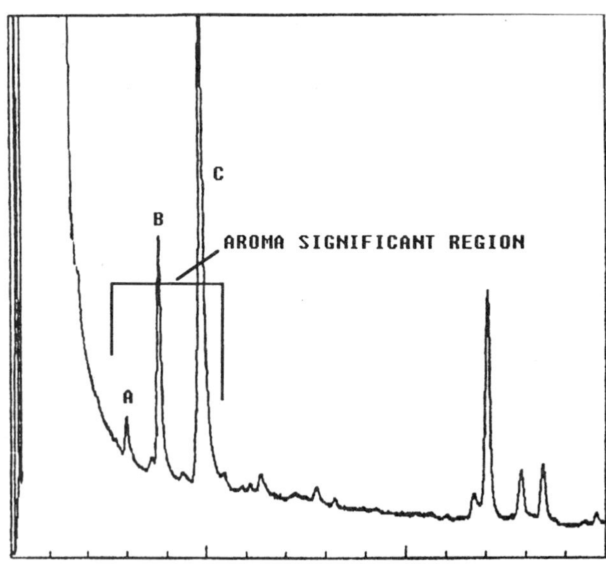

CHROMATOGRAM 1

precolumn effluent directly to the monitor detector. In this case, 3 µl of methylene chloride rice extract is injected under spitless conditions and separated on the 12 m × 0.53 mm ID nonpolar precolumn (12 QC5/BP1 – 1.0 SGE). This trace shows some of the uninteresting, later-eluting components that must be contended with but does not present a true picture of the extent of high-boiling co-extracts. In reality, when these separations are carried out under SDGC conditions (without a backflush option), it is necessary to perform a high-temperature bake-out of the column between runs; resulting in a typical analysis time of 45–60 minutes. This is inconvenient, since olfactory detector evaluation confirmed that the 2-AP peak eluted within the first 3 minutes of the precolumn separation. As a result of the olfactory detector profiling work, the region of the precolumn separation between 2.65 and 5.75 minutes was isolated for subsequent MDGC work-up.

2. Precolumn Separation Minus Broad Heartcut and Backflush

Based on the initial precolumn profile work-up with the monitor detector (FID) and olfactory detector, the same injection and precolumn separation was carried out but with heartcut and precolumn backflush options activated. The heartcut was taken between 2.65 and 5.75 minutes and incorporates what ap-

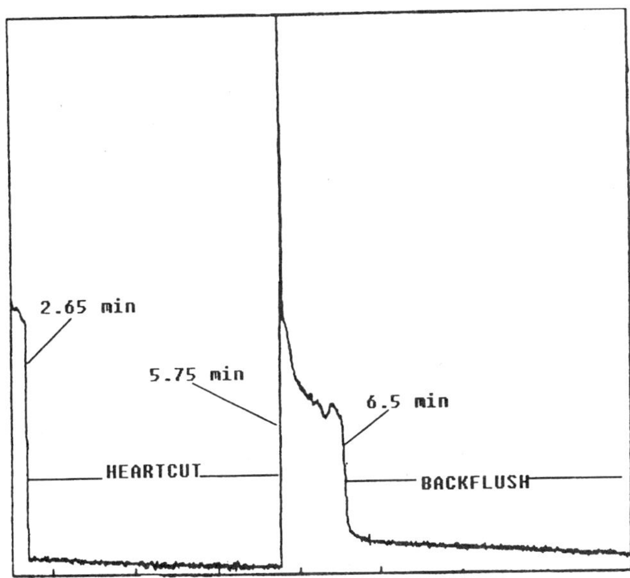

CHROMATOGRAM 2

pears to be six resolved or partially resolved peaks. Since it is only necessary to backflush for a length of time approximately equal to that allowed for forward migration, backflush activation at 6.5 minutes permits a reduction in analysis time to a maximum of 13 minutes. This is true regardless of the relative volatilities of the backflushed high boilers or the column oven temperature. In reality, the precolumn carrier gas flow rate in the backflush direction is usually higher than in the forward direction, resulting in even greater reductions in the required time of analysis. In this particular case, backflush was complete in approximately 10 minutes.

3. Analytical Column Separation of Heartcut/Cryotrap Transfer

The separation of the heartcut and cryotrapped zone shown above was carried out on a 25 m × 0.53 mm ID polar analytical column (25QC5/BP20 – 1.0 – SGE) and initially detected at a second FID. Two regions of interest are denoted in this trace, the first being the methylene chloride cryotrap breakthrough band between 3.75 and 6.75 minutes. Although this region is somewhat unsightly, it is of no particular importance to the separation under development. The second region denoted consists of the actual heartcut and cryotrapped components that were extracted from the ground rice sample. It is

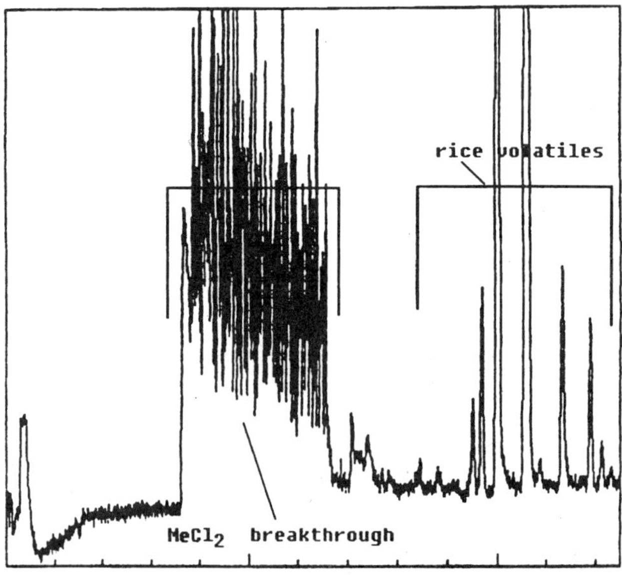

CHROMATOGRAM 3

interesting to note that what appeared to be six components on the nonpolar precolumn separation is shown to be at least 11 baseline resolved peaks on the polar analytical column. Taking into account the required time for the precolumn backflush and the analytical column separation, the overall analysis time in this case was 13 minutes.

4. Expansion of Chromatogram 3: Isolating on the Aroma Critical Region

Denoted in this trace are indicators as to where in the precolumn separation each of the peaks originated (e.g., in the region of peak A, B, or C). These illustrate the expected retention-order reversals when comparisons are made of these separations on the polar analytical column to those of the nonpolar precolumn. Also denoted in this chromatogram are brackets marking the regions of separation where significant aroma notes were detected at the olfactory detector operating in parallel. In this case there were found to be three distinct and separate aroma notes that did not appear to be closely tied to the strongest responses, which were generated at the second FID. The middle note was found to be very strong and based on its aroma character was identified as 2-AP. This identification was subsequently confirmed in a separate off-line GC-MS work-up.

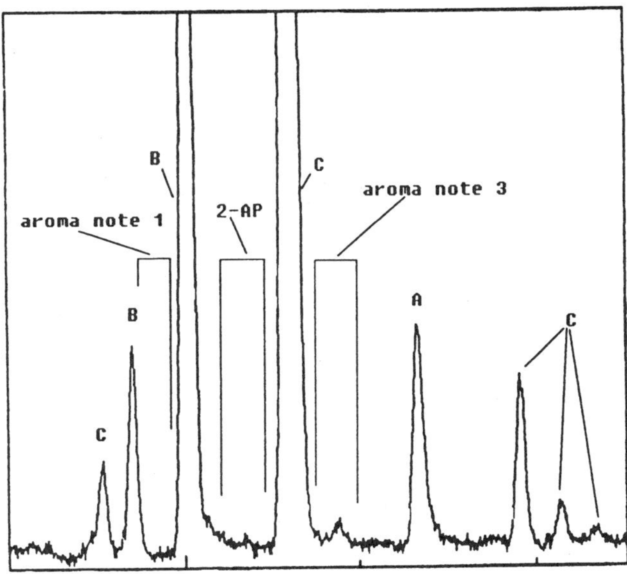

CHROMATOGRAM 4

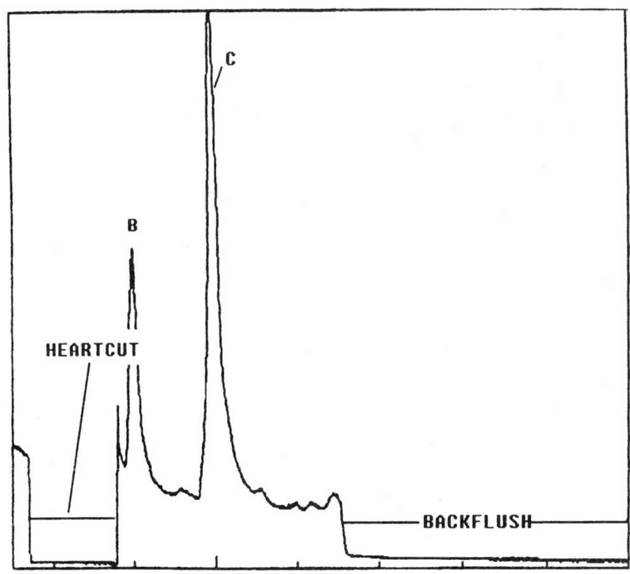

CHROMATOGRAM 5

5. Precolumn Separation Minus Refined Heartcut and Backflush

Based on the previous separation results, this heartcut was taken between 2.65 and 3.75 minutes, which isolated on the region encompassing peak A only. This refined heartcut was taken in an effort to simplify the analytical column separation and focus on just the region of the precolumn separation corresponding to the 2-AP aroma note. Obviously, the regions surrounding peaks B and C are now shown diverted to the monitor detector.

6. Analytical Column Separation of Refined Heartcut/Cryotrap Transfer

This separation of the heartcut and cryotrapped zone shown in the previous section is illustrative of two common characteristics of MDGC separations and aroma profiling. First, it illustrates how the heartcut function can be effectively used to refine a chromatographic separation by stripping away potential interference peaks. Second, it indicates how the sensitivity of the human olfactory response very often outstrips that of highly sensitive electronic detectors. In this case, the injected level of 2-AP was well below its detection limit

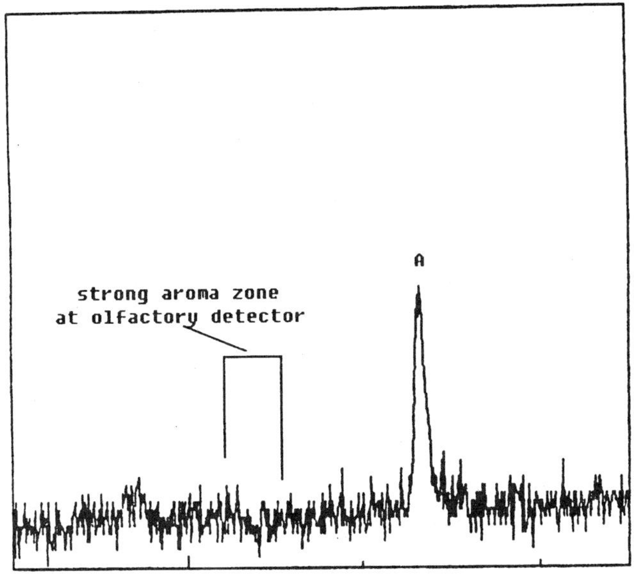

CHROMATOGRAM 6

on the FID in spite of a very strong olfactory response detected at the olfactory detector for the same level.

7. Analytical Column Separation with PID Detection

The run parameters used in this case were essentially the same as those that were adopted for the previous run. The primary differences between the two were the substitution of a PID for the FID and chromatographic separation from an isothermal versus the previous oven temperature–programmed profile. The end result of these two changes was the adoption of the final form of the analytical procedure, featuring near-baseline separation of low ppb level 2-AP from a 10-minute isothermal separation performed from the spitless injection of crude solvent extract from 0.3 g of ground rice. Incorporation of MDGC-based separation and detector strategies made possible the development of a procedure that met the very stringent goals set out at the beginning of the project, goals that would have been impossible to meet if limited to an SDGC approach. A comparison of this chromatogram and that shown in the

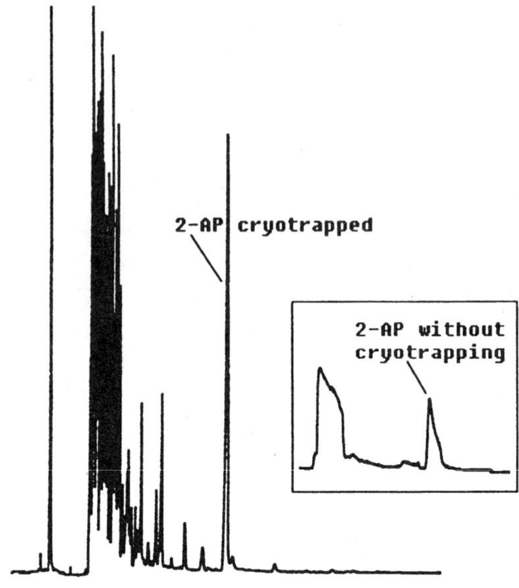

CHROMATOGRAM 7

inset illustrates the impact on resolution and sensitivity that the cryotrap function provides. Except for the fact that the inset chromatogram was generated without the cryotrap function, each of these runs was carried out under the same conditions. The band broadening illustrated in the inset chromatogram resulted from the combination of a large-volume injection, under spitless conditions, at an elevated isothermal column oven temperature—the same conditions that make possible the rapid analysis and turnaround time in the cryotrapped version of the analysis.

VII. OPTIMIZED MDGC CONFIGURATIONS FOR AROMA PROFILING

As demonstrated in the last chromatogram above, the final solution to a difficult aroma analysis may involve creative applications of a combination of MDGC separation and detector strategies. These strategies can represent a variety of hardware configurations—from relatively simple single-oven to highly integrated and complex dual-oven, multidetector configurations. The level of complexity required for an aroma profile system is, in turn, dependent largely on the goals and flexibility requirements of the projects to which the system is applied. The configuration examples presented in this section are representative of the range of options that can be called on to meet these goals and requirements.

A. Single-Oven MDGC Without Direct MS Interfacing

It is a common misconception that true MDGC separations require that both of the series coupled columns must be housed in separate, independently controlled column ovens. Although such a configuration certainly results in a more flexible MDGC system, it is just as certainly not an essential requirement. In fact, as long as one is mindful of the temperature limitations of the respective column phases, very elegant MDGC-based separations can be developed onto the relatively simple, single-oven platform (Fig. 2). Arguably, from a chromatographic separations standpoint there are limitations imposed by this simplified approach. These limitations result when the heartcut, cryotrap refocusing operation forces the second column separation to start from an elevated temperature. Depending on the time width of these MDGC operations, this can result in the second column separation being forced to restart from a considerably elevated temperature, thereby losing the separation aid provided by a lower temperature start. However, it is usually the case that through the application of increased forethought in the early stages of method development, this disadvantage can be largely offset. Among the actions that can be taken in this regard is the careful matching of column length and film thickness between the two columns. Typically, this involves adopting relatively short, thin-film precolumns and relatively long, thick-film anaytical columns. This strategy enables the reduction of the residence time in the precolumn and ensures that transfers to the analytical column are made at the lowest possible temperature.

A second strategy that achieves a very similar result is the establishment of higher carrier gas flow rates through the precolumn relative to those of the analytical column. From a hardware standpoint, this can be achieved by the incorporation of a midpoint split vent into the juncture between the two columns. This strategy can be effective regardless of the relative dimensions or flow capacities of the columns—whether matched 0.53 mm ID capillary or grossly mismatched packed to capillary configurations are used. Where the application permits, a third strategy involves simply breaking the MDGC operations into smaller, more manageable segments. This might involve making a series of short heartcut, cryotrap operations in a temperature-programmed chromatographic run rather than a single extended operation of this type. This action enables the more volatile components in earlier eluting heartcut bands to begin their separation on the analytical column while subsequent transfers are being set up for less volatile, later-eluting components.

The configuration shown in Figure 2 reflects another common characteristic of MDGC-based systems. Like all of the subsequent configurations presented in this section, it is constructed around higher-capacity, lower-efficiency 0.53 mm ID columns coupled in series. This is made possible as a result of the increased separating power of the MDGC techniques. It is easy to find examples of chromatographic separations that are difficult or impossible to achieve under the limitation of SDGC conditions in spite of the utilization of long, narrow-bore, high-efficiency capillary columns. It is often the case, however, that these difficult separations can be achieved fairly easily under MDGC conditions through the application of heartcut transfers between lower-efficiency, large-bore columns representing different selectivities. Instead of relying on the brute force separation power of a single high-efficiency SDGC column, it is possible to take advantage of the combination of the mechanical isolation process enabled by the heartcut option in combination with the selectivity difference between the two-column phases to achieve the desired separation. This approach is clearly advantageous since it enables the use of more robust high-flow, high-capacity columns while at the same time achieving improved separations. An additional advantage gained through this approach is the fact that the higher flow rates tolerated by these larger-bore columns represent a better match to the higher flow requirements of the common headspace-sampling devices. These include the various dynamic headspace samplers, such as purge and trap (36), thermal desorption, and short-path thermal desorption, as well as static headspace auto samplers. It should also be noted that the basic MDGC configuration shown in Figure 2 incorporates the series coupled PID and sniff port, which was used to advantage in the previously described separation of 2-AP. As was shown at that time, such an approach results in the generation of virtually simultaneous responses from a highly sensitive electronic detector (PID) and a sensory detector (sniff port). However, this configuration is limited in that there is no direct access to mass spectral data for identification of peaks shown to be of significance from an aroma standpoint. This deficiency is eliminated in the expanded configuration, which is presented in the following section and illustrated in Figure 3.

B. Dual-Oven MDGC-Based Techniques with Direct MS Interfacing

In spite of its limitations, the basic aroma-profiling system presented in the previous section can be a very effective tool in developing detailed aroma profile information regarding a complex volatiles mixture. However, a number of modifications can be made to this basic configuration to increase the efficiency

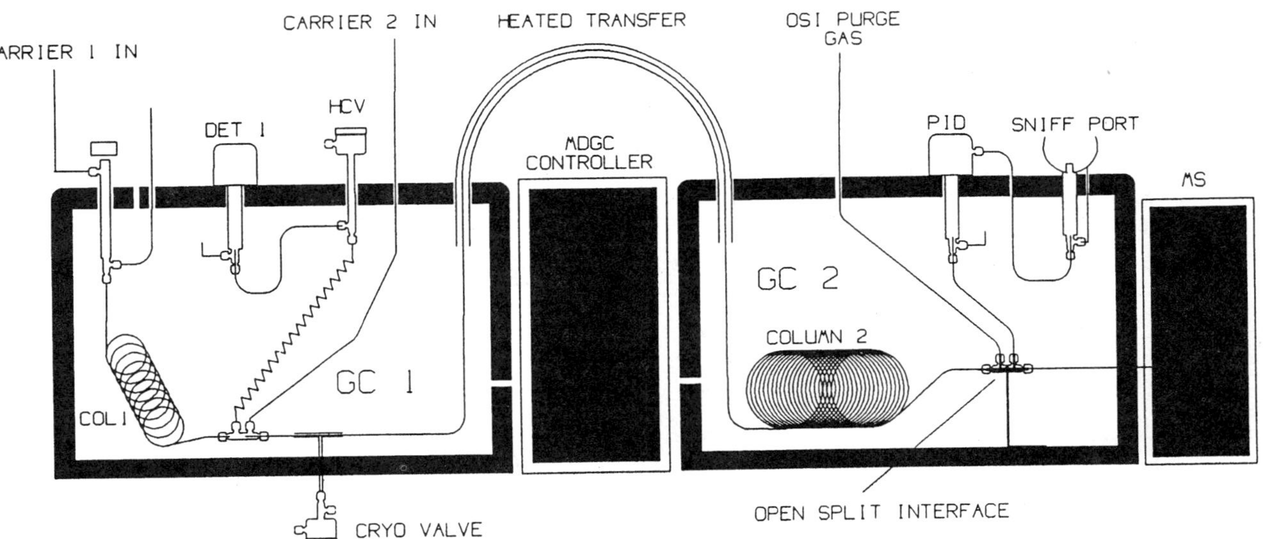

FIGURE 3 Dual-oven MDGC configuration. Schematic diagram illustrating the key elements of an expanded, dual-oven, Deans switch–based MDGC system. This configuration is illustrative of a more complex and highly integrated MDGC system. This system is optimized for the aroma-profiling application and includes direct MS interfacing.

of the MDGC-based aroma-profiling technique. The expanded aroma-profiling system presented in Figure 3 represents the opposite extreme in terms of both system flexibility and complexity. In spite of the added complexity, however, this expanded system still shares a number of features with the basic system, including a dual 0.53 mm ID column-based MDGC system and its utilization of series coupled PID and olfactory detectors (J. Valukas and R. Pandya, personal communication). In this case, however, the system has been expanded considerably to increase its flexibility and expand the range of information that can be extracted from each chromatographic separation. The most obvious expansion is the incorporation of dual gas chromatographs operating as part of an integrated system. This modification permits the two columns to be housed in separate GC ovens maintained under independent temperature-controlled profiles. This serves to increase system flexibility by reducing the critical nature of the configuration decisions made during the early stages of methods development. The two columns are linked by way of a length of uncoated but deactivated fused silica tubing, which is passed through a heated interface link. The heated interface used to link the two GC ovens should represent one of two possible hardware approaches: either a rigid through-wall device or a flexible heated interface line. The rigid mounted through-wall approach is typically a tubular passage that is machined into or encased in a brass heater block. This approach carries the advantage of superior temperature control, both from the standpoint of uniformity of heat distribution and the buffering of heat cycling. Alternately, the flexible heated interface offers the advantages of ease of installation and manipulation by eliminating the requirement that the two GC ovens be physically positioned adjacent to each other. Linked GC systems have been successfully constructed in which the linked instruments are physically located back to back on adjoining lab benches. Adverse effects on chromatographic performance resulting from the reduced precision of temperature control in the flexible interface are minimized through the use of uncoated fused silica transfer lines operating at elevated temperatures. The residence times within the transfer line will be extremely short (e.g., approximately 6 seconds on 1.5 m of 0.53 mm ID fused silica transfer line operating at a linear velocity of 25 cm/sec at the interface). Under these conditions, the chromatographing components traverse the transfer line very quickly and are refocused when they contact the stationary phase at the front of the analytical column. The refocusing effect is enhanced by the fact that at the time of transfer the analytical column oven will normally be operating at a temperature lower than that of the precolumn oven.

The second major modification represented in the expanded aroma-profiling configuration is the addition of an open split interface (OSI) to the exit of the analytical column (Fig. 4). This modification enables the simultaneous

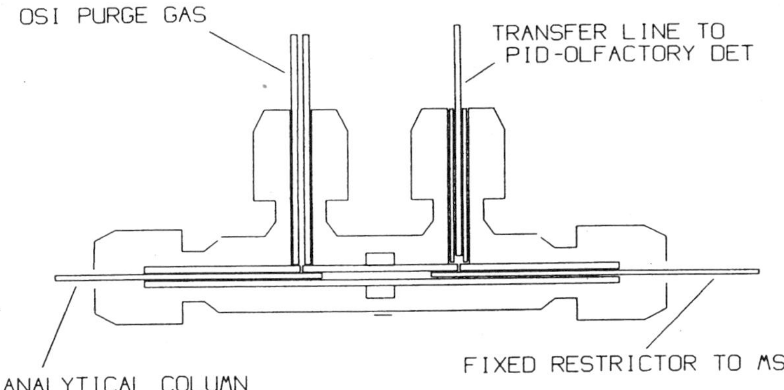

FIGURE 4 Open split interface detail. Diagram illustrating cut-away details of the open split interface shown in the expanded MDGC configuration in Figure 3.

generation of mass spectral profiles in addition to the PID and aroma profiles of the basic system. This is achieved by simply diverting the OSI purge gas flow through a length of fused silica transfer line to the series coupled PID and olfactory detectors. This configuration is particularly convenient for the aroma-profiling application from a number of other aspects. First, the open split interface permits the use of the higher-flow, higher-capacity megabore column configurations, preserving the various advantages as presented in the previous section. These advantages are preserved while ensuring that the exit of the analytical column is maintained at atmospheric pressure, thus assuring optimized chromatographic performance regardless of the high vacuum at the mass spectrometer. The use of the open split interface also makes possible the establishment of some degree of variability in the split ratio between the PID/olfactory and MS pathways. By incorporating a flow switch valve into the purge gas feed line to the OSI, it is possible to toggle between high and low purge rates, thereby changing the analytical column effluent split ratio. With this process it is possible to switch between a maximum of approximately 40–50% and a minimum of approximately 5% transfer to the mass spectrometer.

In addition to these two modifications, there are a number of "variations on the theme" substitutions that can be integrated into these expanded aroma-profiling systems as a means of customizing for particular requirements. These include techniques such as the substitution of a series coupled PID-olfactory detector for the FID monitor detector, enabling a rapid precolumn aroma profile screen to precede the refined MDGC separations. Taking advantage of the rapid aroma screen permits somewhat improved efficiency in these aroma investigations by providing a quick indication of those precolumn effluent regions of primary importance from an aroma standpoint. Adopting this detector configuration also opens up the possibility of modifying the detector strategy employed for the analytical column. In this case, an FPD, chemiluminescence, or NPD detector could be substituted for the olfactory detector, providing the powerful combination of a series-coupled highly sensitive general first detector and a highly selective second detector.

Obviously, these are only a few of the configurations and substitutions that are possible for customizing MDGC systems for aroma profile analysis. However, they do provide an indication of the range of options possible for MDGC systems applied to this specialized field.

VIII. FUTURE OF MDGC IN AROMA PROFILING

Aroma analysis presents a unique set of challenges to the analyst charged with developing analytical methods for its study. These challenges result from the combination of a high degree of sensitivity and selectivity, which is characteristic of the human olfactory response. New and emerging technologies such as neural network–based detector technologies and other chemometric-based pattern recognition techniques offer promise as useful tools for the rapid quality control screening of samples for composite aroma quality. It is expected that these technologies will continue to emerge as important analytical tools in the arsenal of the fragrance analyst. However, it is unlikely that there are techniques on the near horizon that offer the kind of detailed aroma-specific information that is accessible through the combination of MDGC-based separation and detector strategies. It is expected that for the foreseeable future, MDGC technology will continue to be relied on for the critical details regarding the basic building blocks of this important area of volatile analysis.

ACKNOWLEDGMENTS

The author wishes to express appreciation to Dr. Wolfgang Bertsch and Dr. Alfred Huthig Publishers for permission to use referenced material (1) and to Cheryl Earp of RiceTec Inc. for reference samples of Basmati rices from international sources and Helen Wright for patience and diligence in preparing this manuscript.

REFERENCES

1. W. Bertsch, Methods in high resolution gas chromatography. 1. Two dimensional techniques, *HRC & CC 1*:85 (1978).
2. R. E. Kaiser, Analytik im Umweltschutz, *Z. Anal. Chem. 272*:186 (1974).
3. J. C. Giddings, Sample dimensionality: a predictor of order-disorder in component peak distribution of multidimensional separation, *J. Chromatogr. A 703*:3 (1995).
4. B. M. Gordon, M. S. Uhrig, M. F. Borgerding, H. L. Chung, W. M. Coleman, J. F. Elder, J. A. Giles, D. S. Moore, C. E. Rix, and E. L. White, Analysis of flue-cured tobacco essential oil by hyphenated analytical techniques, *J. Chromatogr. Sci. 26*:174 (1988).
5. B. M. Gordon, C. E. Rix, and M. F. Borgerding, Comparison of state-of-the-art column switching techniques in high resolution gas chromatography, *J. Chromatogr. Sci. 23*:1 (1985).
6. T. H. Wang, H. Shanfield, and A. Zlatkis, Analysis of trace volatile organic compounds in coffee by headspace concentration and gas chromatography–mass spectrometry, *Chromatographia 17*:411 (1983).
7. W. V. Ligon and R. J. May, Target compound analysis by two-dimensional gas chromatography–mass spectrometry, *J. Chromatogr. 294*:77 (1984).
8. T. H. Parliment and M. D. Spencer, Application of simultaneous FID/NPD/FPD detectors in the capillary gas chromatographic analysis of flavors, *J. Chromatogr. Sci. 19*:435 (1981).
9. J. Butler, High temperature tandem PID/NPD/FID for characterization of petroleum hydrocarbons by GC, *Am. Lab. (Dec.)*:20 (1994).
10. H. J. Stan and D. Mrowetz, Residue analysis of organophosphorus pesticides in food with two-dimensional gas chromatography using capillary columns and flame photometric detection, *HRC & CC 6*:255 (1983).
11. V. Tachotikul and T. C. Hsieh, Volatile flavor components in crayfish waste, *J. Food Sci. 54*:1515 (1989).
12. R. J. Phillips, A. Gratzfeld-Husgen, Sensory evaluation of chromatographic peaks using capillary columns and thermal conductivity detection, Hewlett-Packard Instrument Company Application Note 228-38, 1984.
13. J. N. Driscoll, Review of photoionization detection in gas chromatography: the first decade, *J. Chromatogr. Sci. 23*:488 (1985).
14. M. L. Langhorst, Photoionization detection sensitivity of organic compounds, *J. Chromatogr. Sci. 19*:98 (1981).
15. N. Johansen, M. Plam, and M. Legier, Detection of sulfur compounds in hop oils with a novel sulfur-selective detector for gas chromatography, *Brewers Digest (April)*:36 (1990).
16. R. L. Benner and D. H. Stedman, Universal sulfur detection by chemluminescence, *Anal. Chem. 61*:1268 (1989).
17. E. A. Smith, E. Chambers IV, and S. Colley, Development of vocabulary and ref-

erences for describing off-odors in raw grains, *Cereal Food World 39*:495 (1994).

18. L. M. Seitz and D. B. Saur, Detection of specific compounds that indicate off-odors in grains, Proceedings of 79th annual meeting of the AACC, Nashville, TN, 1994.
19. P. A. Tice and C. P. Offen, Odors and taints from paperboard food packaging, *Tappi J. 77*:149 (1994).
20. V. Laksanalamai and S. Ilangantileke, Comparison of aroma compound (2-acetyl-l-pyrroline) in leaves from Pandan and Thai fragrant rice, *Cereal Chem. 70*:381 (1993).
21. R. G. Buttery, L. C. Ling, and T. R. Mon, Quantitative analysis of 2-acetyl-l-pyrroline in rice, *J. Agric. Food Chem. 34*:112 (1986).
22. C. F. Lin, T. C.-Y. Hsieh, and B. J. Hoff, Identification and quantification of the "popcorn"-like aroma in Louisiana aromatic della rice, *J. Food Sci. 55*:1466 (1990).
23. V. Tanchotikul and T. C.-Y. Hsieh, An improved method for quantitification of 2-acetyl-l-pyrroline a "popcorn"-like aroma in aromatic rice by high-resolution gas chromatography/mass spectrometry/selected ion monitoring, *J. Agric. Food Chem. 39*:944 (1991).
24. R. G. Berger, F. Drawert, H. Kollmannsberger, S. Nitz, and B. Schrufstetter, Novel volatiles in pineapple fruit and their sensory properties, *J. Agri. Food Chem. 33*:232 (1985).
25. R. G. Buttery, L. C. Ling, B. O. Juliano, and J. G. Turnbaugh, Cooked rice aroma and 2-acetyl-l-pyrroline, *J. Agric. Food Chem. 31*:823 (1983).
26. D. W. Wright, K. O. Mahler, and L. B. Ballard, The application of an expanded multidimensional GC system to complex fragrance evaluations, *J. Chromatogr. Sci. 24*:60 (1986).
27. D. W. Wright, K. O. Mahler, L. B. Ballard and E. Dawes, The application of multidimensional techniques to the rapid pyrolysis-GC profiling of synthetic polymers, *J. Chromatogr. Sci. 24*:13 (1986).
28. D. W. Wright, Assaying for trace impurities in high purity vinyl chloride using HRGC and MDGC, Proceedings of Pittsburgh Conference, Atlanta, Georgia, 1989.
29. ASTM Method D-5507-94, Determination of trace impurities in monomer grade vinyl chloride by capillary column/multidimensional gas chromatography, ASTM, 1994.
30. D. W. Wright, K. O. Mahler, and John Davis, The application of multidimensional techniques to the analysis of sub-ppb levels of vinyl chloride monomer in polyvinylchloride, *J. Chromatogr. Sci. 30*:291 (1992).
31. G. Schomberg, H. Husmann, and E. Hubinger, Multidimensional capillary gas chromatography-enantiomeric separations of selected cuts using a chiral second column, *HRC & CC 7*:404 (1984).
32. D. R. Deans, A new technique in heartcutting in gas chromatography, *Chro-*

matographia 1:18 (1968).
33. D. W. Wright, A multidimensional conversion system for capillary GC, *Am. Lab. 17*:74 (1985).
34. A multidimensional GC conversion system for packed and capillary columns, Technical bulletin GC 16, Scientific Glass Engineering, Inc, 1984.
35. K. A. Krock, N. Ragunthan, and C. L. Wilkins, Parallel cryogenic trapping multidimensional gas chromatography with directly linked infrared and mass spectral detection, *J. Chromatogr. 645*:153 (1993).
36. J. D. Green, Direct sampling method for gas chromatographic headspace analysis on glass capillary columns, *J. Chromatogr. 210*:25 (1981).

6

Enantiomers: Why They Are Important and How to Resolve Them

ALEXANDER BERNREUTHER
Joint Research Centre, Environment Institute, Ispra, Italy

ULRICH EPPERLEIN AND
BERNHARD KOPPENHOEFER
University of Tübingen, Tübingen, Germany

I. ENANTIOSPECIFIC ODOR DIFFERENCES

A. Theoretical Background

1. The Sense of Smell

Each individual has a unique, genetically determined scent. This olfactory identity is coupled with a remarkable ability to distinguish thousands of odors. The basic anatomy of olfaction has been understood for long time. In mammals, an odor is first detected in the upper region of the nose at the olfactory epithelium. In this region, millions of neurons (signaling cells) provide a direct physical connection between the external world and the brain. From one end of each neuron, cilia (hairlike sensors) extend outward into the nasal cavity. As part of the cilia, receptors can bind odorants. At the other end of the neuron cell, an axon (fiber) runs into the olfactory bulb in the brain. In the bulb (the connection of nose and brain), axons converge at the glomeruli; from there signals are relayed to other regions of the brain, including the olfactory cortex, which then projects to higher sensory centers in the cerebral cortex, the area of the brain that controls thoughts and behaviors (1).

When an odor interacts with an olfactory receptor, signaling proteins (G proteins) are activated to initiate a cascade of events resulting in the transmission on an electrical impulse along the olfactory sensory axon. Around 1000 different receptors are encoded by 1000 different genes. This means that nearly 1% of all genes are devoted to the detection of odors, making this the largest gene family thus far identified in mammals. At least 10,000 odors can be detected; consequently, each of the 1000 different receptors must respond to several odor molecules, and each odor must bind to several receptors. It is believed that various receptors respond to discrete parts of an odorant's structure and that an odorant consists of several functional groups each of which activates a characteristic receptor. To distinguish the smell, the brain must then determine the precise combination of receptors activated by a particular odorant. Theoretically, mammals should be able to detect an extraordinarily large number of odors. Because odors interact with multiple receptors rather than with individual ones, the possible combinations exceed by several orders of magnitude the number of odors that animals can actually detect. The remaining question—how the olfactory cortex is decoding the signals provided by the olfactory bulb—is one of the central and most elusive problems in neurobiology (1).

2. Prerequisites of an Odorous Molecule

Sensorily active compounds have to fulfill several molecular and physical prerequisites to initialize an olfactory receptor signal (2,3):

1. A certain vapor pressure for the ability to reach the olfactory epithelium
2. A minimal solubility in water to penetrate the aqueous layer of the membrane as well as a low polarity (surface-active properties; highly polar compounds are odorless)
3. A lipophilic behavior to penetrate the fatty layer of the neuronal cells

4. A molecular weight that is not too high (the highest molecular weight of an odorant is 294)

However, several organic compounds that exhibit all of these properties still do not initialize any olfactory impression. For instance, vanillin has a sweet-floral flavor; its isomer isovanillin, differing only in the spatial arrangement of the same substituents, does not smell. A weakly polar region and a strongly hydrophobic region in the molecule, associated with a certain molecular shape, are most probably the minimum requirements of sensory activity.

3. Olfactory Theories

Today we witness an intense era of molecular biology research in various fields, including receptor ligand interaction and signal transmission. It is important to keep this perspective while looking back to the more or less empirical models of olfaction established in the past. On the other hand, we should not forget that only the signaling process via G proteins (4) is relatively well known, whereas the mechanisms of recognition of an odorant by one or several receptors (5) are still not fully elucidated.

The very first olfactory theory is more than 2000 years old. The Roman doctor Galenus discovered the olfactory nerves, and the Roman poet and philosopher Titus Lucretius Carus described various odorants. According to Carus's theory, pleasant odorants had a spherical shape, whereas stinking substances were acute and prickly particles; an olfactory sensation would need molecules that are able to pass through a slot of the complementary sensory organ (see Ref. 3).

More than 20 different theories have since been developed. Some of these are clearly not valid, such as the penetration and puncturing theory of Davies (6), the chromatographic theory (7), and the information theory (8). Other hypotheses, created for an empirical description of the olfactory system of insects, cannot be transferred from the pheromone field to olfaction by mammals. Only receptor-related theories may be complementarily used in different fields of research (9).

The vibrational theory of Wright (10,11) is based on the assumption that a certain odor is recognized as such by distinct molecular vibrations in the frequency range of 50–400 cm^{-1} (infrared range), the olfactory cell being stimulated by a synchronous "throbbing" of the odorous molecule and the receptor site. For example, compounds having a musky smell were related to four characteristic bands of absorbance frequency (9). To overcome the apparent shortcoming in explaining odor differences of mirror image isomers (in the following called "enantiomers"), Wright suggested that enantiomeric molecules have the same vibrational frequencies only if they are not perturbed by an external agency and that such a perturbation could arise from a close approach of a stimulus molecule to a chiral receptor site (12). This idea is inspired by Hayward's theory of dispersion-induced optical activity in olfaction (13).

The principle "similar profile, similar odor" stands behind the profile functional group theory established by Beets (14). Here the functional group with the highest tendency to interact with a receptor site would orient itself towards the receptor, similarities in the profile of the rest of the odorous molecule thus determining similarities in odor; specialized receptors do not occur in this picture.

Following the principles established for substrate recognition by enzymes, Amoore (15) developed his stereochemical theory. He suggested complementary acceptor sites ("pits" and "sockets") for particularly shaped regions of odorant molecules. Five "primary odors" (camphoraceous, musty, minty, floral, ethereal) could be associated with five groups of compounds classified on the basis of their molecular shape and dimensions, while functional groups were not taken into consideration. For mixed odors, the odorant would fit into two or more different types of receptors. A modified theory presumes that olfactory substances supposed to cause an "anosmic defect" would interact with specific receptor sites and thus produce the primary odors.

Randebrock postulated a molecular theory (16) based on the assumption that the odorant would specifically interact with an amide group of the α-helix of a receptor protein located in the olfactory cilia. Here, the hydrogen-bonding network constituted by three continuous chains around the α-helix would form a vibrational system that could be thermally excited. These vibrations were influenced by attached odorous substances in two directions, longitudinal as well as transversal, depending on two factors: (a) the molecular mass of the odorant and (b) the direction of the interaction.

4. Enantioselectivity

Chiral recognition of substrates is one of the primary criteria of biological activity. One of the pioneers in this field was Pasteur, who also postulated asymmetrical olfactory nerves for the first time (17). Enantiodiscrimination of volatile compounds was later found in many organisms, including bacteria, gametes (19), spiders, insects (20), fish (21), frogs, mole rats (22), and deer (23); mammalian taste, too, can distinguish the enantiomers of a certain chiral compound (e.g., a D- from an L-amino acid (24).

The olfactory epithelium being chiral as a sheer consequence of the molecular composition of biological tissue invokes a natural ability to differentiate between two enantiomers. In other words, the specific receptor-odorant interaction on the epithelium follows from the different stabilities of the respective diastereomeric receptor-ligand complexes. On the other hand, only intimate contact, e.g., operating in enzymatic reactions, is associated with accordingly high differences in free interaction energies of the protein with the two enantiomers of a substrate. In contrast, the typically small differences in odor of enantiomers were sometimes mistakenly attributed to impurities (25). It is fair to say that these subtle differences in biological action tend to vary case by case, leaving much room for speculation on a subject that is still not fully understood.

In a recent work, Polak et al. (26) tested the human odor responses to α-ionone enantiomers, some human subjects being much more sensitive to (R)-(+) than to (S)-(–) and vice versa. In 63 subjects the (R)/(S) threshold concentration ratio varied more than 4 orders of magnitude. It was postulated that odor discrimination of α-ionone enantiomers involves at least two receptor types of opposite enantioselectivity and that their distribution varies independently in human population.

There are several cases known where a given enantiomeric pair is most likely recognized by more than one receptor. For instance, the major part of a panel smelled both enantiomers of carvone, but 8% suffered from chiral anosmia (odor blindness) (27,28). As these individuals could not smell the (R)-(–)-enantiomer, it is believed that they lacked the appropriate receptor. This statement may be underlined by another example: while the (+)-enantiomer of 5α-androst-16-en-3α-ol exhibits a sweaty-urine muscone-type odor with a threshold of approximately 1 ppb, the corresponding (–)-enantiomer is nearly odorless. Only 10% of a panel could detect a very weak musk odor at the 1000 ppm level (29). Another case of chiral anosmia is encountered when both enantiomers fake the same odor. Specific chiral anosmia and parosmia (weak odor perception) are apparently widespread phenomena, even among experienced perfumers (30). So far, close to 100 different anosmia (achiral and chiral) have been documented in the literature (31).

In a huge survey, more than 1.5 million participants tested six different odors (32,33). Only 70.5% of women and 62.8% of men were able to detect 5α-androst-16-en-3-one (sweat). Similar results were obtained for galaxolide (musk), which could be smelled by only 74.6% of women and 66.7% of men. In contrast, isoamyl acetate (banana), eugenol (cloves, spicy), mercaptans (natural gas, obnoxious sulfur), and a rose fragrance were detected by 97% of the test population. These facts support the hypothesis that at least anosmia are inherited. Indeed, it had been demonstrated that the ability to smell androstenone is genetically determined (34).

Last but not least, we cannot rule out a significant contribution of the phospholipid component of the olfactory receptor membrane to the discrimination of odorant enantiomers; the stereoselectivity of a monolayer constituted of a chiral phosphocholine is well established (35).

B. Historical Overview

The first hint that enantiomers of odorous compounds might differ in their smell dates back to 1874 (36). The odor of two essential oils containing (+)- and (–)-borneol, respectively, revealed distinct differences, as outlined in Table 1. The last decade of the nineteenth century witnessed a general tendency to treat this problem from an increasingly scientific perspective.

A major shortcoming of the early research in this discipline was the lack of good qualitative and quantitative criteria. In 1925, Richter (18) attempted to improve this situation by introducing a terminology suited to describe differences in odor. One year later, von Braun and Haensel (55) criticized earlier reports in as much as these had erroneously compared a single enantiomer with the racemate instead of with the antipode. Moreover, it is desirable to have the two enantiomers isolated from the same source, although this is normally not easily accomplished. In the absence of the sharp analytical tools available today (as compared with polarimetric measurements), many of the results reported up to the 1960s suffer from possible interference of odorous impurities with the odor of the test compounds. In some cases, the authors failed to consider all possible stereoisomers (46,49). Another group of molecules investigated does not smell because of the high molecular weight of over 400 (49), far beyond the aforementioned limit of 294 (see Sec. I.A).

A prominent compound listed in Table 1 is α-ionone. The ample difference in optical rotations reported for the enantiomers (+348° and –406°, respectively) (50) leaves enough room for impurities that supposedly alter the respective original odors of the two enantiomers. Some years later, α-ionone was tested again (51), but with optically purer antipodes (–401° and –408°, respectively). However, the intriguing observation that the racemate smells more intensely than either of the single enantiomers could be an artifact. There is only one other example (E-α-irone) known where a racemate smells more intensely than the single enantiomers (53).

Another dubious report deals with 2-phenyl-4-pentenoic acid (54). It appears improbable that only the racemic mixture has a smell, while the single enantiomers are practically odorless. Provided that these observations are correct, Beets (56) assumes that the two antipodes present in the racemate might interact in a synergistic way with more than one receptor at the same time.

In 1961 (57) and 1962 (58) compounds of high but opposite enantiomeric purity were synthesized from the same source (citronellol from (+)- and (–)-pinane, linalool from (+)- and (–)-α-pinene) for the first time. Later

TABLE 1 Historical Overview of Reported Enantiospecific Odor Differences

Compound	Odor description	Year (Ref.)
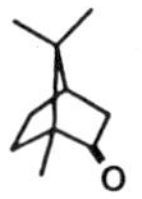 Camphor	No odor differences found.	1863 (37)
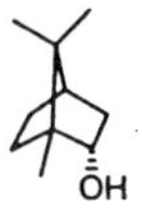 Borneol	Borneocamphor oil [contains (+)-borneol] and ngaicamphor oil [contains (–)-borneol] were found to smell differently. The odor of the first is weak camphorlike and unpleasant peppery; the odor of the latter is camphor and turpentinelike (38). Possibly the first indication of odor differences of enantiomers.	1874 (36)
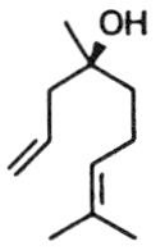 Homolinalool	Active is more intensive than racemate.	1896 (39)
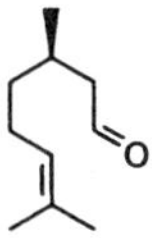 Citronellal	(S)-(–) somewhat sweater than (R)-(+). According to von Braun and Kaiser (40), possible isopulegol traces.	1897 (41)
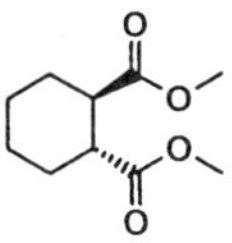 Dimethyl E-hexahydrophthalate	(–) rather strong, but (+) nearly odorless. No odor differences found by Posvic (42). According to von Braun and Kaiser (40), insufficient purification of the enantiomers.	1899 (43)
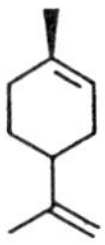 Limonene	(+) isolated from caraway oil smells different than that synthesized from tetrabromide. Doubtful literature source.	1899 (44)

TABLE 1 Continued

Compound	Odor description	Year (Ref.)
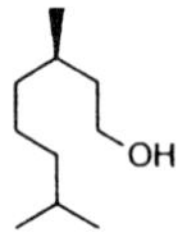 3,7-Dimethyloctanol	(+) fresher and more penetrating than racemate	1923 (40)
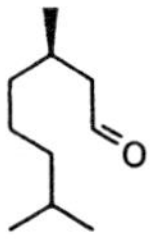 3,7-Dimethyloctanal	Racemate is similar to citronellal, with lemon note, more pleasant and more intensive than (+). (+) is similar to citral, with lemon note.	1923 (40)
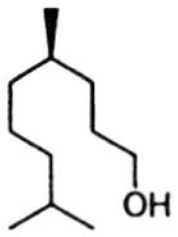 4,8-Dimenthylnonanol	Racemate is more intensive and harsher than (+).	1923 (40)
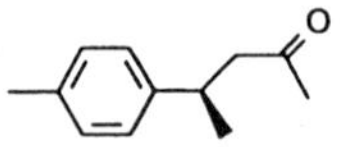 Curcumone	Racemate: strong curcuma-flavor, weaker and finer (sweeter) than active. Active: strong curcuma-flavor, more herblike and less pleasant than racemate	1924 (45)
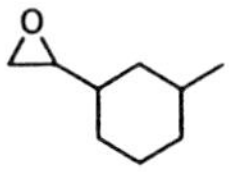 1-(1,2-Epoxyethyl)-3-methylcyclohexane	Racemate: more intensive and more pungent note than (–). (–) milder than racemate. Possible diastereomers might not be taken into account.	1925 (46)
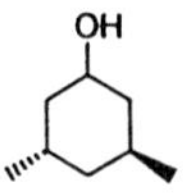 3,5-Dimethylcyclohexanol	(+) fresher, more powerful. (–) milder, heavier. Synthesized from E-3,5-dimethylcyclohexanone.	1927 (47)

TABLE 1 Continued

Compound	Odor description	Year (Ref.)
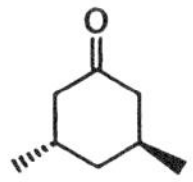 E-3,5-Dimethyl cyclohexanone	(+) minty, ester-like (amyl ester note). (–) minty, faintly reminiscent of isopulegone. Diastereomeric (Z) reminiscent of camphor and thujone.	1927 (47)
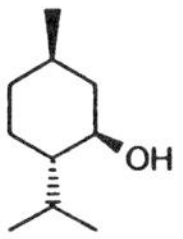 Menthol	(+) is fainter than (–), but of same general character.	1931 (48)
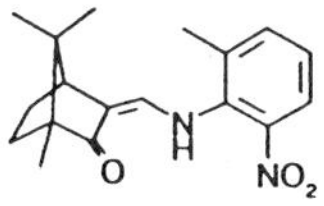 3-Nitro-o-toluidino methylenecamphor	(–) more intensive than racemate. Racemate more intensive than (+)	1939 (49)
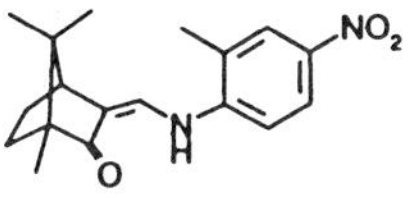 5-Nitro-o-toluidino methylenecamphor	(–) more intensive than racemate. Racemate more intensive than (+)	1939 (49)
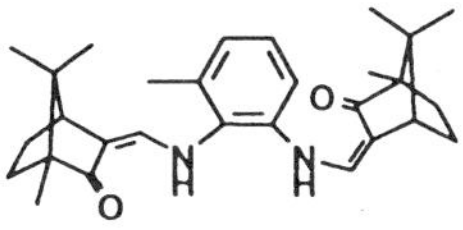 2,3-Toluylene bis(amino methylenecamphor)	(–) more intensive than racemate. Racemate more intensive than (+). Possible formation of diastereomers might not be taken into account, since two molecules of camphor were bound.	1939 (49)
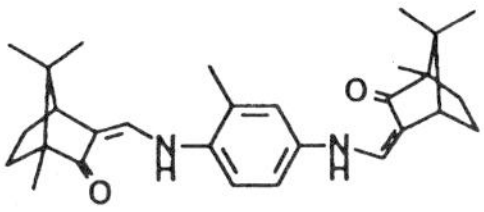 2,5-Toluylene bis(amino methylenecamphor)	(–) more intensive than racemate. racemate more intensive than (+) Possible formation of diastereomers might not be taken into account, since two molecules of camphor were bound.	1939 (49)

TABLE 1 Continued

Compound	Odor description	Year (Ref.)
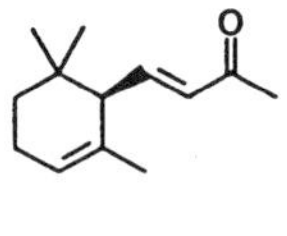 α-Ionone	Distinct odor difference between (+) and (−). Active weaker (0.002–0.008 μg/liter air) racemate more intensive (0.00025–0.0005 μg/liter air).	1943 (50) 1947 (51)
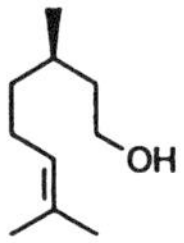 Citronellol	No odor differences found between the single enantiomers. Racemate is less pleasant and less "expensive" than the single enantiomers.	1946 (52)
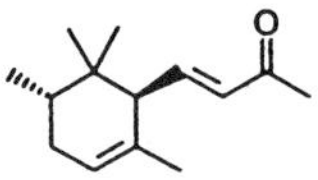 E-α–Irone	Racemate is more intensive than active.	1953 (53)
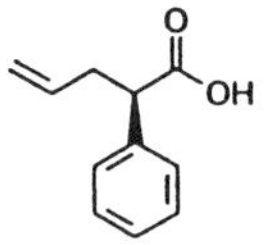 2-Phenyl-4-pentenoic acid	(+) practically odorless. (−) practically odorless. Racemate clear honeytype odor. It is rather improbable that only the racemic mixture is odorous (see text for details).	1961 (54)

many chiral flavor compounds were synthesized and sensorily evaluated following these principles.

One frequently cited example is carvone. In 1971, several groups of researchers (27,59,60) independently reported on odor differences of the carvone enantiomers. While the characteristic difference in the odors of carvone enantiomers was reported for the first time in 1968 (61), there was still a possibility that these differences originated from impurities, resulting from the different origins of the two enantiomeric samples. In an elegant experimental scheme (see Fig. 1), Friedman and Miller (27) interconverted synthetic (R)- and (S)-limonene, thus deliberately triggering its odor characteristics and at the same time excluding trace impurities as the major cause of the observed

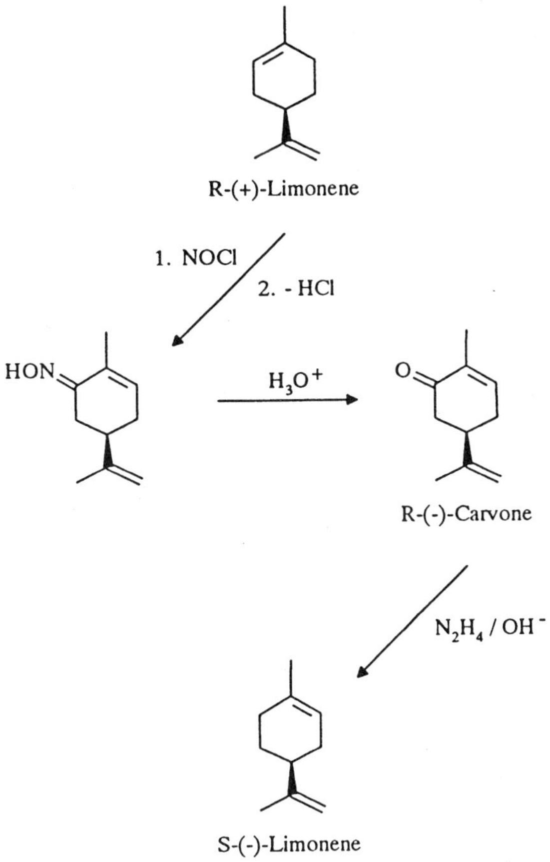

R-(+)-Limonene

1. NOCl
2. - HCl

HON

H_3O^+

O

R-(-)-Carvone

N_2H_4 / OH^-

S-(-)-Limonene

Figure 1 Interconversion of both enantiomers of limonene via carvone clearly demonstrates that differences in odor are not to be traced back to impurities.

odor characteristics. More recently, (R)-carvone was reported to cause a strongly stereospecific allergy, while the (S)-enantiomer has no effect (62).

C. Examples

Following a seminal paper in 1977 by Theimer et al. (63), a landmark example of total olfactory enantioselectivity was reported by Ohloff in 1980 (64). Both enantiomers of the steroid androsta-4,16-dien-3-one were synthesized. A panel of 100 subjects described the odor of the "natural" (+)-enantiomer—with the very low threshold of 1 ppb—as urinous, sweaty, woody and musky, while the "unnatural" (–)-enantiomer was described as odorless, even at very high concentrations. In a subsequent report by Ohloff et al. (29), these results were confirmed with a 30-subject panel. In addition, two more steroids with maximum odor difference were found. It is interesting to note that Prelog and coworkers (65–67) performed a sensory evaluation of the "natural" isomers of these and other steroids as early as 1945, but missed the question of odor differences between "natural" and "unnatural" enantiomers. Also, in 1980 Ohloff et al. (68) reported on the total olfactory enantioselectivity of two norlabdane derivatives. More compounds were later added to the list (Table 2).

In several examples the odors of enantiomers differ not only qualitatively, but also quantitatively. Moreover, some optically active flavor compounds exhibit differences only in threshold concentrations. Several examples are listed in Table 3. Some of these show remarkable differences, such as nootkatone, the flavor impact of grapefruit (a sesquiterpenoic ketone): the threshold of the natural enantiomer is 2000 times lower (72). The enantiomers of a decalin derivative were found to differ at least 10,000 times in the threshold [determination via sniffing GC (73)].

Unfortunately, threshold values often cannot be compared due to different measurement conditions. Some authors reported only relative odor intensities or sniffing GC results (83), others used different solvents such as buffers (28). Therefore, standardization and harmonization of human olfactory thresholds is absolutely necessary for a better comparison of the reported data. Such compilations already exist, but only very few chiral compounds are listed (84). There is still a need for systematic investigations to overcome these problems.

It is a well-known fact that the sense of smell in dogs is much more sensitive than that in humans, but one should not forget that this phenomenon is strongly dependent on the particular odorant. For instance, the dog's threshold for butyric acid is one million times lower than that of humans, but for a typical flavor compound such as α-ionone, a difference of only 2500 times was reported (11). This indicates that in some cases human olfactory receptors are more specialized to specific compounds than to standard compounds such as butyric acid; in other words, some molecules interact more intensely with the receptors than others. In this context it may be relevant that (R)-(+)-nicotine caused an unpleasant odor sensation to both smokers and nonsmokers, while only smokers perceived the (S)-(–)-enantiomer as pleasant (85).

Some rare examples are found in the literature where the enantiomers

Table 2 Maximum Qualitative Odor Differences

Compound	Odor description	Ref.
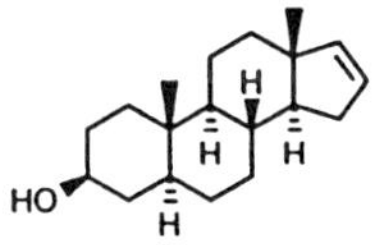 5α-Androst-16-en-3β-ol	(3S,5S,8S,9S,10R,13R,14S)-(+) sweaty-urine, very weak (3R,5R,8R,9R,10S,13S,14R)-(−) odorless	29
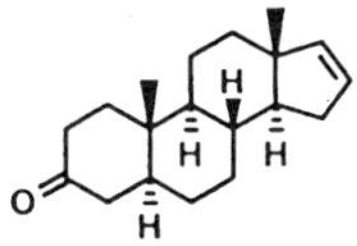 5α-Androst-16-en-3-one	(5S,8S,9S,10R,13R,14S)-(+) sweaty-urine, weak muscone-type odor with a sandalwood-like basic note (5R,8R,9R,10S,13S,14R)-(−) odorless	29
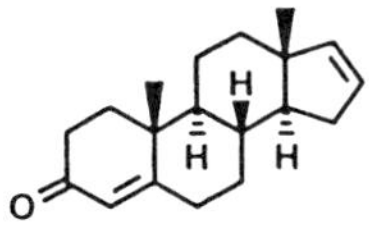 Androsta-4,16-dien-3-one	(8S,9S,10R,13R,14S)-(+) urinous, sweaty, woody, musk (8R,9R,10S,13S,14R)-(−) odorless	64
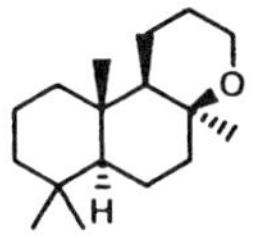 8,13-Epoxy-14,15,16-trinorlabdane	(5S,8S,9R,10S)-(+) odorless (5R,8R,9S,10R)-(−) musty menthol-like odor, woody-balsamic note, camphoraceous, fruity, odor is distinct from ambergris	68, 69
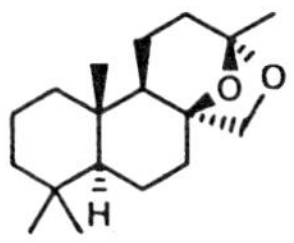 8,13:13,20-Diepoxy-14,15-dinorlabdane	(5S,8R,9R,10S,13R)-(−) odorless (5R,8S,9S,10R,13S)-(+) woody character, ambergris tonality, odor is distinct from ambergris	68, 69
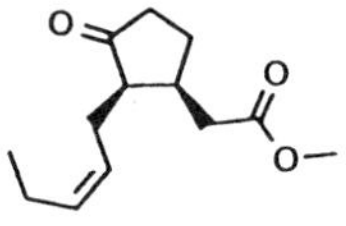 Methyl Z-epijasmonate	(1R,2S)-(+) strong jasmine odor (1S,2R)-(−) odorless	70

TABLE 2 Continued

Compound	Odor description	Ref.
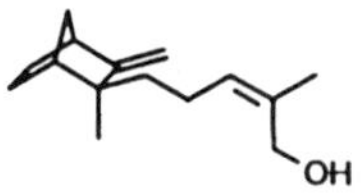 Z-β–Santalol	(–) typical sandalwood scent (+) odorless	71
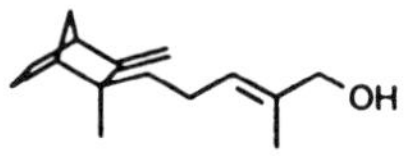 E-β–Santalol	(–) sandalwoodlike, weaker than Z-(–) (+) odorless	71
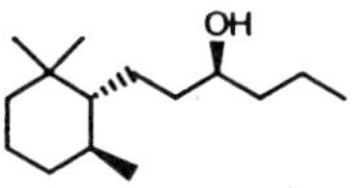 Norlimbanol	(5S,6S,9S)-(+) powdery, woody, with animal tonality (5R,6R,9R)-(–) odorless	3

did not show any odor difference (see Table 4). The first case was camphor, published in 1863 (37). The complete absence of any odor difference between the camphor enantiomers was reconfirmed in 1977 (63). This feature is most probably closely related to the molecular structure, as Table 4 contains some compounds structurally related to camphor (e.g., methylborneol). On the other hand, some structures are associated with a surprising lack of olfactory enantioselectivity (e.g., 3-mercapto-1-hexanol and 5-hexanolide), although similar compounds are known to exhibit distinct odor differences (see Table 5). Interestingly, some 2-(alkoxy)pyrazines (alkoxy = 2-butoxy and 2-pentoxy, respectively) showed no odor differences, while for higher homologs (alkoxy = 2-heptoxy and 2-octoxy, respectively) significant threshold differences were noted (79).

In Figure 2, a sensory evaluation of all possible stereoisomers of menthol is shown (90; R. Hopp, personal communication). Here, each class chosen from 25 odor classes is quantitatively described on a scale of 0 to 5 (1 = very low; 5 = very high) designed to demonstrate enantiospecific flavor differences of the menthol isomers. This is a very good example to show the importance of standardized odor descriptions for better comparability.

Menthol has three stereogenic centers in the carbon skeleton of the cyclo-

TABLE 3 Quantitative Odor Differences of Enantiomers

Compound	Threshold	Ref.
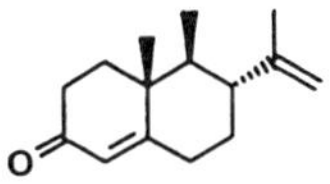 Nootkatone	(4R,5S,7R)-(+) 600–1000 ppb (4S,5R,7S)-(–) 400000–800000 ppb	72
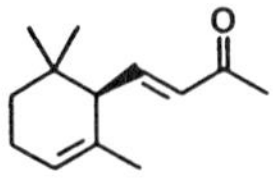 α-Ionone	(R)-(+) 0.5–5 ppb (S)-(–) 20–40 ppb	74
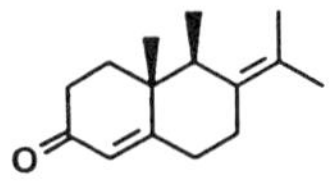 α-Vetivone	(4R,5S)-(+) 600–1000 ppb (4S,5R)-(–) 6000–15000 ppb	72
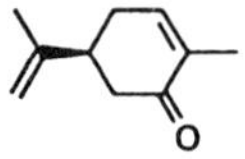 Carvone	(S)-(+) 85–130 ppb (R)-(–) 2 ppb	27
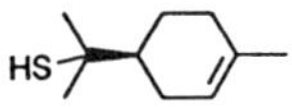 p-1-Menthene-8-thiol	(R)-(+) 0.00002 ppb (S)-(–) 0.00008 ppb	75
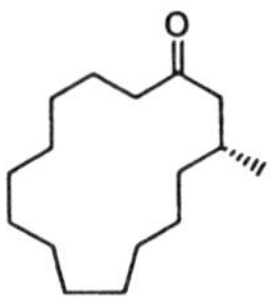 Muscone	(R)-(–) 61 ppb (S)-(+) 233 ppb	76
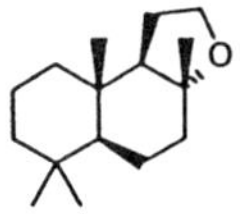 Ambrox	(3aR,5aS,9aS,9bR)-(–) 0.3 ppb (3aS,5aR,9aR,9bS)-(+) 2.4 ppb	77

Table 3 Continued

Compound	Threshold	Ref.
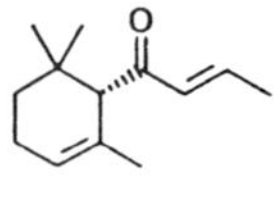 α-Damascone	(S)-(–) 1.5 ppb (R)-(+) 100 ppb In contrast to a prior publication, no threshold difference was found [1 ppb for each enantiomer (74)].	76
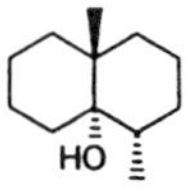 Geosmin	(4R,4aR,8aS)-(+) 0.078 ppb (4S,4aS,8aR)-(–) 0.0095 ppb Mean thresholds of 50 panelists with 6 repetitions each.	78
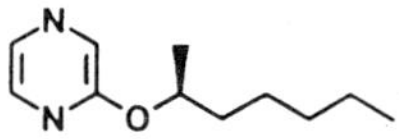 2-(2-Heptoxy)pyrazine	(R)-(+) 200 ppb (S)-(–) 70 ppb	79
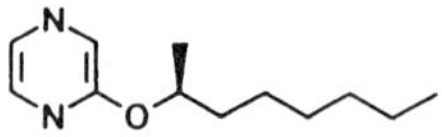 2-(2-Octoxy)pyrazine	(R)-(–) 90 ppb (S)-(+) 30 ppb	79
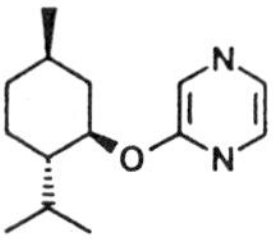 2-Menthoxypyrazine	(1'R,2'S,5'R)-(–) 2 ppb (1'S,2'R,5'S)-(+) 10 ppb	79
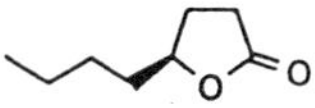 4-Octanolide	(R)-(+) 7 ppb (S)-(–) 1 ppb	80
4-Decanolide	(R)-(+) 1.5 ppb (S)-(–) 5.6 ppb	80

TABLE 3 Continued

Compound	Threshold	Ref.
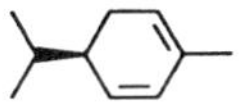 α-Phellandrene	(R)-(–) 300–700 ppb (S)-(+) 100–300 ppb	81
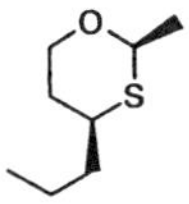 Z-2-Methyl-4-propyl-1,3-oxathiane	(2S,4R)-(+) 2 ppb (2R,4S)-(–) 4 ppb	82

Threshold values determined in aqueous solutions.

hexane ring, thus it occurs in four pairs of enantiomers. (–)-Menthol, the main component of peppermint and cornmint oils, is more abundant in nature than the (+)-antipode. The oxidation products menthone and isomenthone as well as (–)-menthyl acetate are main components of several essential oils from the *Mentha* species (38); their enantiospecific odor differences were also described (90).

As a class of very important and powerful flavors, chiral sulfur-containing compounds are outlined in Table 5. Some of these occur in tropical fruits (e.g., passion fruits), especially the oxathiane derivatives (82,91), 3-mercapto-hexanol (88), and its acetate (92). The thiomenthones and their acetates are important constituents of buchu leaf oils responsible for their characteristic black current odor. Buchu leaf oils are often used for commercial cassis flavors (38). The (R)-enantiomer of the structurally related compound *p*-1-menthene-8-thiol is responsible for the typical grapefruit flavor (together with nootkatone). It is one of the most powerful flavors with an extremely low odor threshold: 0.02 ng/liter water for the natural (R)-enantiometer and 0.08 ng/liter water for the (S)-enantiomer, which exhibits an obnoxious odor (75).

Table 6 shows the enantiospecific sensory evaluation of several examples of aliphatic esters of 2-alkanols. Mosandl and Deger (98) systematically investigated acetates, butanoates, hexanoates, and octanoates of a homolog series of secondary alcohols (2-butanol to 2-nonanol). Many of these esters were found in the flavor of banana and other fruits. In recent reports, the enantiomeric distribution of a great deal of these compounds was addressed (99–102).

Table 4 Compounds Exhibiting No Enantiospecific Odor Differences

Compound	Ref.	Compound	Ref.
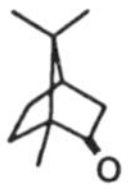 Camphor	37	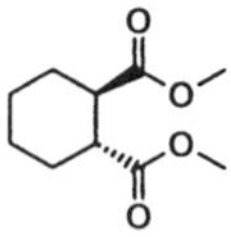 Dimethyl E-hexahydrophthalate	42
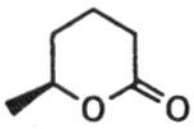 5-Hexanolide	86	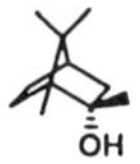 2-Methylborneol	87
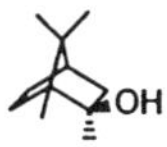 2-Methylisoborneol	87	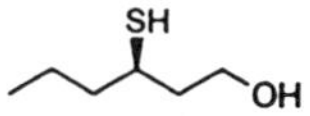 3-Mercaptohexanol	88
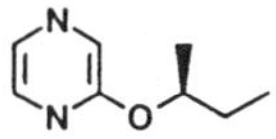 2-(2-Butoxy)pyrazine	79	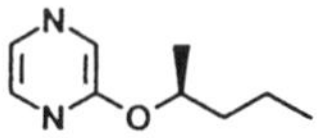 2-(2-Pentoxy)pyrazine	79
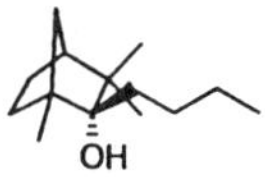 2-Butylfenchol	89	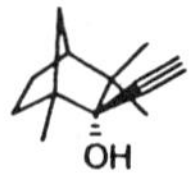 2-Ethynylfenchol	89

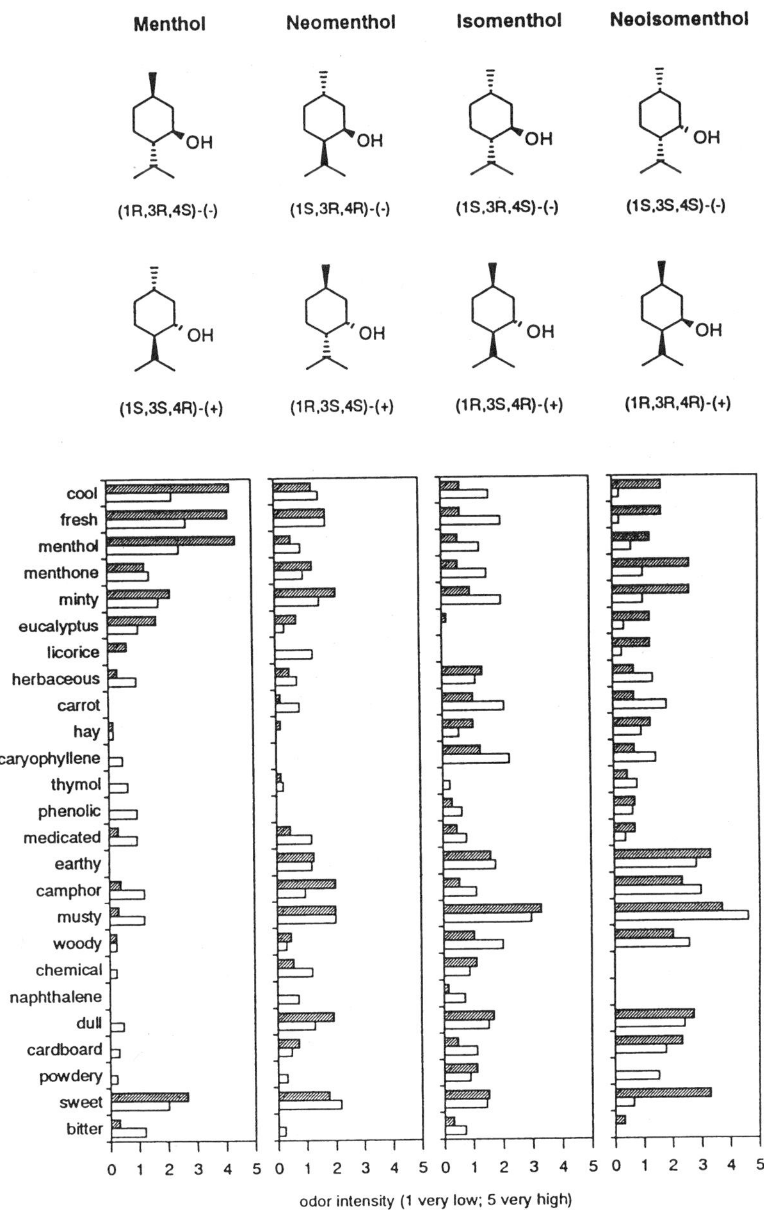

FIGURE 2 Sensory evaluation of all possible stereoisomers of menthol.

TABLE 5 Sensory Evaluation of Sulfur-Containing Flavor Compounds

Compound	Odor description	Ref.
3-Mercaptohexanol	Intensive sulfur-note No odor differences found	88
3-Mercaptohexyl acetate	(R) penetrating, reminiscent of tropical fruits (S) penetrating sulfurous, herbaceous	92
3-Mercaptohexyl butanoate	(R) intensive of tropical fruits (passion fruit) (S) sulfurous, oniony, later unspecific fruity	92
3-Mercaptohexyl hexanoate	(R) herbaceous, fresh sulfur note (S) sulfurous, burnt	92
3-Methylthiohexanol	(R) herbaceous, weak (S) exotic, fruity	88
3-Methylthiohexyl acetate	(R) fruity (stronger than homolog butanoate and hexanoate) (S) intensive sulfurous, herbaceous	92
3-Methylthiohexyl butanoate	(R) very weak, unspecific fruity (S) oniony, later weak fruity	92
3-Methylthiohexyl hexanoate	(R) very weak, unspecific fruity (S) weak oniony, roasty	92

TABLE 5 Continued

Compound	Odor description	Ref.
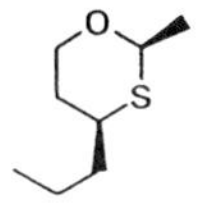 Z-2-Methyl-4-propyl-1,3-oxathiane	(2S,4R) typical sulfurous with rubbery onion note, reminiscent of grapefruit peel, mango, and passion fruit (2R,4S) weaker than the enantiomer, no pronounced sulfur character, possessing a fresh note with more iris character	82
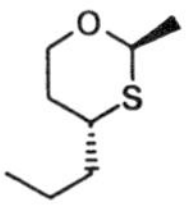 E-2-Methyl-4-propyl-1,3-oxathiane	(2R,4R) green-grass root, earthy red radish note (2S,4S) sulfurous, slightly bloomy-sweet, less intensive than enantiomer	91
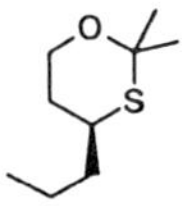 2,2-Dimethyl-4-propyl-1,3-oxathiane	(R) slight, fruity, soft lemon note (S) typical carrot note, sweet	91
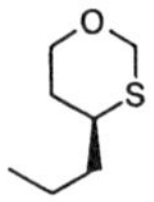 4-Propyl-1,3-oxathiane	(R)-(+) artificial fruity, fatty with slight grapefruit note (S)-(–) artificial, unpleasant sulfurous note, burnt gumlike	91
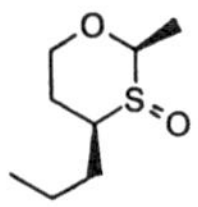 2-Methyl-4-propyl-1,3-oxathiane-S-oxide I	(2R,3R,4S) intensive, pungent green foul sulfur note (H_2S) (2S,3S,4R) intensive, exotic fruity note, highly volatile	93
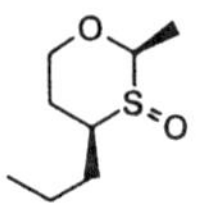 2-Methyl-4-propyl-1,3-oxathiane-S-oxide II	(2R,3S,4S) grassy, green unpleasant, sticky sulfur note (2S,3R,4R) intensive, green sulfur note, reminiscent of fresh rhubarb	93

Table 5 Continued

Compound	Odor description	Ref.
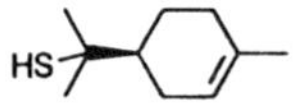 *p*-1-Menthene-8-thiol	(R) pleasant, fresh grapefruit juice (S) extremely obnoxious sulfur note	94
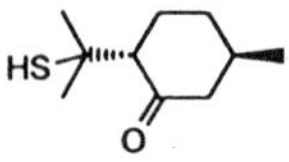 E-Thiomenthone	(1R,4R) oniony, moldy, slightly fruity, tropical fruits (1S,4S) tropical fruits, buchu leaf oil, more intensive than enantiomer	95,96
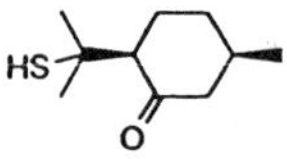 Z-Thiomenthone	(1R,4S) rubber, mercaptane note, is opulegone note, burnt, sulfurous, unpleasant (1S,4R) black currant leaves, tropical note of passion fruit, most intensive fruity note	95,96
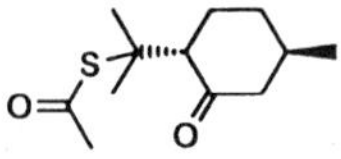 E-Thiomenthone acetate	(1R,4R) musty, sulfury note, intensive (1S,4S) green, black currant, exotic, intensive, and penetrating note	97
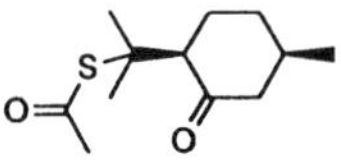 Z-Thiomenthone acetate	(1R,4S) delicate, fruity, sweet (1S,4R) strong, sweet, slightly pungent	97

D. Critical Remarks

In the following, prerequisites for successful scientific investigations of enantiospecific odors are summarized to emphasize their importance:

1. Chemical and optical purity is absolutely necessary (30) (in some cases this is a very difficult task, because of ultra-trace impurities, which still can influence the odor even if not detected with modern analytical methods).
2. Both enantiomers must derive from the same source (see also Fig. 1) (3).

TABLE 6 Sensory Evaluation of Aliphatic Esters of 2-Alkanois

Compound	Odor description	Ref.
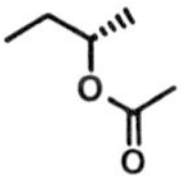 2-Butyl acetate	(S)-(+) intensive fruity ester note, slightly volatile (R)-(–) musty, herbaceous, slightly volatile	98
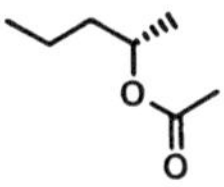 2-Pentyl acetate	(S)-(+) unspecific chemical (R)-(–) similar to enantiomer, but weaker	98
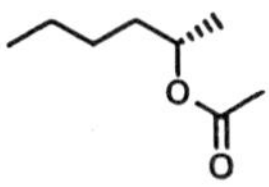 2-Hexyl acetate	(S)-(+) weak, unspecific ester note (R)-(–) weak flowery	98
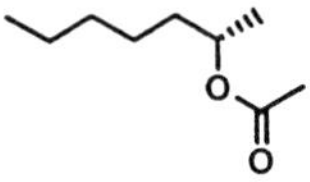 2-Heptyl acetate	(S)-(+) weak, pure fruit note (R)-(–) penetrating sweat note	98
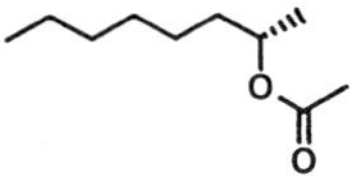 2-Octyl acetate	(S)-(+) fine, pure fruity (R)-(–) herbaceous, weak fruity	98
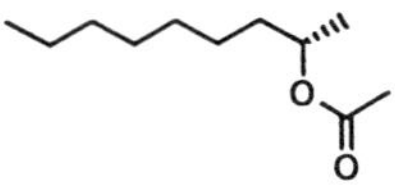 2-Nonyl acetate	(S)-(+) typical fruity note (R)-(–) flowery, more intense than enantiomer	98
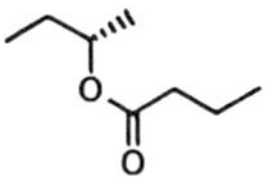 2-Butyl butanoate	(S)-(+) intensively fruity, sweet ester note (R)-(–) flowery, musty, weaker than enantiomer	98

TABLE 6 Continued

Compound	Odor description	Ref.
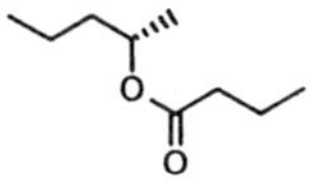 2-Pentyl butanoate	(S)-(+) fruity, easily volatile, sweaty aftersmell (R)-(–) spicy, smoky	98
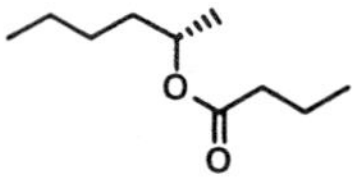 2-Hexyl butanoate	(S)-(+) pure fruity (R)-(–) weak fruity, herbaceous	98
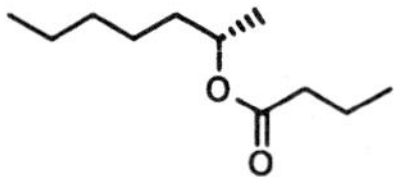 2-Heptyl butanoate	(S)-(+) distinct fruity aroma note (R)-(–) fruity-sweet ketone note	98
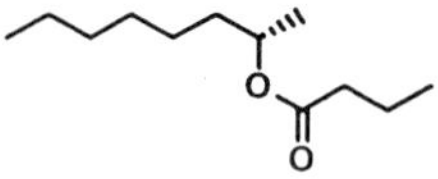 2-Octyl butanoate	(S)-(+) weak fruity (R)-(–) weak flowery note	98
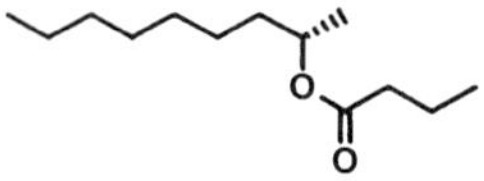 2-Nonyl butanoate	(S)-(+) first unspecific, then somewhat spicy (R)-(–) unspecific, weak flowery	98
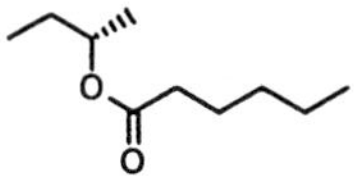 2-Butyl hexanoate	(S)-(+) intensive fruity penetrating note (R)-(–) herbaceous, weaker than enantiomer	98
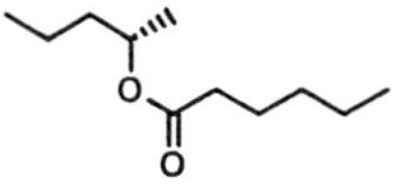 2-Pentyl hexanoate	(S)-(+) pleasant fruity note (R)-(–) flowery fragrance note	98

TABLE 6 Continued

Compound	Odor description	Ref.
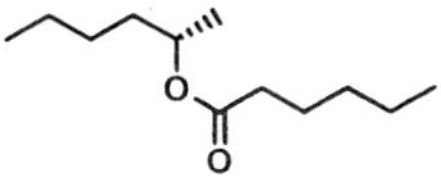 2-Hexyl hexanoate	(S)-(+) spicy (R)-(–) sweet, flowery	98
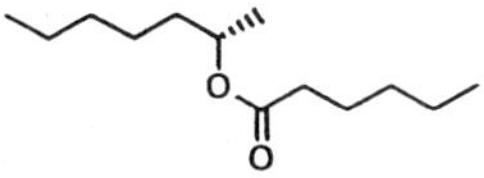 2-Heptyl hexanoate	(S)-(+) distinct fruity ester note (R)-(–) fruity sweet ketone note	98
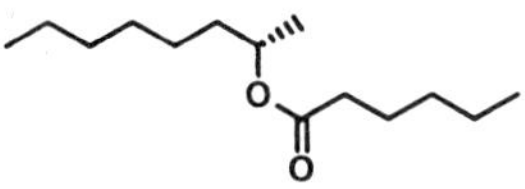 2-Octyl hexanoate	(S)-(+) intensive pure fruit note, reminiscent of raspberries (R)-(–) herbaceous, green	98
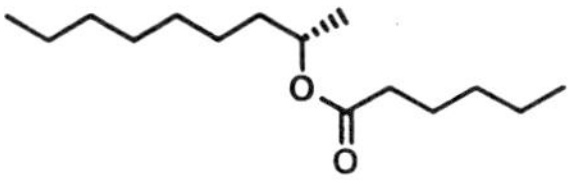 2-Nonyl hexanoate	(S)-(+) flowery sweet (R)-(–) weak fruity, slightly earthy note	98
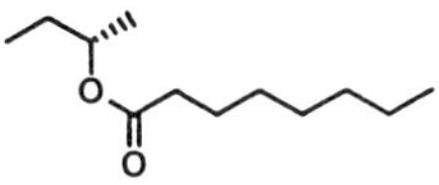 2-Butyl octanoate	(S)-(+) distinct ester note (R)-(–) first sweet, then smoky	98
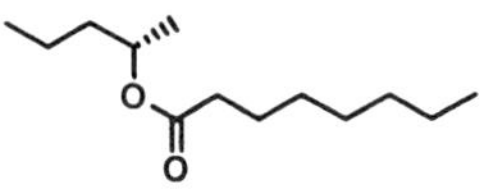 2-Pentyl octanoate	(S)-(+) weak fruity (R)-(–) unspecific, very weak	98
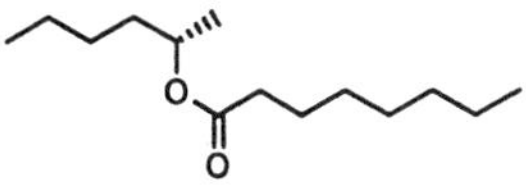 2-Hexyl octanoate	(S)-(+) weak spicy (R)-(–) very weak sweet, flowery	98

TABLE 6 Continued

Compound	Odor description	Ref.
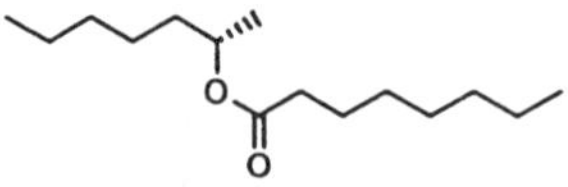 2-Heptyl octanoate	(S)-(+) moldy, musty, unspecific (R)-(–) very weak herbaceous, unspecific	98
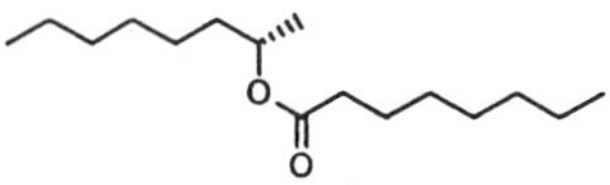 2-Octyl octanoate	(S)-(+) first fine fruity, then intensive lovage note (R)-(–) weak fruity, unspecific note	98
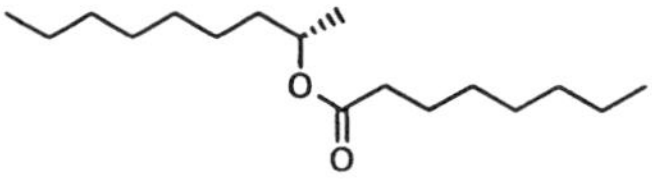 2-Nonyl octanoate	(S)-(+) weak unspecific note (R)-(–) weak unspecific note, but distinguishable	98

3. Standardized odor descriptors are desirable (90).
4. Standardized threshold determination is necessary (84) (only aqueous solutions or in air, at room temperature, with a certain humidity, etc.).
5. Odor qualities depend also on the concentration of the compound in a solvent (80) (at different concentrations, different odor quality might occur).
6. A panel of at least five subjects (preferably well-trained experts) should evaluate the sensory qualities of flavors, because of the individuality of odor perception (26) (achiral and chiral anosmia and parosmia have to be taken into account as well as the psychological state of the subjects).
7. The time between the sensory evaluation of enantiomers should be long enough to avoid overlapping of odor sensations, some compounds effect a remaining odor impression (sustain up to 1 hour), therefore, olfactory receptors may be blocked (3).
8. Sniffing GC should be applied on a multidimensional system to avoid accidental co-elution of odorous trace compounds (see Sec. II.B), and, taking into account the former statement, enantiomers have to be separated with at least one minute difference in retention times.

II. ANALYSIS OF CHIRAL FLAVOR COMPOUNDS

A. Methodology

The most popular approach to the separation of enantiomeric pairs involves diastereomorphous interaction with a chiral environment. In the early days, this task was conveniently accomplished by derivatization of the analyte with a chiral auxiliary, followed by separation of the diastereomers in an archiral environment, e.g., by chromatographic or electrophoretic methods. Likewise, the diastereomers were dissolved in an achiral solvent and analyzed by nuclear magnetic resonance (NMR) spectroscopy. It turned out that this methodology suffered from several drawbacks, the most serious being the lack of complete enantiomeric purity of the chiral derivatization agent (CDA). Thus, a small signal assigned to the minor diastereomer may originate from both sources—the analyte and the auxiliary—without further identification.

More recently, several methods involving reversible weak interactions with a chiral environment were introduced. Here, a lack of complete enantiomeric purity does not show in a signal that may be erroneously attributed to the minor enantiomer of the analyte; instead, such a deviation will typically result in a decrease in the degree of discrimination. As compiled in Table 7, these methods comprise chiral stationary phases, mobile phase additives, buffer additives, solvating agents, and lanthanide shift reagents.

In the following sections, the most important techniques used for the analysis of flavors and fragrances are briefly summarized (103).

1. Chiroptical Methods

There are several chiroptical methods used in analytical chemistry, such as polarimetry, circular dichroism (CD), optical rotatory dispersion (ORD), and methods based on vibrational optical activity. In the past, polarimetry was the method of choice for flavor analysis, for single compounds, and for complex mixtures such as essential oils. Polarimetry is still part of routine analysis to determine the optical purity of flavor compounds as well as quality control of flavors and essential oils. Admittedly, polarimetry is a convenient method, but its use is restricted by relatively large sample amounts required for correct measurements. In addition, there are several factors affecting the accuracy of optical rotation determination, such as the temperature applied, the nature and the purity of the solvent used, as well as traces of optically active or inactive impurities originally present in the analyte. More recently, the chiroptical methods have increasingly been supplemented and replaced by chromatographic methods. Since the 1980s, polarimetry and circular dichroism (CD)

TABLE 7 Enantioselective Analytical Techniques

Analytical technique	Abbreviation
Nuclear magnetic resonance spectroscopy	NMR
High-performance liquid chromatography	HPLC
Gas chromatography	GC
Supercritical fluid chromatography	SFC
Thin-layer chromatography	TLC
Countercurrent chromatography	CCC
Capillary electrophoresis	CE

Chiral principle	Abbreviation	Analytical technique
Chiral derivatization agents	CDA	NMR, HPLC, GC, SFC, TLC, CCC, CE
Chiral stationary phases	CSP	HPLC, GC, SFC, TLC, CE
Chiral mobile phase additives	CMA	HPLC, TLC, CCC, CE
Chiral buffer additives	CBA	HPLC, CE
Chiral solvating agents	CSA	NMR
Chiral lanthanide shift reagents	CLSR	NMR

have also been used as detectors for high-performance liquid chromatography (HPLC) (104–107) and even for gas chromatography (GC) (108).

2. Nuclear Magnetic Resonance Spectroscopy

NMR performed in an achiral solvent typically does not differentiate between enantiomers; in first order, resonances of enantiotopic nuclei are isochronous. The determination of enantiomeric composition by NMR, therefore, requires one of the three possible methodologies outlined in Table 7 (CDAs, CLSRs, or CSAs). These are widely used in research, albeit less in routine analysis, of flavors.

3. Electrophoresis

In the past few years, capillary electrophoresis (CE) became very popular, especially for the analysis of drugs, pharmaceutical metabolites, pesticides, and other nonvolatile compounds (e.g., amino acids, carbohydrates). Unfortunately, there are several obstacles to its application to flavor compounds, such as low solubility in aqueous solvents and lack of chromophores suitable for UV detection.

4. Chromatography

The three basic chromatographic methods (GC, HPLC, and TLC) are applied to the analysis of flavors and fragrances in an uneven proportion. The use of TLC in this field is mainly restricted to achiral routine analysis. For preparative enantiomer separation, HPLC and supercritical fluid chromatography (SFC), rather than GC, offer the advantage of larger sample throughput. For analytical purposes, GC is the first choice; thus, a more detailed presentation of important GC techniques is given in the following section.

B. Gas Chromatographic Techniques Used for Enantiomer Separation

An increasing number of publications deal with the GC separation of enantiomers (see also Sec. II.C). The majority of these report on the development and application of methods to flavors and fragrances. The precise knowledge of enantiomeric ratios of flavor compounds has become of interest, for instance, in the authenticity control of foodstuffs and essential oils as well as in the composition and preparation of fragrances and perfumes.

As mentioned previously, the use of chiral stationary phases (CSP) of high (but to necessarily absolute) enantiomeric purity is superior to the conversion of enantiomers into diastereomeric derivatives by an optically pure CDA.

1. Chiral Derivatization Agents Used in GC

For a long time, derivatization of enentiomers to diastereomers, originally developed by Bailey and Hass (109), was the only method available. Here, alcohols were derivatized with 2-acetyl lactic acid and acids with (–)-menthol. The volatile diastereomeric esters formed were partially separated by rectification. The first specific use of this indirect method in GC was reported by Casanova and Corey (110), separating racemic camphor via cyclic acetals after derivatization with (R,R)-2,3-butanediol.

In principle, this methodology is applicable to a wide range of chiral compounds, such as alcohols, aldehydes, ketones, carboxylic acids, esters, lactones, and even hydrocarbons. More than 100 different CDAs have been used to far in gas chromatography. The most important reagents are listed in Table 8.

Most of the applications to flavor compounds were published (120–123) before the advent of cyclodextrin-based CSPs. In view of the prohibitive cost of the latter method, the indirect method is still in use

TABLE 8 Chiral Derivatization Agents Used for Enantioselective Flavor Analysis by GC

Chiral derivatization agent	Analytes	Ref.
2-Butanol	Hydroxycarboxylic acids	111
2,3-Butanediol	Ketones, hydrocarbons (after oxidation to ketones)	110
1-Phenyl ethyl amine	Alkylcarboxylic acids	112
Trolox™ methyl ester	Sec. alcohols, 2-alkyl-1-alkanols	113
Acetyl lactyl chloride	Sec. alcohols, lactones (after ring opening with or without reduction to diols	114
Menthylchloroformate	Sec. alcohols, hydroxycarboxylic acid esters	115
2-Methoxy-2-trifluoromethyl-2-phenylacetyl chloride	Sec. alcohols, ketols, hydroxycarboxylic acid esters, lactones (after ring opening)	116
Tetrahydro-5-oxo-2-furan-carboxylic acid chloride	Sec. alcohols, hydroxycarboxylic acids, lactones (after ring opening)	117
Dimethyl tartrate	Aldehydes, ketones	118
1-Phenylethyl isocyanate	Sec. alcohols, alkylcarboxylic acids, hydroxycarboxylic acids, lactones (after opening, with or without reduction to diols)	119

Source: Ref. 103.

where only a few analyses have to be done. The diastereomeric derivatives can be analyzed on almost all achiral stationary phases available for routine purposes, such as polysiloxanes and polyglycols. For the precise determination of enantiomeric purity, however, the inherent disadvantages of the indirect method led to continuous replacement by the direct method, i.e., the direct analysis of the sample on a CSP. One should not forget, however, that there are still certain enantiomeric pairs that cannot be resolved on a CSP (113,124,125).

2. Chiral Stationary Phases

The most important chiral stationary phases used in gas chromatography (Fig. 3) can be divided into three main classes (guided by the *principle* separation mechanism): amide phases (*hydrogen bonds*, dipole, and van der Waals interactions), metal complex phases (*complexation*, dipole and van der Waals interactions) and cyclodextrin phases (*inclusion*, dipole, and van der Waals interactions). Other CSPs developed are merely of scientific interest.

L-Chirasil-Val

XE-60-L-Valine-(R)-α-phenylethylamide

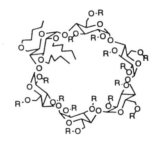

Nickel(II) bis(heptafluorobutyryl-1R-camphorate)

2,3,6-Tri-O-pentyl-α-cyclodextrin

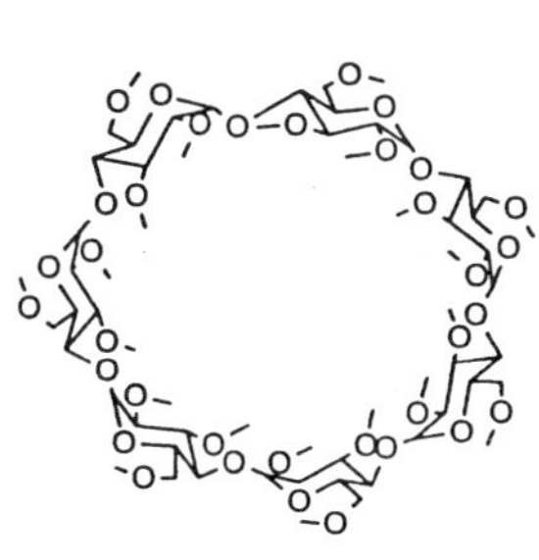

2,3,6-Tri-O-methyl-β-cyclodextrin

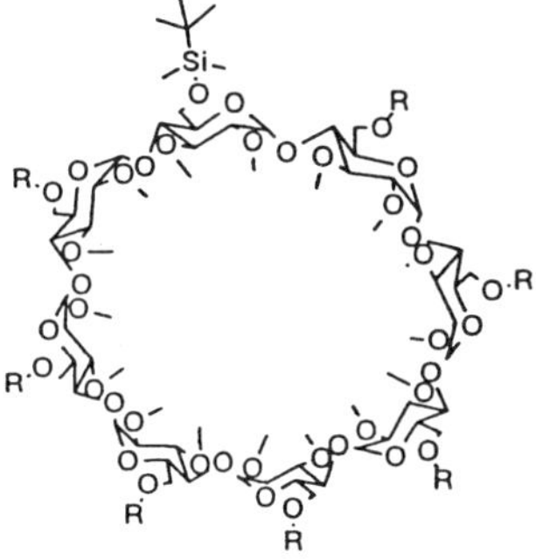

2,3-Di-O-methyl-6-O-tert.-butyldimethylsilyl-γ-cyclodextrin

FIGURE 3 Some typical examples of CSPs used in GC.

Amide Phases

The landmark paper in enantiomer separation by GC was published by Gil-Av et al. in 1966 (126); baseline separation was achieved for most derivatives of enantiomeric pairs of proteinogenic amino acids. The enantiomer separation was verified using a column coated with a mirror image stationary phase. In the early days of enantioselective GC, mainly amino acid derivatives and similar compounds were analyzed, while flavor and fragrance compounds were out of scope because of the lack of functional groups that were deemed a perquisite for the separation.

Among a great variety of CSPs developed of the amide type, the commercially available polymeric phases L- (127) and D-Chirasil-Val (128) and XE-60-(S)-Valine-(S)-(–PEA) (129) are used frequently. These CSPs have been applied occasionally in the field of flavors and pheromones (130) (see also Sec. II.B.4).

The separation power of these amide phases for enantiomers is sometimes higher than that of cyclodextrin phases, albeit strongly dependent on the presence of certain functional groups in the analyte structure. Even though compounds with hydrogen-bonding capability still exhibit medium polarity, the parent analytes, in particular amino acids, are often highly polar and nonvolatile. Therefore, achiral derivatization is often required. On well-deactivated capillaries, however, hydroxyl groups may be left underivatized, leading to an increase in separation factors (α) (131). While for many important flavor compounds, such as hydrocarbons, amide phases are not suitable, others like γ-lactones could be separated completely (132) or partially (133).

Metal Complex Phases

The first attempts to use chiral metal coordination compounds as enantioselective stationary phases for GC enantiomer separation were undertaken by Schurig and Gil-Av in 1971 (134). The first successful separation was published by Schurig in 1977 (135) for 3-methylcyclopentene; chalcogran as the first pheromone was separated by Koppenhoefer et al. in 1980 (136). Later, several flavor compounds (e.g., 1-octen-3-ol, menthone, linalyl acetate, oxanthianes) were separated into enantiomeric pairs (103). One of the most efficient CSPs of this type is nickel(II)-bis-[1R-3-heptafluorobutanoyl camphorate], either dissolved in OV-101 (137) or, in order to overcome the drawbacks of low thermal stability, covalently bound to a dimethylpolysiloxane (138).

Cyclodextrin Phases

Since 1987, the field of enantiomer separation has been influenced by the ever-increasing popularity of the cyclodextrin-based CSPs. Cyclodextrins are cyclic glucans (cyclomaltooligoses) with at least 6–12 D-glucopyranose units in α-1,4-glycosidic connection. In analytical chemistry, α-,β-, and γ-cyclodextrins are applied, containing 6, 7, and 8 glucose units, respectively. Almost all different chromatographic and electrophoretic methods (HPLC, SFC, GC, TLC, CZE, ITP, MEKC, EC) benefit from this trend (103).

In the early 1960s, peracetylated and perpropionylated α- and β-cyclodextrins were used above their melting points (>220°C) as stationary phases in packed GC columns for the separation of fatty acid methyl esters (139). In 1983, the first application of a cyclodextrin phase to the separation of enantiomers by GC was reported by Koscielski et al. (140). These authors separated the enantiomers of α- and β-pinene, respectively, on celite coated with an aqueous formamide solution of α- and β-cyclodextrins in packed column gas solid chromatography (GSC).

In 1988, Schurig and Nowotny reported on permethylated β-cyclodextrin dissolved in different polysiloxanes, mainly polycyanopropyl phenyl vinyl methyl siloxane (OV-1701) (141). Meanwhile, this CSP has been made available as a polysiloxane-anchored immobilized phase (142). At about the same time, several peralkylated and acylated/alkylated cyclodextrins were introduced by König et al. (143), forming a liquid coating at normal GC operating temperatures (40–220°C); these cyclodextrin derivatives were later diluted by the polysiloxane OV-1701 (144).

A great variety of CSPs based on cyclodextrins, some of them very efficient for flavor analysis, were proposed during the following years by many researchers (145–147). Remarkable separations can be carried out, for instance, on heptakis(2,3-di-*O*-acetyl-6-*O*-tert-butyldimethylsilyl)-β-cyclodextrin dissolved in OV-1701 (148). Meanwhile, nearly every chiral flavor compound has been made amenable to enantiomer separation by GC, although a researcher in this field will find it difficult to search the most suitable CSP for a given separation problem. This issue of *information crisis* will be further addressed in Section II.C.

3. Instrumentation

As compared to routine analysis of flavors and fragrances, the separation of enantiomers requires a more sophisticated instrumentation. Quality problems may arise from overlapping of the additional peaks, leading to wrong peak assignments, and from misrepresentation of enantiomer ratios (ee). In a typical flavor analysis, a single GC system equipped with an unspecific detector such as a flame ionization detector (FID) will not cope with the demand for high-precision determination of ee. Even though coinjection of the analytes may be applied, dependent on the availability of reference compounds, correct quantitation remains difficult. Therefore, a so-called multidimensional gas chromatographic system (MDGC) composed of an achiral precolumn and a chiral main column should be used (106,149–151); moreover, sample preparation is easier and, hence, less time consuming.

A promising although costly alternative involves coupling of a single-column system to a mass spectrometer as detector that is, for instance, run in the selected ion-monitoring mode (SIM) (152–154). Of course, combining the two methods, i.e. coupling of an MDGC system to an MS instrument, will further improve the reliability and accuracy of the results, especially in trace analysis (102,107,153,155). Given a sufficient concentration of a flavor component of interest, an Fourier transform infrared spectrometer (FTIR) may also serve as a GC detector (156). It has been reported that some homologs of a compound class are not separable on a given CSP (101); in other instances, a reverse in the elution order was observed (107). Setting up a new analysis, e.g., by switching to a novel CSP, involves elaborate tests for each analyte of interest. For instance, a certain chiral compound may change the elution order of the enantiomers when a different type of cyclodextrin is applied (145). Last but not least, the structure and percentage of the polysiloxane used for mixing with a cyclodextrin derivative may largely influence the enantioselectivity of such phases (see Ref. 103 for details).

4. Objectives and Applications

Detailed knowledge of the enantiomer composition of chiral compounds is a key to answering many questions. For a better understanding of biochemical pathways and biosynthesis of flavor compounds and pheromones, such data are indispensable. From an industrial perspective, process analysis of enantiomeric purity of microbiologically produced or asymmetrically synthesized flavors are the main tasks of flavor analysts. Another major issue in quality control is the proof of authenticity and origin of flavors, fragrances, and essential oils by the above-mentioned methods (101,103,157–160). In the following, a couple of typical examples are presented to underline the importance of the methodology.

Allmendinger and Koppenhoefer (132) checked the enantiomer composition of commercially available (S)-(+)-terpinen-4-ol on Chirasil-L-Val (see Sec. II.B.2). They found about 15% of the (R)-(−)-enantiomer (see Fig. 4).

Galfré et al. (161) separated all enantiomeric pairs of irone stereoisomers (Z-α, E-α, β, Z-γ, E-γ; see Fig. 5). Application of this analytical method to industrially produced Orris oils of various origins allowed the differentiation between natural and nonnatural qualities (see Table 9). A typical example is shown in Figure 6. Olfactory characterization of the pure enantiomers was also reported (161,162).

A method of detecting added reconstituted mandarin oil in genuine cold-

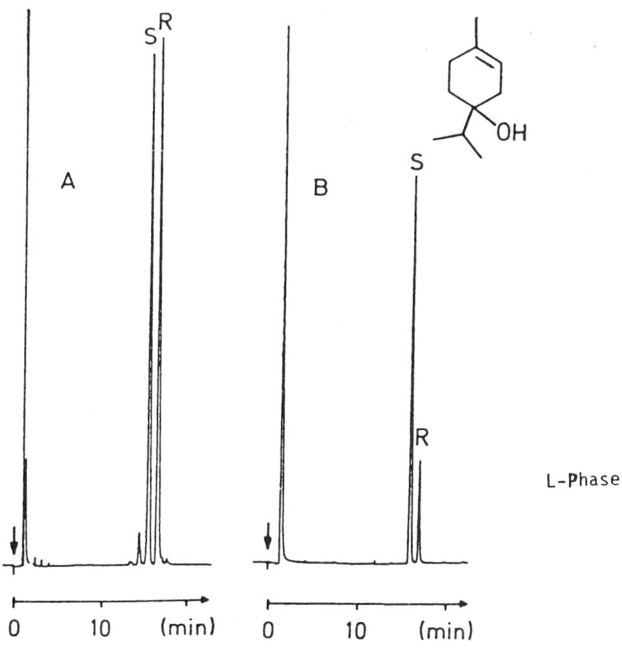

FIGURE 4 Separation of terpinen-4-ol enantiomers on L-Chirasil-Val (glass capillary 20 m × 0.25 mm i.d.; 70°C; 0.4 bar H_2). (A) Racemic mixture; (B) commercially available (S)-(+)-enantiomer. (From B. Koppenhoefer and H. Allmendinger, unpublished.)

pressed mandarin essential oils by determination of the enantiomer distribution of limonene was described by Dugo et al. (Table 10) (163). The chromatograms in Figure 7 show the enantiomer separation of limonene of mixtures of cold-pressed mandarin oils with 5% (A) and 10% (B) reconstituted oils, respectively.

Enantiomer separation of monoterpenoid peppermint constituents of two peppermint oils of different origin as well as the respective racemic standards are shown in Figure 8 (W. A. König, personal communication).

The occurrence of (–)-bicyclogermacrene in a liverwort (*Scapania uliginosa*) and of (+)-bicyclogermacrene in the essential oil of marjoram (*Majorana hortensis*) was investigated by König (personal communication). The racemic standard was derived from isolation of the bicyclogermacrene enantiomers of the respective essential oils by means of preparative GC. The results are presented in Figure 9.

Being an important class of flavors, γ- and δ-lactones are widespread in

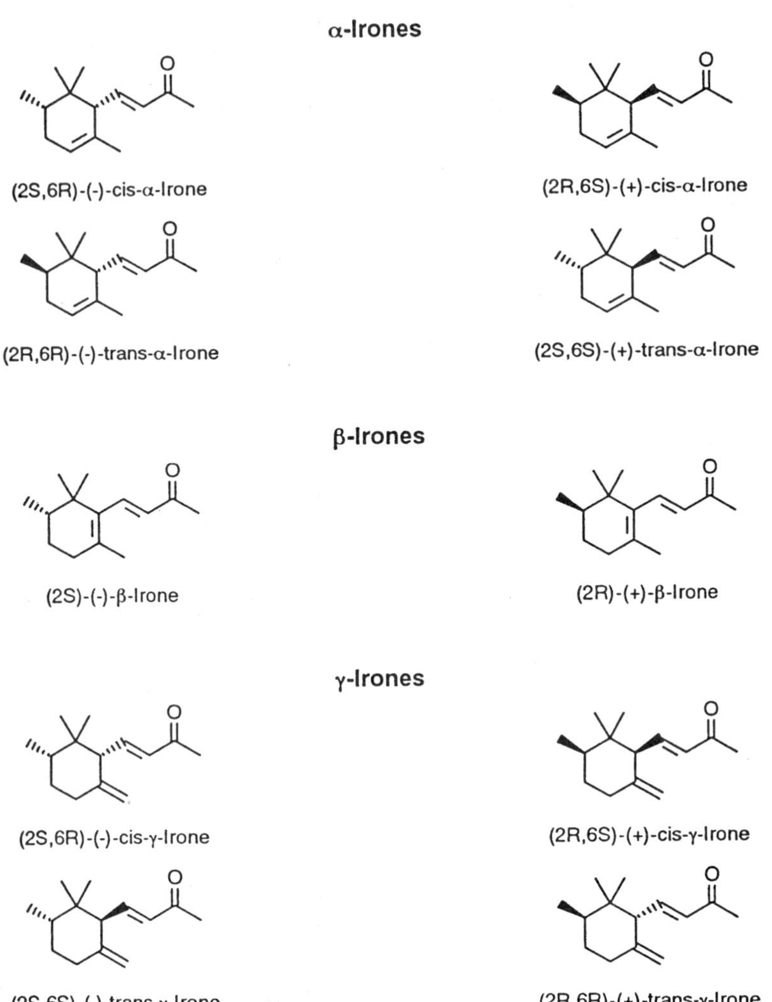

FIGURE 5 Ten possible stereoisomers (five enantiomeric pairs) of irone.

foodstuffs. Accordingly, several publications deal with their enantioseparation (e.g., Refs. 106,107,164). Bernreuther et al. (106) used MDGC for enantioselective analysis of γ-lactones from genuine fruit flavors (101,106). The enantioseparation of γ-decalactone from a peach flavor extract is presented in Figure 10.

TABLE 9 Irone Enantiomer Distributions (%) in Orris Butters and Absolutes of Different Origins

Batch number	Product type	(+) *trans*-α	(−) *trans*-α	(+) *cis*-α	(−) *cis*-α	(+) *cis*-γ	(−) *cis*-γ
1	Germanica butter	99.5	0.5	8.8	91.2	31.2	68.8
2	Germanica butter	99.5	0.5	9.3	90.7	32	68
3	Germanica butter	99	1	10	90	36.2	63.8
4	Germanica butter	95	5	7.8	92.2	28	72
5	Germanica butter	99	1	8.2	91.8	32.5	67.5
6	Germanica butter	95	5	9	91	27.6	72.4
7	Pallida butter	99	1	99	1	99	1
8	Pallida butter	99	1	81.6	18.4	99	1
9	Pallida butter	99	1	69	31	96	4
10	Germanica absolute	67	33	12.5	87.5	34.7	65.3
11	Germanica absolute	67.5	32.5	18.3	81.7	39	61
12	Germanica absolute	100	ca. 0	9.8	90.2	36	64
13	Pallida absolute	90	10	66.9	33.1	96.4	3.6
14	Pallida absolute	98	2	80.5	19.5	100	ca. 0
15	Pallida absolute	99	1	85.4	14.6	98	2
	Average:						
	Germanica butter	97.83	2.16	8.85	91.15	31.25	68.75
	Pallida butter	99	1	83.2	16.8	98	2
	Germanica absolute	78.16	21.83	13.53	86.46	36.56	63.43
	Pallida absolute	95.67	4.33	77.6	22.4	98.13	1.87

Source: Ref. 161.

Simultaneous determination of γ- and δ-lactones in dairy products under MDGC conditions was performed by Lehmann et al. (164). As typical examples, the enantioseparation of γ- and δ-lactones from a parmesan cheese and a country butter are shown in Figure 11. Genuine lactones of dairy products preferably occur as (R)-enantiomers.

The aliphatic terpenoid alcohol linalool is widely abundant in essential oils (e.g., rosewood oil, lavender oil) as well as in many fruit flavors. The enantiodifferentiation of linalool in an essential oil of lavender (155) is shown in Figure 12 (101). Genuine lavender oils contain (R)-linalool in a high enantiomeric purity (155,165).

The combination of enantioselective GC with sniffing GC is especially useful in the characterization of odors of single enantiomers. Fischer and Hammerschmidt (166) investigated the important flavor compounds 2,5-di-

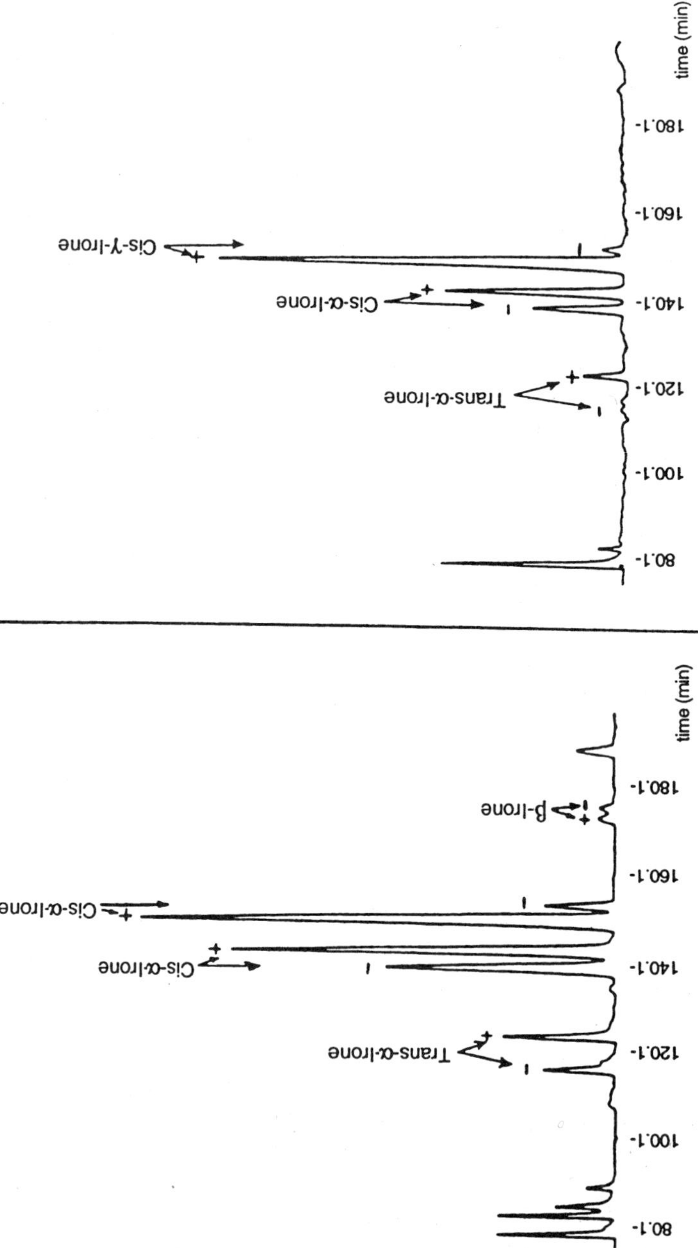

FIGURE 6 Enantiomer analysis of irone stereoisomers in Orris oils (ex *Iris pallida*) on octakis (6-O-methyl-2,3-di-O-pentyl)-γ-cyclodextrin/OV-1701 (1:1) (fused silica capillary 25 m × 0.25 mm i.d.; 90°C; 0.7 bar He) (161). (Left) nonnatural origin; (right) natural origin. (Courtesy of Allured Publishing Corporation, Carol Stream, IL.)

TABLE 10 Limonene Enantiomeric Ratios (%) in Samples of Genuine Cold-Pressed Mandarin Essential Oil and Those Containing 5% and 10% Reconstituted Oil

			99% confidence limits			
	x̄	s	Min	Max		
Genuine oil						
(−)-Limonene	2.2	0.14	1.8	2.6		
(+)-Limonene	97.8	0.14	97.4	98.2		
Reconstituted oil 5%						
	1	2	3	4	5	6
(−)-Limonene	3.3	3.3	3.1	3.1	2.8	3.0
(+)-Limonene	96.7	96.7	96.9	96.9	97.2	97.0
	7	8	9	10	11	12
(−)-Limonene	3.0	3.4	3.0	3.0	3.2	3.1
(+)-Limonene	97.0	96.6	97.0	97.0	96.2	96.9
Reconstituted oil 10%						
	13	14	15	16	17	18
(−)-Limonene	3.9	3.7	4.0	3.9	3.9	3.8
(+)-Limonene	96.1	96.3	96.0	96.1	96.1	96.2

Source: Ref. 163.

methyl-4-hydroxy-3[2*H*]-furanone (furaneol®) and 2,5-dimethyl-4-methoxy-3[2*H*]-furanone (mesifuran) with octakis(2,6-di-O-pentyl-3-trifluoroacetyl)-γ-cyclodextrin as CSP. By the same technique, the sensory properties of this and other furanoic compounds were characterized by Bruche et al. (167,168). The aforementioned irones were also olfactorily analyzed via sniffing GC (161). Further applications of enantioselective GC/olfactometry are published for terpenoid compounds (169), 2-alkyl-branched esters abundant in apple flavor (154), secondary alkyl-branched acids (170), aerangis-lactones (171), sulfur-containing compounds (172), and amberlike odors (73).

C. Electronic Information Retrieval

1. Rapid Access to Information

As flavor compounds are volatile by nature, GC is the method of choice for the determination of enantiomeric composition. With the present state of

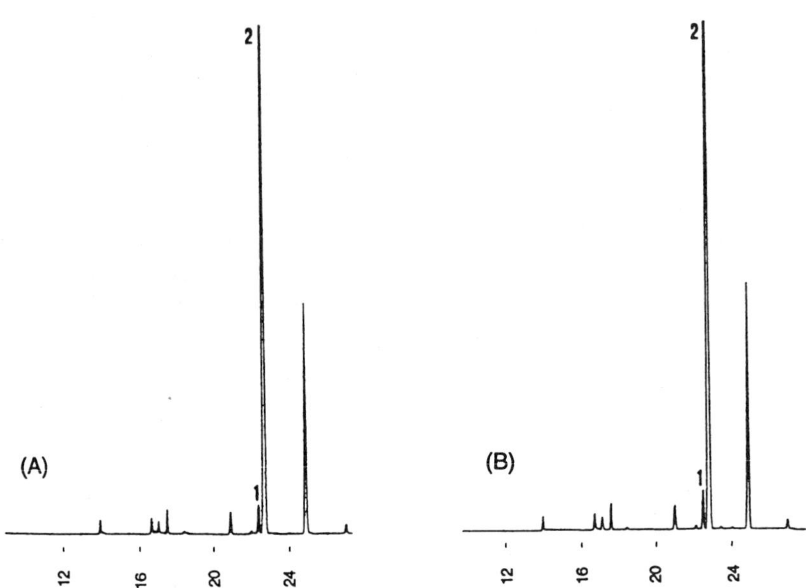

FIGURE 7 Enantiomer analysis of limonene in mixtures of cold-pressed mandarin oil on heptakis (2,3,6-tri-O-methyl)-β-cyclodextrin/OV-1701 (30:70) (fused silica capillary 25 m × 0.25 mm i.d.; 8 min at 80°C, then to 105°C at 1.2°C/min; 0.65 bar H_2) (163). (A) 5% of reconstituted oil; (B) 10% of reconstituted oil. (Courtesy of Allured Publishing Corporation, Carol Stream, IL.)

knowledge, the mechanisms of enantiomer separation by GC have been only tentatively elucidated; unusual chromatographic behavior, such as the change of the elution order in homologue series of flavor compounds (107) and the reverse of the elution order of enantiomers at different temperatures (173), invoke further complication. In view of the large number of CSPs on the market, the search for an optimum or at least satisfactory solution for a given separation task is bound to end up in what some analyst recently called an "information crisis."

Indeed, the amount of data published on this subject is growing rapidly, doubling every 2–3 years. To cope with this informational explosion, the graphic molecule database Chirbase/GC was created (174), paralleling Chirbase/LC (175). According to release 4/95, Chirbase/GC contains 5,651 enan-

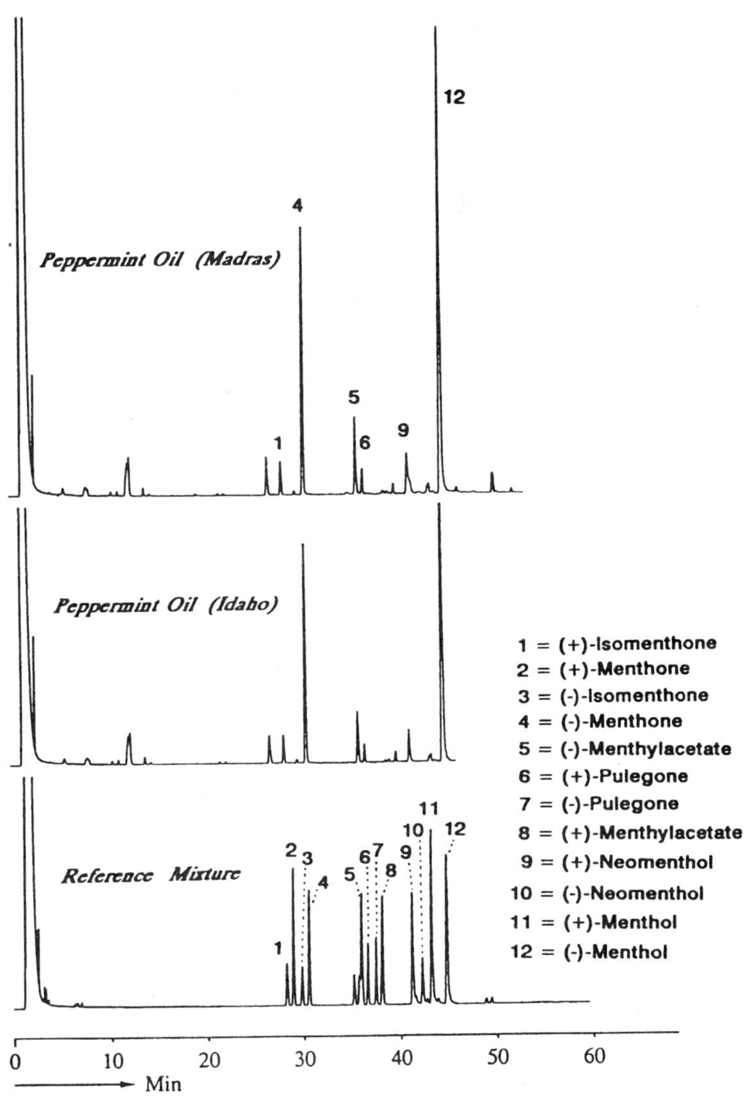

FIGURE 8 Enantioselective separation of peppermint oil constituents as well as racemic mixtures on octakis (2,6-di-O-methyl-3-O-pentyl)-γ-cyclodextrin/OV-1701 (50:50) (fused silica capillary 25 m × 0.25 mm i.d.; 60°C to 120°C at 1°C/min) (Courtesy of W. A. König, Hamburg, Germany.)

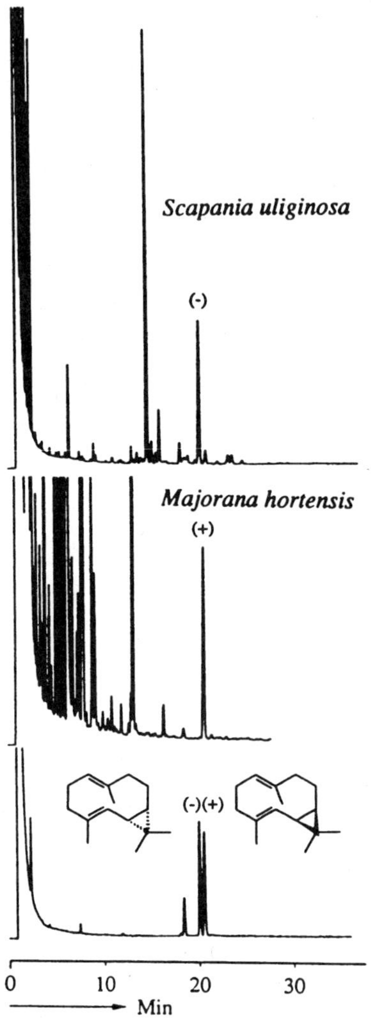

FIGURE 9 Enantiomer separation of bicyclogermacrene in a liverwort and in marjoram oil as well as a racemic mixture on octakis (2,6-di-O-methyl-3-O-pentyl)-γ-cyclodextrin/OV-1701 (20:80) (fused silica capillary 25 m × 0.25 mm i.d.; 115°C). (Courtesy of W. A. König, Hamburg, Germany.)

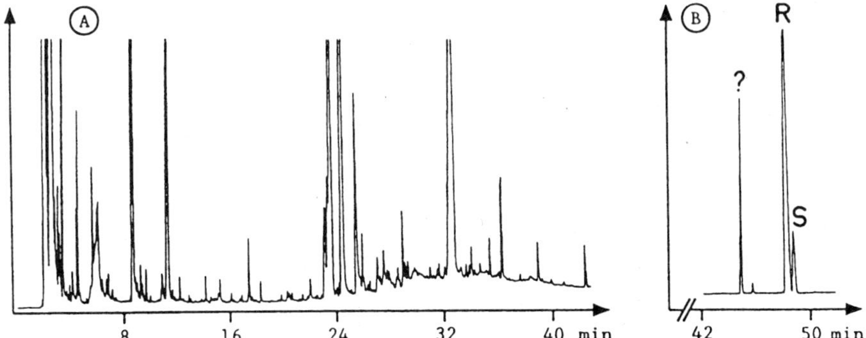

FIGURE 10 Enantioselective MDGC of γ-decalactone in a peach flavor extract (101). (A) Precolumn separation of peach aroma compounds on SE-54 (fused silica capillary 25 m × 0.25 mm i.d.; 80°C to 280°C at 5°C/min; N_2). (B) Main column separation of γ-decalactone on hexakis (3-O-acetyl-2,6-di-O-pentyl)-β-cyclodextrin (Lipodex B) (pyrex glass capillary 25 m × 0.25 mm i.d.; 10 min at 100°C, then to 180°C at 2°C/min).

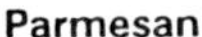

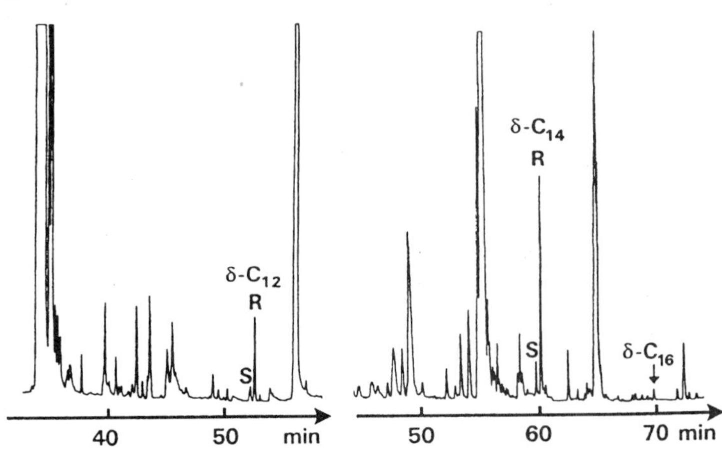

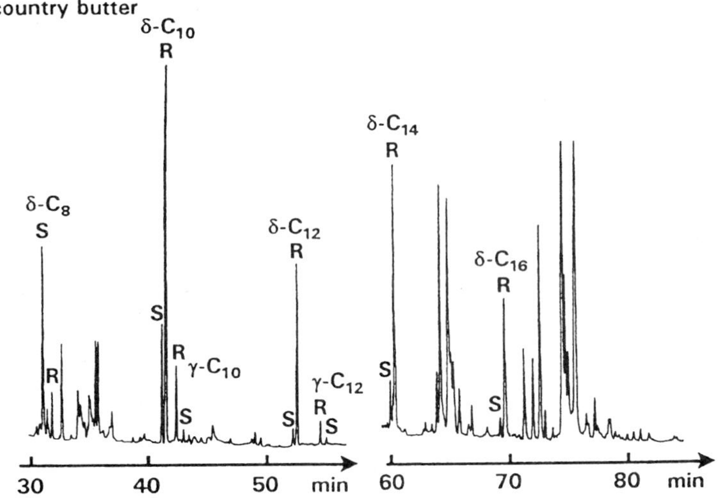

FIGURE 11 Enantioselective MDGC of γ- and δ-lactones in dairy products (precolumn: duran glass capillary OV-1701-vi; 30 m × 0.32 mm i.d.; different temperature programs for short-chained and long-chained lactones are used; H_2.) C_8-C_{12}-Lactones: heptakis (2,3-di-O-acetyl-6-O-tert-butyl-dimethylsilyl)-β-cyclodextrin/OV-1701 (fused silica capillary 30 m × 0.25 mm i.d.; 2 min at 45°C, then to 120°C at 20°C/min, held for 15 min, then to 125°C at 3°C/min and to 175°C at 1.5°C/min, then finally to 200°C at 5°C/min). C_{13}-C_{18}-Lactones: heptakis (2,3-di-O-acetyl-6-O-tert-butyl-dimethylsilyl)-β-cyclodextrin/PS 255 (duran glass capillary 25 m × 0.23 mm i.d.; 2 min at 45°C, then to 120°C at 20°C/min, held for 35 min, then to 160°C at 2°C/min and to 200°C at 1°C/min.) (From Ref. 164.)

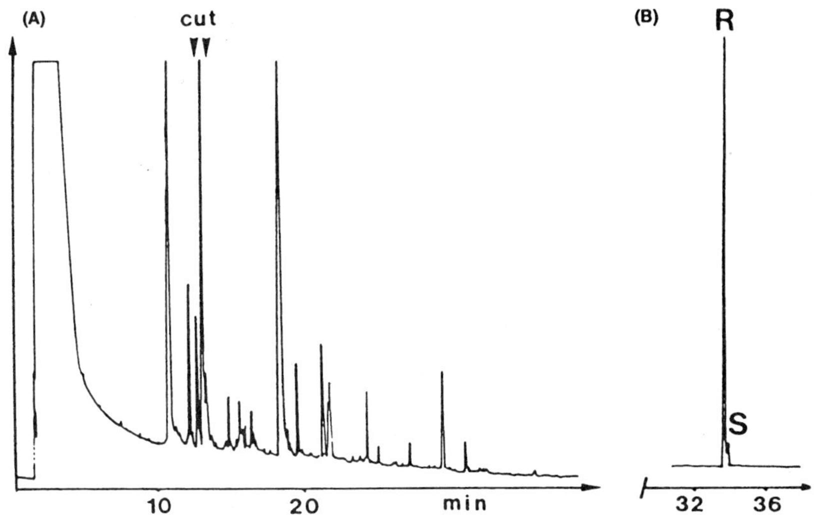

FIGURE 12 Enantioselective MDGC-MS of linalool in lavender oil. (A) Precolumn separation of lavender aroma compounds on DB-5 (fused silica capillary 30 m × 0.25 mm i.d.; 60°C to 300°C at 5°C/min; He). (B) Main column separation of linalool on heptakis (2,3,6-tri-O-pentyl)-β-cyclodextrin (Lipodex C) (fused silica capillary 25 m × 0.25 mm i.d.; 20 min at 60°C, then to 120°C, at 2°C/min). (From Ref. 101.)

tiomeric pairs, 15,900 separations, and 518 CSPs, 103 of which have been made commercially available.

Each database entry of Chirbase/GC contains 33 fields, including fields for the molecular structures, numeric fields for separation data [separation factor (α), peak resolution (R), net retention times (t'_{R1}) and (t'_{R2}), and capacity factors (k'_1) and (k'_2)]; moreover, there are text fields containing bibliographic data, compound names, suppliers of CSPs, stereochemical descriptors, separation conditions, and standard comments. Each field may be retrieved and sorted by the built-in capability of the database software ChemBase and ISIS, respectively. The special features of the database management software, in particular the structure and substructure querying functions, allow the planning of most promising separation experiments for a given pair of enantiomers. In many relevant examples, the target structure or at least an analogous structure can be retrieved in the database. In any case, Chirbase/GC supports the selection of suitable derivatization reactions and optimum chromatographic operation conditions.

2. Search Example: Limonene

(R)-(+)-limonene is found with a concentration of over 90% in citrus peel oils, (S)-(–)-limonene in oils from the Mentha species and conifers. Racemic limonene is called dipentene. Limonenes are commercially used as fragrance materials for perfuming household products (38).

The odor quality of limonene being critically dependent on its enantiomer composition, a large number of separation experiments by GC are reported in the literature. Due to its abundance in a great variety of essential oils, this is one of the most widely investigated compounds (see also Table 12, rank 3).

Limonene as a typical terpene hydrocarbon is lacking functional groups, thus, it cannot be resolved into enantiomers on CSPs of the amide type. Hence, myriads of cyclodextrin CSPs have been investigated, although with varying success. Separation is due to shape selectivity brought about by numerous van der Waals interactions of the analyte with the interstitious and probably also with the cavity of the cyclodextrin molecules. On this basis, it is difficult to establish straightforward rules for the selection of a most suitable CSP for this compound.

To find all relevant information in Chirbase/GC, a query input for limonene is done by structure, name, or molecule number. Within seconds, 98 entries are found in Chirbase/GC (Version 4/95). The one with the highest separation factor (α) is depicted in Figure 13. A quick overview of all separation factors will yield Table 11. A comprehensive display of the whole database content would exceed the space limit of this chapter by several orders of magnitude. Thus, only selected database fields can be shown here. Some entries deserve further comments, as follows.

By far the best separation factors (α) were reported by König et al. on CSPs based on 6-O-methyl-2,3-O-pentyl-γ-cyclodextrin (Table 11, entries 1–3) for slight variations in the separation conditions (176,177). In this case, the β-analogue is far less efficient in terms of the separation factor (Table 11, entry 26); however, it is still valuable for peak identification because the elution order of the two enantiomers is reversed as compared to the corresponding γ-derivative (176). Lindström et al. addressed the separation problem in a unique way by introducing underivatized α-cyclodextrin as a CSP for the determination of monoterpene hydrocarbons of spruce phloem (178).

Molecular modeling experiments on chiral recognition in GC were performed by Kobor et al. (179) for 2,3-di-O-methyl-6-O-tert.butyldimethylsilyl-β-cyclodextrin and permethylated-β-cyclodextrin (both diluted in OV-1701) as selectors. They concluded that the less flexible 2,3-di-O-methyl-6-O-tert.butyldimethylsilyl-β-cyclodextrin seems advantageous for certain enan-

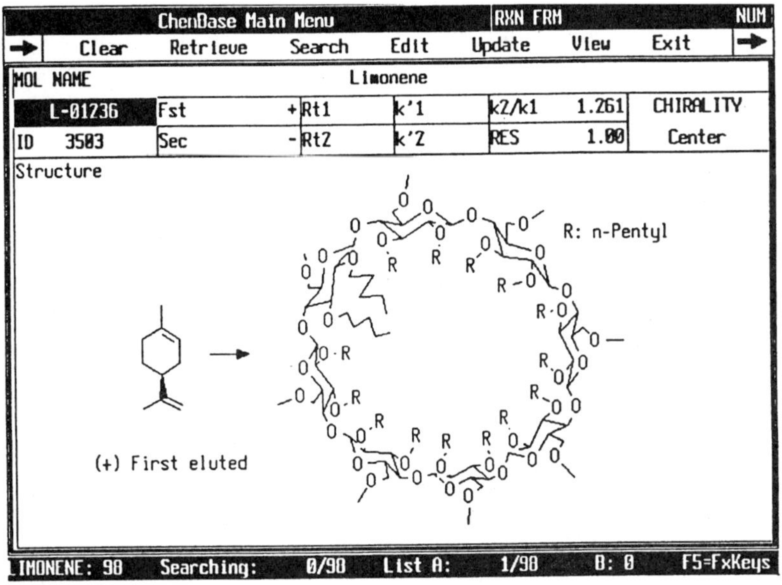

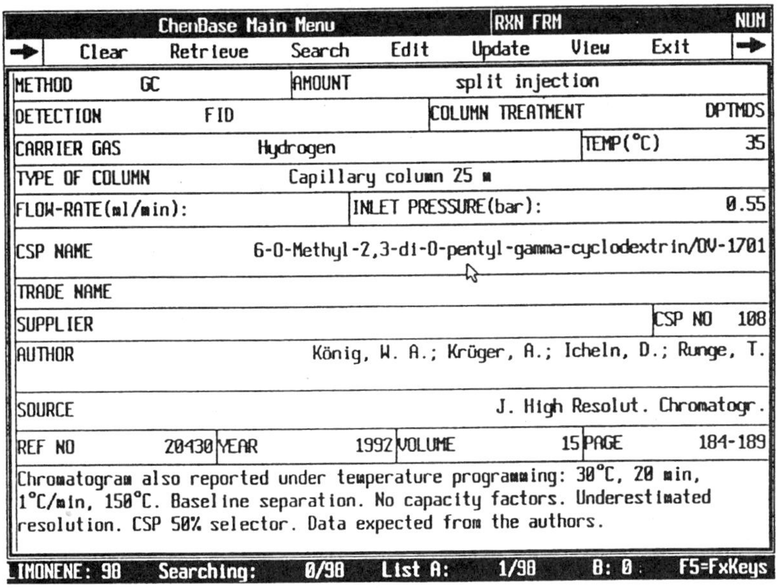

ChemBase Main Menu | RXN FRM | NUM

Clear | Retrieve | Search | Edit | Update | View | Exit

MOL NAME	Limonene				
L-01236	Fst +	Rt1	k'1	k2/k1 1.261	CHIRALITY
ID 3503	Sec -	Rt2	k'2	RES 1.00	Center

Structure

R: n-Pentyl

(+) First eluted

LIMONENE: 98 Searching: 0/98 List A: 1/98 B: 0 F5=FxKeys

ChemBase Main Menu | RXN FRM | NUM

Clear | Retrieve | Search | Edit | Update | View | Exit

METHOD	GC	AMOUNT	split injection
DETECTION	FID	COLUMN TREATMENT	DPTMDS
CARRIER GAS	Hydrogen	TEMP(°C)	35
TYPE OF COLUMN	Capillary column 25 m		
FLOW-RATE(ml/min):		INLET PRESSURE(bar):	0.55
CSP NAME	6-O-Methyl-2,3-di-O-pentyl-gamma-cyclodextrin/OV-1701		
TRADE NAME			
SUPPLIER		CSP NO	108
AUTHOR	König, W. A.; Krüger, A.; Icheln, D.; Runge, T.		
SOURCE	J. High Resolut. Chromatogr.		
REF NO 20430	YEAR 1992	VOLUME 15	PAGE 184-189

Chromatogram also reported under temperature programming: 30°C, 20 min, 1°C/min, 150°C. Baseline separation. No capacity factors. Underestimated resolution. CSP 50% selector. Data expected from the authors.

LIMONENE: 98 Searching: 0/98 List A: 1/98 B: 0 F5=FxKeys

FIGURE 13 Upper and lower output screen of Chirbase/GC; first hit of a search for limonene.

TABLE 11 Enantiomer Separation of Limonene by GC Selected from Chirbase/GC

No.	CSP name	α	R	First	T	Gas
1	6-O-Methyl-2,3-di-O-pentyl-γ–CD/OV-1701	1.261	1.00	R	35	H_2
2	6-O-Methyl-2,3-di-O-pentyl-γ–CD	1.185	5.00	a	a	H_2
3	6-O-Methyl-2,3-di-O-pentyl-γ–CD/OV-1701	1.180	1.00	R	45	H_2
4	α-CD	1.123	0.85	S	25	He*
5	2,3-Di-O-methyl-6-O-tert.butyldimethylsilyl-β–CD/SE-52	1.110	5.36	a	70	H_2
6	α-CD/formamide/Chromosorb W	1.100	a	S	30	a
7	α-CD/formamide/Chromosorb W NAW	1.090	a	S	30	Ar
8	2,3-Di-O-methyl-6-O-tert.butyldimethylsilyl-β-CD/SE-54	1.079	2.50	S	120	H_2
9	2,3-Di-O-methyl-6-tert.butyldimethylsilyl-β–CD/OV-1701	1.078	1.50	S	80	H_2
10	2,3-Di-O-methyl-6-O-tert.butyldimethylsilyl-β–CD/OV-1	1.055	a	a	120	H_2
11	2,6-Di-O-methyl-3-O-pentyl-γ–CD	1.046	a	a	70	a
12	2,3-Di-O-methyl-6-O-tert.butyldimethylsilyl-β–CD/PS-086	1.046	a	a	120	H_2
13	2,3-Di-O-methyl-6-O-tert.butyldimethylsilyl-β–CD/OV-1701	1.044	a	a	120	H_2
14	3,6-Di-O-pentyl-2-O-methyl-β–CD	1.043	a	a	40	a
15	2,3,6-Tri-O-methyl-β–CD	1.037	2.01	S	70	H_2
16	2,3-Di-O-methyl-6-O-pentyl-β–CD	1.032	a	a	50	a
17	Permethyl-(S)-hydroxypropyl-α–CD	1.030	a	a	70	N_2
18	Permethyl-(S)-hydroxypropyl-β–CD	1.030	a	a	100	N_2
19	Permethyl-(S)-hydroxypropyl-β–CD	1.030	a	a	30	N_2
20	Permethylated-β–CD-5-oct-1-enyl-siloxane	1.030	1.50	a	70	H_2
21	2,3,6-Tri-O-methyl-β–CD	1.030	1.40	S	70	a
22	2,3,6-Tri-O-methyl-β–CD/OV-1701	1.030	1.00	a	90	H_2
23	2,3,6-Tri-O-methyl-β–CD	1.030	0.35	S	50	H_2
24	2,3,6-Tri-O-methyl-β–CD 0.08m/OV-1701	1.029	a	S	80	a
25	3,6-Di-O-methyl-2-O-pentyl-γ–CD	1.027	a	a	50	a
26	6-O-Methyl-2,3-di-O-pentyl-β–CD/OV-1701	1.026	a	S	35	H_2
27	2,3,6-Tri-O-pentyl-β–CD	1.020	a	a	90	N_2
28	2,3,6-Tri-O-pentyl-α–CD	1.020	a	a	80	N_2
29	2,3,6-Tri-O-pentyl-γ–CD	1.020	a	a	70	N_2
30	2,3-Di-O-methyl-6-O-tert.butyldimethylsilyl-α–CD/SE-54	1.019	a	a	120	H_2

Table 11 Continued

No.	CSP name	α	R	First	T	Gas
31	2,6-Di-O-pentyl-3-O-methyl-β–CD	1.019	1.00	S	60	H_2
32	2,3,6-Tri-O-pentyl-β–CD	1.018	a	S	70	H_2
33	2,6-Di-tert.-butyldimethylsilyl-γ–CD 22%/SE-52	1.015	a	a	35	H_2
34	2,6-Di-O-tert.-butyldimethylsilyl-γ–CD 22%/SE-52	1.013	a	a	75	H_2
35	2,3,6-Tri-O-methyl-β–CD/OV-1701	1.010	a	a	100	N_2
36	2,3-Di-O-methyl-6-O-pentyl-γ–CD	1.009	a	a	50	a
37	2,6-Di-O-methyl-3-O-pentyl-β–CD 10%/OV-225	—	2.30	a	TP	a
38	2,6-Di-O-methyl-3[O-pentyl-β–CD 10%/OV-1701	—	2.20	a	TP	a
39	2,6-Di-O-methyl-3-O-pentyl-β–CD 10%/PS-086	—	1.90	a	TP	a
40	2,6-Di-O-methyl-3-O-pentyl-β–CD 10%/PS-347.5	—	1.40	a	TP	a
41	2,3,6-Tri-O-methyl-β–CD/OV-1701	a	1.00	S	50	H_2
42	2,6-Di-O-pentyl-3-O-methyl-γ–CD	a	1.00	S	60	H_2
43	2,3,6-Tri-O-methyl-β–CD/OV-1701	a	1.00	S	50	H_2
44	2,3,6-Tri-O-methyl-β–CD 10%/OV-1701	a	1.00	S	50	a
45	2,3,6-Tri-O-methyl-β–CD/DB-1701	a	1.00	S	55	a
.						
.						
.						
63	β-CD/celite/formamide	1.000	—	a	60	He
64	γ-CD/celite/formamide	1.000	—	a	60	He
65	2,6-Di-O-pentyl-3-O-methyl-β-CD 30%/OV-1701	1.000	—	a	a	a
66	2,3,6-Tri-O-pentyl-β–CD 30%/OV-1701	1.000	—	a	a	a
67	2,3,6-Tri-O-*n*-butylarbamate amylose/OV-61	1.000	—	a	a	H_2
68	3,6-Di-O-pentyl-2-O-methyl-γ–CD	1.000	—	a	70	a
69	3,6-Di-O-methyl-2-O-pentyl-β–CD	1.000	—	a	70	a
70	2,6-Di-O-pentyl-3-O-trifluoracetyl-α–CD	1.000	—	a	110	He
71	2,6-Di-O-pentyl-α–CD	1.000	—	a	110	He
72	2,3-Di-O-methyl-6-O-tert.butyldimethylsilyl-γ–CD/SE-54	1.000	—	a	120	H_2
73	2,6-Di-O-pentyl-3-O-butyryl-γ–CD	1.000	—	a	50	He

TABLE 11 Continued

No.	CSP name	α	R	First	T	Gas
74	Permethyl-(S)-2-hydroxypropyl-α–CD	1.000	—	a	100	N_2
75	Permethyl-(S)-2-hydroxypropyl-γ–CD	1.000	—	a	100	N_2
76	2,6-Di-O-pentyl-β–CD	1.000	—	a	100	N_2
77	2,6-Di-O-pentyl-γ–CD	1.000	—	a	100	N_2
78	2,6-Di-O-pentyl-3-O-trifluoroacetyl-β–CD	1.000	—	a	100	N_2
79	2,6-Di-O-pentyl-3-O-trifluoracetyl-γ–CD	1.000	—	a	100	N_2
80	2,3,6-Tri-O-methyl-β–CD/DB-1701	1.000	—	a	100	N_2
81	Polydimethylsiloxane funct. with L-valine-tert.-butylamide	1.000	—	a	100	N_2
82	Other batch of L-Chirasil-Val	1.000	—	a	100	N_2
83	2,3,6-Tri-O-pentyl-α–CD	1.000	—	a	100	N_2
84	2,6-Di-O-pentyl-3-O-acetyl-α–CD	1.000	—	a	100	N_2
85	2,3,6-Tri-O-pentyl-β–CD	1.000	—	a	100	N_2
86	2,6-Di-O-pentyl-3-O-acetyl-β–CD	1.000	—	a	100	N_2
87	Wall-immobilized, 1:4 allylpermethyl-β–CD:PS537	1.000	—	a	100	N_2
88	2,6-Di-O-pentyl-6-O-propylcarbamate-β–CD	1.000	—	a	80	N_2
89	2,6-Di-O-pentyl-6-O-propylarbamate-α–CD	1.000	—	a	80	N_2
90	2,6-Di-O-pentyl-6-O-propylcarbamate-γ–CD	1.000	—	a	70	N_2
91	2,6-Di-O-pentyl-6-O-isopropylcarbamate-β–CD	1.000	—	a	80	N_2
92	2,6-Di-O-pentyl-6-O-isopropylcarbamate-α–CD	1.000	—	a	80	N_2
93	2,6-Di-O-pentyl-6-O-isopropylcarbamate-γ–CD	1.000	—	a	80	N_2
94	2,6-Di-O-pentyl-6-O-phenylcarbamate-β–CD	1.000	—	a	80	N_2
95	2,6-Di-O-pentyl-6-O-phenylcarbamate-α–CD	1.000	—	a	80	N_2
96	2,6-Di-O-pentyl-6-O-phenylcarbamate-γ–CD	1.000	—	a	80	N_2
97	2,6-Di-O-pentyl-3-O-acetyl-γ–CD	1.000	—	a	80	N_2
98	3,6-Di-O-ert.-butyldimethylsilyl-2-O-methyl-γ–CD 22%/SE-52	1.000	—	a	a	H_2

α, Separation factor, $\alpha = k'_2/k'_1$ with k′ = net capacity factor; R, peak resolution, $R = 2\cdot(tr_2 - tr_1)/(w_1 + w_2)$. First, configuration of the first eluted enantiomer; T, column temperature; TP, temperature programming; Gas, carrier gas; *, carrier gas saturated with water vapor; a, not reported; —, for separation factor α: not defined, in case of temperature programming; for peak resolution R: no resolution.

tiomer separations, especially for nonpolar analytes (179) (Table 11, entry 9); more recent examples for the same system include entries 8, 10, 12, and 13 in Table 11 (180). In addition to investigations by Venema et al. on the effect of size and position of the alkylated substituents on the separation ability of modified β-cyclodextrins (181), König and coworkers compared the selectivity of a complete set of regio-selectively methylated and pentylated β- and γ-cyclodextrins (182) (Table 11, entries 11, 14, 16, 25, 36). Bicchi and coworkers compared the separation abilities of 2,6-di-O-methyl-3-O-pentyl-β-cyclodextrin and permethylated β–cyclodextrin and established the influence of factors like the structure of the cyclodextrin derivatives, the polysiloxane ratio, and the minimum operating temperature on the reproducibility and lifetime of the columns (183) (Table 11, entries 38, 65, 66). According to this report, limonene was only poorly separated on 2,6-di-O-methyl-6-O-tert.butyldimethylsilyl-γ-cyclodextrin mixed with achiral SE-52, whereas entries 65 and 66 in Table 11 indicate the lack of resolution for two trialkyl β–cyclodextrin derivatives.

Quite a few publications did not allow extraction of the separation factor (α), particularly when a temperature program was applied. In these cases, the resolution factor (R) is considered a valuable measure to estimate the degree of separation under given conditions (see entries 37–45 in Table 11; entries 46–62, lacking both quantities, have been omitted from the table). In contrast, experiments with a clearly negative outcome are still valuable information (Table 11, entries 63–98) as they prevent the reader from spending time and money on experiments that do not work. Nonetheless, we find it amazing how many researchers do spend their resources on such trials, as they are not aware of the great amount of information collected in Chirbase/GC.

Research in this field is still proliferating for several reasons. Besides the scientific challenge of driving through the sheer endless permutations of cyclodextrin substitution patterns, there is an economic need for finding columns that do an acceptable job for a many compounds as possible. In this context, a search for a given CSP or a substructure thereof will also be of great interest to many users. First of all, browsing through the CSP database will not only serve to quickly identify CSP numbers but also gives the user an unprecedented overview of the large collection of CSPs on the market. As to the separations performed on a given CSP or class of CSPs, there are several more efficient routes through Chirbase to fulfill this task, e.g., search by CSP structure or a substructure, CSP name or a substring of this name, by CSP number, by author, etc. Moreover, this information may be used in a combined search, together with a given analyte or an analyte class (as defined by a substructure).

3. Data Collection and Validation

As compared to the retrieval step, the input of these data is far from being a trivial task. For Chirbase/GC, 87 journals are scrutinized page by page on a regular basis, in addition to monographs, posters, and private communications (altogether more than 400 different sources of information). Quite often the crucial information is hidden in a footnote, and most often it is incomplete. We do acknowledge a positive response from hundreds of authors to whom requests for information missing in the original paper had been sent by letter. From this rather tedious process it turned out that enantiomer separation has matured from the early stage of development into a stage of widespread application. Therefore, the information collected in Chirbase has gained a great practical value for everyone working in this field.

4. Standard Column Versus Optimized Conditions

In the early days, some experts hoped for a standard CSP that would accomplish all relevant separation tasks. Due to its widespread commercial availability, permethyl-β–cyclodextrin derivatives were considered promising candidates. In fact, several analytes could be separated on this class of CSPs, although with limited success. With restriction to the widely used OV-1701–type cyclodextrin CSPs, satisfactory separations occur less often than expected. The selection of dedicated columns for each analyte provides a striking advantage for the separation factors achieved. This is demonstrated for important flavor compounds as listed in Table 12. A total of 38 flavor compounds made it to the top 75 analytes (selected from 5651 individual analyte structures contained in Chirbase/GC, Version 4/95); the ranking is based on the number of citations for each structure in the database. The most frequently separated flavor compound limonene, ranking at position 3 of all analytes separated into enantiomers by GC, reflects the strong attention devoted to this field. On the other hand, this raises the issue of whether resources for method development could have been saved by a better awareness of the possibilities offered by information retrieval in this database.

III. CONCLUSIONS

The human brain still outperforms contemporary computers when it comes to recognition and associative tasks. In the present context, unfortunately, scientists have not yet been able to establish models appropriate to predict the de-

TABLE 12 Selection of Flavor Compounds from the Top 75 Analytes in Chirbase/GC[a]

Abundance	Rank	Compound	α_{max}	α_{pmb}
98	3	Limonene	1.261	1.030
84	5	γ-Decalactone	1.163	1.013
80	6	1-Phenylethanol	1.210	1.082
77	8	α-Pinene	2.200	1.060
73	9	Menthol	1.092	1.039
67	10	γ-Nonalactone	1.101	n.p.
61	12	γ-Octalactone	1.115	n.p.
58	13	γ-Undecalactone	1.103	n.p.
53	15	Linalool	1.080	1.056
53	16	β-Pinene	1.500	n.p.
52	17	Carvone	1.090	1.000
51	21	γ-Dodecalactone	1.050	n.p.
45	25	γ-Hexalactone	1.221	n.p.
45	26	Camphene	3.260	n.p.
44	27	γ-Heptalactone	1.186	1.030
43	29	1-Phenyl-1-propanol	1.070	1.040
43	30	γ-Valerolactone	1.439	n.p.
40	33	Methyl mandelate	1.120	1.024
40	34	2-Ethylhexanoic acid	1.037	1.036
38	36	δ-Decalactone	1.056	n.p.
37	38	Camphor	1.236	n.p.
37	39	3-Octanol	1.150	n.p.
34	44	1-Phenyl-2-propanol	1.067	1.021
34	45	Menthone	1.185	n.p.
33	49	δ–Nonalactone	1.159	n.p.
32	50	α-Terpineol	1.059	1.028
31	52	β-Butyrolactone	1.620	1.320
31	54	2-Octanol	1.109	1.020
30	55	1-Terpinen-4-ol	1.082	1.016
30	59	δ–Octalactone	1.550	n.p.
28	63	α-Ionone	2.020	1.173
27	67	Piperitone	1.123	n.p.
27	68	Pulegone	1.177	1.010
27	69	Lactic acid methyl ester	1.469	1.111
27	70	Isoborneol	1.085	1.040
27	71	2-Butanol	1.108	1.081

TABLE 12 Continued

Abundance	Rank	Compound	α_{max}	α_{pmb}
26	74	*cis*-Pinane	1.118	1.118
26	75	2-Hexanol	1.180	n.p.

[a]Comparison of most suitable CSP and a standard CSP. α_{max}, best α value in Chirbase/GC; α_{pmb}, best α value in Chirbase/GC, obtained on permethyl-β-CD/OV-1701 columns; n.p., not published.

gree of enantiomer separation of a given analyte on any of the numerous stationary phases described in the literature. In this situation, the brute force of state-of-the-art computational equipment is required for long-term storage and fast retrieval of the growing mountain of information published in this field. In a promising ongoing project, we are working on associative computational methods linked to the database.

Indeed, there is an intriguing analogy between the artificial neural networks used in these studies and the biological neural networks that are trained to recognize molecular structures by odor. Merging the two scientific disciplines will certainly shed new light on the old question of how odor is brought about and how it may be predicted for a new molecular structure. As a first step in a presumably long journey, we need precise qualitative and quantitative data on the odor of as many compounds as possible, determined with panels as large as necessary. Needless to say, these compounds should be of exceedingly high and well-established chemical and enantiomeric purity. At the same time, all data available must be stored in electronic form, preferentially as a graphic molecule database. Chirbase/Flavor is another proliferating project in our group to accomplish this task.

ACKNOWLEDGMENT

We are grateful to all authors contributing to this chapter by sending separation examples in form of personal communications and reprints, and also to hundreds of authors who responded to our letters asking for additional data on separations published in the literature. A. B. is indebted to the British Library for rapid and convenient document supply. B. K. and U. E. wish to thank Fonds der Chemischen Industrie and the Deutsche Forschungsgemeinschaft in Germany for financial support.

REFERENCES

1. R. Axel, The molecular logic of smell, *Sci. Am. 273:*130 (1995).
2. G. Ohloff, Chemistry of the sense of smell, *Chem. Zeit 5:*114 (1971).
3. G. Ohloff, *Riechstoffe und Geruchssinn—Die molekulare Welt der Düfte*, Springer, Berlin, 1990.
4. A. G. Gilman, G proteins and dual control of adenylate cyclase, *Cell 36:*577 (1984).
5. H. Breer, K. Raming, and J. Krieger, Signal recognition and transduction in olfactory neurons, *Biochem. Biophys. Acta 1224:*277 (1994).
6. J. T. Davies, A theory of the quality of odours, *J. Theor. Biol. 8:*1 (1965).
7. M. M. Mozell and M. Jagodowicz, Chromatographic separation of odorants by the nose: retention times measured across in vivo olfactory mucosa, *Science 181:*1247 (1973).
8. R. M. Hainer, A. G. Emsile, A. Jacobson, *Ann. N. Y. Acad. Sci. 58:*158 (1964).
9. F. J. Ritter, General introduction and overview, in *Chemical Ecology: Odour Communication in Animals* (F. J. Ritter, ed.), Elsevier, Amsterdam, 1979, p. 1.
10. R. H. Wright, Odor and molecular vibration: neural coding of olfactory information, *J. Theor. Biol. 64:*473 (1977).
11. R. H. Wright, *The Sense of Smell*, CRC Press, Boca Rota, FL, 1982.
12. R. H. Wright, Odor and molecular vibration: optical isomers, *Chem. Senses Flav. 3:*35 (1978).
13. L. D. Hayward, A new theory of olfaction based on dispersion-induced optical activity, *Nature 267:*554 (1977).
14. M. G. J. Beets, in *Molecular Structure and Organoleptic Quality, Monograph 1* (M. Stoll, Ed.), Society of Chemical Industry, London (1957).
15. J. E. Amoore, Progress towards some direct quantitative comparisons of the stereochemical and vibrational theories of odor, *Gustation and Olfaction* (G. Ohloff and A. F. Thomas, eds.), Academic Press, New York, 1971 p. 147.
16. R. E. Randebrock, Odor and constitution, Part IV: an argumentation for the molecular theory of odor, *Parf. Kosmet. 67:*10 (1986).
17. C. R., *Acad. Sci. Paris 46:*615 (1858).
18. F. Richter, Questions about the odor of stereoisomers, *Z. Ang. Chem. 38:*1200 (1925).
19. W. Boland, L. Jaenicke, D. G. Müller, and A. Peters, Differentiation of algal chemoreceptors, *Eur. J. Biochem. 144:*169 (1984).
20. R. M. Silverstein, Enantiomeric composition and bioactivity of chiral semiochemicals in insects, *Chemical Ecology: Odour Communication in Animals* (F. J. Ritter, ed.), Elsevier, Amsterdam, 1978, p. 133.
21. J. G. Brand, B. P. Bryant, R. H. Cagan, and D. L. Kalinowski, Enantiomeric specifity of alanine taste receptor sites in catfish, *Ann. NY Acad. Sci, 510:*193 (1987).
22. G. Heth, E. Nevo, R. Ikan, V. Weinstein, U. Ravid, and H. Duncan, Differential olfactory perception of enantiomeric compounds by blind subterranean mole rats (*Spalax ehrenbergi*), *Experientia 48:*897 (1992).

23. D. Müller-Schwarze, U. Ravid, A. Claesson, A. G. Singer, R. M. Silverstein, C. Müller-Schwarze, N. J. Volkman, K. F. Zemanek, and R. M. Butter, The deer-lactone: source, chemical properties and responses of black-tailed deer, *J. Chem. Ecol. 4:*247 (1978).
24. J. Solms, L. Vuataz, and R. H. Egli, The taste of L- and D-amino acids, *Experientia 21:*692 (1965).
25. P. Weyerstahl, Odor and structure, *J. Prakt. Chem. 336:*95 (1994).
26. E. H. Polak, A. M. Fombon, C. Tilquin, and P. H. Punter, Sensory evidence for olfactory receptors with opposite chiral selectivity, *Behav. Brain Res. 31:*199 (1989).
27. L. Friedman, and J. G. Miller, Odor incongruity and chirality, *Science 172:*1044 (1971).
28. P. Pelosi and R. Viti, Specific anosmia to l-carvone: the minty primary odour, *Chem. Sensed Flav. 3:*331 (1978).
29. G. Ohloff, B. Maurer, B. Winter, and W. Giersch, Structural and configurational dependence of the sensory process in steroids, *Helv. Chim. Acta 66:*192 (1983).
30. E. T. Theimer and M. R. McDaniel, Odor and optical activity, *J. Soc. Cosmet. Chem. 22:*15 (1971).
31. L. Träger, *Chemie in der Kosmetik heute*, Hüthig, Heidelberg, 1995.
32. B. Gibbons, The intimate sense of smell, *Natl. Geogr. 170:*324 (1986).
33. A. N. Gilbert and C. J. Wysocki, The smell survey, *Natl. Geogr. 172:*514 (1987).
34. C. J. Wysocki and G. K. Beauchamp, Ability to smell androstenone is genetically determined, *Proc. Natl. Acad. Sci. USA 81:*4899 (1984).
35. S. Pathirana, W. C. Neely, L. J. Myers, and V. Vodyanoy, Chiral recognition of odorants (+)- and (–)-carvone by phospholipid monolayers, *J. Am. Chem. Soc. 114:*1404 (1992).
36. S. Plowman, The physical and chemical properties of ngai-camphor, *Arch. Pharm. 205:*237 (1874).
37. Chautard, *Jour. de Pharm. 44:*13 (1863).
38. K. Bauer, D. Garbe, and H. Surburg, *Common Fragrance and Flavor Materials. Preparation, Properties and Uses*, VCH, Weinheim, 1990.
39. F. Tiemann and R. Schmidt, About homolinalool, *Chem. Ber. 29:*691 (1896).
40. J. von Braun and W. Kaiser, Odor and molecular asymmetry, *Chem. Ber. B56:*2268 (1923).
41. F. Tiemann and R. Schmidt, About D- and L-configurations in the series of citronellal, *Chem. Ber. 30:*33 (1897).
42. H. Posvic, The odors of optical isomers, *Science 118:*358 (1953).
43. A. Werner and H. E. Conrad, About the optically active trans hexahydrophthalic acids, *Chem. Ber. 32:*3046 (1899).
44. R. Godlewski, *J. Russ. Phys.-Chem. Ges. 31:*210 (1899).
45. H. Rupe and F. Wiederkehr, The constitution of curcumone from the oil of curcuma, *Helv. Chim. Acta 7:*654 (1924).

46. J. von Braun and W. Teuffert, Odor and molecular asymmetry. Part II, *Chem. Ber. B58:*2210 (1925).
47. J. von Braun and E. Anton, Odor and molecular asymmetry: three 1.3-dimethyl-cyclohexanone-5 and four 1.3-dimethyl-cyclohexanole-5. Part IV, *Chem. Ber. B60:*2438 (1927).
48. J. Read and W. J. Grubb, Researches in the menthone series. Part IX. A new optical resolution of dl-menthol and of dl-camphor-10-sulphonic acid, *J. Chem. Soc.* 188 (1931).
49. B. K. Singh and A. B. Lal, Difference in odour of d-, and l- and dl-derivatives of amino- and bisamino-methylenecamphors, *Nature 144:*910 (1939).
50. H. Sobotka, E. Bloch, H. Cahnmann, E. Feldbau, and E. Rosen, Studies on ionone. II. Optical resolution of dl-α-ionone, *J. Am. Chem. Soc. 65:*2061 (1943).
51. Y.-R. Naves, Studies on volatile plant materials. XLVI. Separation of d,l-alpha-ionone, *Helv. Chim. Acta 30:*769 (1947).
52. Y.-R. Naves, The rotary dispersion of citronellol, citronellal and citronellic acid, *Perf. Ess. Oil Rec.* 120 (1946).
53. Y.-R. Naves, About the active racemic iso-α-irones and its derivates, *C. R. Acad. Sci. 237:*1167 (1953).
54. H. Veldstra, private communication to M. G. J. Beets (1961) (see Ref. 56).
55. J. von Braun and W. Haensel, Odor and molecular asymmetry. Part III, *Chem. Ber. B59:*1999 (1926).
56. M. G. J. Beets, Olfactory response and molecular structure, *Handbook of Sensory Physiology. Vol. IV. Chemical Senses. 1. Olfaction* (L. M. Beidler, ed.), Springer, Berlin, 1971, p. 257.
57. R. Rienäcker and G. Ohloff, Optically active β-citronellol from (+)- and (–)-pinane, *Angew. Chem. 73:*240 (1961).
58. G. Ohloff and E. Klein, The absolute configuration of linanlol by connection with the pinane system, *Tetrahedron 18:*37 (1962).
59. T. J. Leitereg, D. G. Guadagni, J. Harris, T. R. Mon, and R. Teranishi, Evidence for the difference between the odours of the optical isomers (+)- and (–)-carvone, *Nature 230:*455 (1971).
60. G. F. Russell and J. I. Hill, Odor differences between enantiomeric isomers, *Science 172:*1043 (1971).
61. E. E. Langenau, Correlation of objective-subjective methods as applied to the perfumery and cosmetics industries, *Am. Soc. Test. Mat. Spec. Techn. Pub. No. 440:*71 (1968).
62. B. M. Hausen, Toothpaste allergy caused by l-carvone, *Akt. Dermatol. 12:*23 (1986).
63. E. T. Theimer, T. Yoshida, and E. M. Klaiber, Olfaction and molecular shape. Chirality as a requisite for odor, *J. Agric. Food Chem. 25:*1168 (1977).
64. G. Ohloff, Stereochemistry-activity relationships in human odor sensation: "The triaxial rule," *Olfaction and Taste VII* (H. van der Starre, ed.), IRL Press Ltd., London, 1980, p. 3.

65. V. Prelog and L. Ruzicka, Two musky smelling stereoids isolated of extracts of the swine testes, *Helv. Chim. Acta 27:*61 (1944).
66. V. Prelog, L. Ruzicka, and P. Wieland, Preparation of the two musky smelling Δ^{16}-androstenols-(3) and related compounds, *Helv. Chim. Acta 27:*66 (1944).
67. V. Prelog, L. Ruzicka, P. Meister, and P. Wieland, Investigations on the relationship between constitution and odor of steroids, *Helv. Chim. Acta 28:*618 (1945).
68. G. Ohloff, C. Vial, H. R. Wolf, K. Job, E. Jégou, J. Polonsky, and E. Lederer Stereochemistry-odor relationships in enantiomeric ambergris fragrances, *Helv. Chim. Acta 63:*1932 (1980).
69. G. Ohloff, B. Winter, and C. Fehr, Chemical classification and structure-odour relationships, *Perfumes* 287 (1991).
70. T. E. Acree, R. Nishida, and H. Fukami, Odor thresholds of the stereoisomers of methyl jasmonate, *J. Agric. Food Chem. 33:*425 (1985).
71. A. Krotz and G. Helmchen, Total synthesis of sandalwood fragrances: (Z)- and (E)-β-santalol and their enantiomers, ent-β-santalene, *Tetrahedron Asymmetry 1:*537 (1990).
72. H. G. Haring, F. Rijkens, H. Boelens, and A. van der Gen, Sesquiterpenoids, *J. Agric. Food Chem. 20:*1018 (1972).
73. N. Neuner-Jehle and F. Etzweiler, The measuring of odors, *Perfumes. Art, Science and Technology* (P. M. Müller and D. Lamparsky, eds.), Elsevier Applied Science, London, 1991, p. 153.
74. P. Werkhoff, W. Bretschneider, M. Güntert, R. Hopp, and H. Surburg, Chirospecific analysis in flavor and essential oil chemistry, Part B: Direct enantiomer resolution of trans-α-ionone and trans-α-damascone by inclusion gas chromatography, *Z. Lebensm. Unters. Forsch. 192:*111 (1991).
75. E. Demole, P. Enggist, and G. Ohloff, 1-p-Menthene-8-thiol: a powerful flavor impact constituent of grapefruit juice (*Citrus paradisi* Macfayden), *Helv. Chim. Acta 65:*1785 (1982).
76. W. Pickenhagen, Enantioselectivity in odor perception, *ACS Symp. Ser. 338:*151 (1989).
77. G. Ohloff, W. Giersch, W. Pickenhagen, A. Furrer, and B. Frei, Significance of the geminal dimethyl group in the odor principle of ambrox, *Helv. Chim. Acta 68:*2022 (1985).
78. E. H. Polak and J. Provasi, Odor sensitivity to geosmin enantiomers, *Chem. Senses 17:*23 (1992).
79. H. Masuda and S. Mihara, Preparation and odor evaluation of both enantiomers of alkoxypyrazines, *Agric. Biol. Chem. 12:*3367 (1989).
80. E. Guichard, Chiral γ-lactones, key compounds to apricot flavor, *ACS Symp. Ser. 596:*258 (1995).
81. I. Blank, A. Sen, and W. Grosch, Sensory study on the character-impact flavour compounds of dill herb (*Anethum graveolens* L.), *Food Chem. 43:*337 (1992).
82. W. Pickenhagen and H. Brönner-Schindler, Enantioselective synthesis of (+)-

and (–)-cis-2-methyl-4-propyl-1,3-oxathiane and their olfactive properties, *Helv. Chim. Acta 67:*947 (1984).

83. F. Drawert and N. Christoph, Significance of the sniffing-technique for the determination of odour thresholds and detection of aroma impacts of trace volatiles, *Analysis of Volatiles* (P. Schreier, ed.), de Gruyter, Berlin, 1984, p. 269.
84. M. Deos, F. Patte, J. Rouault, P. Laffort, and L. J. van Gemert, *Standardized Human Olfactory Threshold*, IRL Press at Oxford University Press, Oxford, 1990.
85. T. Hummel, C. Hummel, E. Pauli, and G. Kobal, Olfactory discrimination of nicotine-enantiomers by smokers and non-smokers, *Chem. Senses 17:*13 (1992).
86. G. Tuyenenburg Muys, B. van der Ven, and A. P. de Jonge, Preparation of optically active γ- and δ-lactones by microbiological reduction of the corresponding keto acids, *Appl. Microbiol. 11:*389 (1963).
87. L. D. Tyler, T. E. Acree, and R. M. Butts, Odor characterization of the synthetic stereoisomers of 2-methylborneol, *J. Agric. Food Chem. 26:*1415 (1978).
88. G. Heusinger and A. Mosandl, Chiral sulfur containing flavour compounds of the yellow passion fruit (*Passiflora edulis f. flavicarpa*). Synthesis of the enantiomers and absolute configuration, *Tetrahedron Lett. 25:*507 (1984).
89. P. Finato, R. Lorenzi, and P. Pelosi, Synthesis of new earthy odorants, *J. Agric. Food Chem. 40:*857 (1992).
90. R. Emberger and R. Hopp, Synthesis and sensory characterization of menthol enantiomers and their derivatives for the use in nature identical peppermint oils, *Topics in Flavour Research*, Eichhorn, Marzling-Hargenham, Germany, 1985, p. 201.
91. A. Mosandl and G. Heusinger, 1,3-Oxathianes, chiral fruit flavour compounds, *Liebigs Ann. Chem.* 1185 (1985).
92. B. Weber, H.-P. Haag, and A. Mosandl, Stereoisomeric flavour compounds: LIX. 3-Mercaptohexyl- and 3-methylthiohexylalkanoates—structure and properties of the enantiomers, *Z. Lebensm. Unters. Forsch. 195:*426 (1992).
93. A. Mosandl, W. Deger, M. Gessner, G. Günther, G. Heusinger, and G. Singer, Structure and analysis of stereoisomeric flavour compounds, *Lebensmittelchem. Gerichtl. Chem. 41:*35 (1987).
94. A. Mosandl, U. Hagenauer-Hener, U. Hener, D. Lehmann, P. Kreis, and H.-G. Schmarr, Chirality evaluation in flavour analysis, *Flavour Science and Technology* (Y. Bessière and A. F. Thomas, eds.), Wiley & Sons, Chichester, New York, 1990, p. 21.
95. T. Köpke and A. Mosandl, Stereoisomeric flavour compounds. Part LIV. 8-Mercapto-p-menthan-3-one—optically pure stereoisomers and chirospecific analysis, *Z. Lebensm. Unters. Forsch. 194:*372 (1992).
96. P. Werkhoff, S. Brennecke, W. Bretschneider, M. Güntert, R. Hopp, and H. Surburg, Chirospecific analysis in essential oil, fragrance and flavor research, *Z. Lebensm. Unters. Forsch. 196:*307 (1993).
97. T. Köpke, H.-G. Schmarr, and A. Mosandl, Stereoisomeric flavour compounds. Part LVII. The stereoisomers of 3-oxo-p-menthane-8-thiol acetate, simultane-

ously stereoanalysed with their corresponding thiols, *Flav. Fragr. J. 7:*205 (1992).

98. A. Mosandl and W. Deger, Stereoisomeric flavour compounds. Part XVII. Chiral carboxylic esters—synthesis and properties, *Z. Lebensm. Unters. Forsch. 185:*379 (1987).
99. M. Gessner, W. Deger, and A. Mosandl, Stereoisomeric flavour compounds. XXI. Chiral aroma compounds in food, *Z. Lebensm. Unters. Forsch. 186:*417 (1988).
100. V. Schubert, R. Diener, and A. Mosandl, Enantioselective multidimensional gas chromatography of some secondary alcohols and their acetates from banana, *Z. Naturforsch. C 46:*33 (1991).
101. A. Bernreuther, Analytik chiraler Aromastoffe anhand multidimensionaler Gaschromatographie mit chiralen Phasen, Thesis, University of Würzburg, Würzburg, 1992.
102. K. S. Kim and A. Bernreuther, Enantioselective analysis of chiral flavour compounds from banana (*Musa sapientum* L.) by multidimensional gas chromatography/mass spectrometry, *Foods Biotechnol. 4:*000 (1996).
103. P. Schreier, A. Bernreuther, and M. Huffer, *Analysis of Chiral Organic Molecules*, de Gruyter, Berlin, 1995.
104. R. E. Synovec and E. S. Yeung, Fluorescence detected circular dichroism as a detection principle in high-performance liquid chromatography, *J. Chromatogr. 368:*85 (1986).
105. R. E. Synovec and E. S. Yeung, Detectors for liquid chromatography, *Anal. Chem. 58:*1237A (1986).
106. A. Bernreuther, N. Christoph, and P. Schreier, Determination of the enantiomeric composition of γ-lactones in complex natural matrices using multidimensional capillary gas chromatography, *J. Chromatogr. 481:*363 (1989).
107. A. Bernreuther, J. Bank, G. Krammer, and P. Schreier, Multidimensional gas chromatography/mass spectrometry: a powerful tool for the direct chiral evaluation of aroma compounds in plant tissues. I. 5-Alkanolides in fruits, *Phytochem. Anal. 2:*43 (1991).
108. J. S. Gaffney, E. T. Premuzic, T. Orlando, S. Ellis, and P. Snyder, Gas chromatography-circular dichroism system for detection of optically active substances, *J. Chromatogr. 262:*321 (1983).
109. M. E. Bailey and H. B. Hass, New methods for resolution of enantiomorphs. I. Rectification, *J. Am. Chem. Soc. 63:*1969 (1941).
110. J. Casanova Jr. and E. J. Corey, Resolution of (±)-camphor by gas-liquid chromatography, *Chem. Ind. (London):*1664 (1961).
111. E. Gil-Av, R. Charles, and G. Fischer, Resolution of amino acids by gas chromatography, *J. Chromatogr. 17:*408 (1965).
112. K.-A. Karlsson and I. Pascher, Resolution and chromatographic configuration analysis of glycol resolving agents, *Chem. Phys. Lipids 12:*65 (1974).
113. W. Walther, W. Vetter, M. Vechi, H. Schneider, R. K. Müller, and T. Netscher,

(S)-Trolox methyl ether: a powerful derivatizing reagent for the GC determination of the enantiomers of aliphatic alcohols, *Chimia 45:*121 (1991).
114. S. Juliá and J. M. Sans, Resolution of racemic modifications by gas-liquid chromatography via the separation of diastereomeric esters. VII. Cyanohydrins, *J. Chromatogr. Sci. 17:*651 (1979).
115. J. W. Westley and B. Halpern, The use of (−)-menthol chloroformiate in the optical analysis of asymmetric amino and hydroxyl compounds by gas chromatography, *J. Org. Chem. 33:*3978 (1968).
116. J. A. Dale and H. S. Mosher, Nuclear magnetic resonance nonequivalence of diastereomeric esters of α-substituted phenylacetic acids for the determination of stereochemical purity, *J. Am. Chem. Soc. 90:*3732 (1968).
117. R. E. Doolittle and R. R. Heath, (S)-Tetrahydro-5-oxo-2-furanecarboxylic acid: a chiral derivatizing agent for asymmetric alcohols, *J. Org. Chem. 49:*5041 (1984).
118. M. Sanz-Burrata, J. Irurre-Pérez, and S. Juliá-Arechaga, Resolution of racemic ketones and aldehyds via diastereomeric acetals by gas-liquid chromatography III. Choice of glycol resolving agents, *Afinidad 27:*705 (1970).
119. W. Pereira, V. A. Bacon, W. Patton, B. Halpern, and G. E. Pollock, The use of R-(+)-1-Phenylethylisocyanate in the optical analysis of asymmetric secondary alcohols by gas chromatography, *Anal. Lett. 3:*23 (1970).
120. A. Mosandl, M. Gessner, C. Günther, W. Deger, and G. Singer, (S)-O-Acetyllactyl chloride—a versatile chiral auxiliary in stereodifferentiation of enantiomeric flavor compounds, *J. High Resol. Chromatogr. 10:*67 (1987).
121. W. Deger, M. Gessner, C. Günther, G. Singer, and A. Mosandl, Stereoisomeric flavor compounds. 18. Enantiodiscrimination of chiral flavor compounds by diastereomeric derivatization, *J. Agric. Food Chem. 36:*1260 (1988).
122. K.-H. Engel, R. A. Flath, W. Albrecht, and R. Tressl, Gas chromatographic separation of diastereomeric dicarbamate derivatives of γ- and δ-lactones, *J. Chromatogr. 479:*179 (1989).
123. M. Huffer and P. Schreier, High-resolution gas chromatographic resolution of chiral primary alcohols and acids as their diastereomeric 1-phenylethyl amides, *J. Chromatogr. 519:*263 (1990).
124. A. Knierzinger, W. Walther, B. Weber, and T. Netscher, A practical method for the stereochemical analysis of acyclic terpenoid carbonyl compounds, *Chimia 43:*163 (1989).
125. D. A. Rimmer and M. E. Rose, Some novel homochiral derivatizing agents for the gas chromatographic analysis of enantiomeric secondary alcohols, *J. Chromatogr. 598:*251 (1992).
126. E. Gil-Av, B. Feibush, and R. Charles-Sigler, Separation of enantiomers by gas-liquid chromatography with an optically active stationary phase, Proceedings 6th International Symposium on Gas Chromatography and Associated Techniques, Rome 1966 (A. B. Littlewood, ed.), Inst. of Petroleum, London, 1967, p. 227.
127. H. Frank, G. J. Nicholson, and E. Bayer, Rapid gas chromatographic separation

of amino acid enantiomers with a novel chiral stationary phase, *J. Chromatogr. Sci. 15:*174 (1977).
128. E. Bayer, H. Allmendinger, G. Enderle, and B. Koppenhoefer, Application of D-Chirasil-Val in the analysis of enantiomers by gas-chromatography, *Fresenius' Z. Anal. Chem. 321:*321 (1985).
129. W. A. König, I. Benecke, and H. Bretting, Resolution of enantiomers of carbohydrates by gas chromatography on a new chiral stationary phase, *Angew. Chem. 93:*688 (1981).
130. W. A. König, *The Practice of Enantiomer Separation by Capillary Gas Chromatography*, Hüthig, Heidelberg, 1987.
131. B. Koppenhoefer, H. Allmendinger, and G. Nicholson, Direct enantiomer resolution of hydroxy and carbonyl compounds by GC on Chirasil-Val, *Angew. Chem. 97:*46 (1985).
132. H. Allmendinger, Chromatographische Enantiomerenanalyse von Hydroxysäuren und Alkoholen aus chemischen und enzymatischen Reaktionen, Thesis, University of Tuebingen, Germany, 1986.
133. J. Bricout, *Flavour Science and Technology* (M. Martens and G. A. Dalen, eds.), Wiley, Chichester, United Kingdom, 1987, p. 87.
134. V. Schurig and E. Gil-Av, Complexation of olefins with planar rhodium(I) co-ordinated compounds, *J. Chem. Soc. Chem. Commun.* 650 (1971).
135. V. Schurig, Enantiomer resolution of a chiral olefin by complexation chromatography on an optically active rhodium(I)-complex, *Angew. Chem. 89:*113 (1977).
136. B. Koppenhoefer, K. Hintzer, R. Weber, and V. Schurig, Quantitative separation of enantiomeric pairs of the pheromone 2-ethyl-1,6-dioxaspiro[4,4]nonane by complexation chromatography on an optically active metal complex, *Angew. Chem. 92:*473 (1980).
137. V. Schurig, Homogeneous coating of glass and fused silica capillary columns with metal coordination compounds for the selective gas chromatographic separation of structural-, stereo- and optical isomers, German Pat. DE 3,247,714 (1983).
138. V. Schurig, D. Schmalzing, and M. Schleimer, Enantiomer separation on immobilized Chirasil-Metal and Chirasil-Dex with gas chromatography and chromatography with supercritical fluids, *Angew. Chem. 103:*994 (1991).
139. D. M. Sand and H. Schlenk, Acylated cyclodextrins as polar stationary phases for gas-liquid chromatography, *Anal. Chem. 33:*1624 (1961).
140. T. Koscielski, D. Sybilska, and J. Jurczak, Separation of α- and β-pinene into enantiomers in gas-liquid chromatography systems via α-cyclodextrin inclusion complexes, *J. Chromatogr. 280:*131 (1983).
141. V. Schurig and H.-P. Nowotny, Separation of enantiomers on diluted permethylated β-cyclodextrin by high-resolution gas chromatography, *J. Chromatogr. 441:*155 (1988).
142. V. Schurig, D. Schmalzing, U. Mühleck, M. Jung, M. Schleimer, P. Mussche, C. Duvekot, and J. C. Buyten, Gas chromatographic enantiomer separation on poly-

siloxane-anchored permethyl-β-cyclodextrin (Chirasil-Dex), *J. High Resolut. Chromatogr. 13:*713 (1990).

143. W. A. König, S. Lutz, P. Mischnick-Lübbecke, B. Brassat, and G. Wenz, Cyclodextrins as chiral stationary phases in capillary gas chromatography I. Pentylated α-cyclodextrin, *J. Chromatogr. 447:*193 (1988).
144. A. Köhnes and H. Römer, Cyclodextrin-derivatives as chiral stationary phases in gas chromatography with fused-silica capillary columns, *CLB Chem. Lab. Biotech. 41:*70 (1990).
145. D. W. Armstrong, W. Li, and J. Pitha, Reversing enantioselectivity in capillary GC with polar and nonpolar cyclodextrin derivative phases, *Anal. Chem. 62:*214 (1990).
146. H.-G. Schmarr, A. Mosandl, and A. Kauzinger, Influence of derivatization on the chiral selectivity of cyclodextrins: alkylated/acylated cyclodextrins and γ-/δ-lactones as an example, *J. Microcolumn Sep. 3:*395 (1991).
147. C. Bicchi, G. Artuffo, A. D'Amato, A. Galli, and M. Galli, Cyclodextrin derivatives in the GC separation of racemic mixtures of volatile compounds: Part IV, *J. High Resolut. Chromatogr. 15:*655 (1992).
148. A. Dietrich, B. Maas, V. Karl, P. Kreis, D. Lehmann, B. Weber, and A. Mosandl, Stereoisomeric flavor compounds: Stereodifferentiation of some chiral volatiles on heptakis(2,3-di-O-acetyl-6-O-tert-butyldimethylsilyl)-β-cyclodextrin, *J. High Resolut. Chromatogr. 15:*176 (1992).
149. G. Krammer, A. Bernreuther, and P. Schreier, Multidimensional gas chromatography, *GIT Fachz. Lab. 34:*306 (1990).
150. U. Palm, C. Askari, U. Hener, E. Jakob, C. Mandler, M. Gessner, A. Mosandl, W. A. König, P. Evers, and R. Krebber, Stereoisomeric flavour compounds XLVII. Direct chirospecific HRGC analysis of natural δ-lactones, *Z. Lebensm. Unters. Forsch. 192:*209 (1991).
151. P. Werkhoff, S. Brennecke, and W. Bretschneider, Progress in the chirospecific analysis of naturally occurring flavour and fragrance compounds, *Chem. Mikrobiol. Technol. Lebensm. 13:*129 (1991).
152. K. Haase-Aschoff, I. Haase-Aschoff, and H. Laub, Chiral analysis and evaluation of 2-methylbutyric acid and its esters in fruit and fruit products, *Lebensmittelchemie 45:*107 (1991).
153. G. Schmidt, G. Full, P. Winterhalter, and P. Schreier, Synthesis and enantiodifferentiation of isomeric theaspiranes, *J. Agric. Food Chem. 40:*1188 (1992).
154. V. Karl, A. Dietrich, and A. Mosandl, Stereoisomeric flavour compounds. LXIV: The chirospecific analysis of 2-alkyl-branched flavour compounds from apple headspace extracts and their sensory evauation, *Phytochem. Anal. 4:*158 (1993).
155. A. Bernreuther and P. Schreier, Multidimensional gas chromatography/mass spectrometry: a powerful tool for the direct chiral evauation of aroma compounds in plant tissues. II. Linalool in essential oils and fruits, Phytochem. Anal. 2:167 (1991).
156. G. Full, A. Bernreuther, G. Krammer, and P. Schreier, Foodstuff analysis. On-

line-HRGC-FTIR for direct enantiodifferentiation of aroma compounds from complex matrices, *Labo (7-8):*30 (1991).

157. P. Werkhoff, S. Brennecke, W. Bretschneider, M. Güntert, R. Hoppe, and H. Surburg, Chirospecific analysis in essential oil, fragrance and flavor research, *Z. Lebensm. Unters. Forsch. 196:*307 (1993).
158. A. Mosandl, Capillary gas chromatography in quality assessment of flavours and fragrances, *J. Chromatogr. 624:*267 (1992).
159. W. A. König, *Gas Chromatographic Enantiomer Separation with Modified Cyclodextrins*, Hüthig, Heidelberg, 1992.
160. C. Bicchi, V. Manzin, A. D'Amato, and P. Rubiolo, Cyclodextrin derivatives in GC separation of enantiomers of essential oil, aroma and flavour compounds, *Flav. Fragr. J. 10:*127 (1995).
161. A. Galfré, P. Martin, and M. Petrzilka, Direct enantioselective separation and olfactory evaluation of all irone isomers, *J. Ess. Oil Res. 5:*265 (1993).
162. C. Chapuis and R. Brauchli, Preparation of optically active flowery and woody-like odorant ketones via Corey-Chaykovsky oxiranylation: irones and analogues, *Helv. Chim. Acta 76:*2070 (1993).
163. G. Dugo, I. S. d'Alcontres, A. Cotroneo, and P. Dugo, On the genuineness of citrus essential oils. Part XXXV. Detection of added reconstituted mandarin oil in genuine cold-pressed mandarin essential oil by high resolution gas chromatography with chiral capillary columns, *J. Ess. Oil Res. 4:*589 (1992).
164. D. Lehmann, B. Maas, and A. Mosandl, Stereoisomeric flavour compounds. LXIX: stereodifferentiation of δ(γ)-lacones C_8-C_{18} in dairy products, margerine and coconut, *Z. Lebensm. Unters. Forsch. 201:*55 (1995).
165. V. Schubert and A. Mosandl, Chiral compounds of essential oils. VIII: Stereodifferentiation of linalool using multidimensional gas chromatography, *Phytochem. Anal. 2:*171 (1991).
166. N. Fischer and F.-J. Hammerschmidt, A contribution to the analysis or fresh strawberry flavour, *Chem. Mikrobiol. Technol. Lebensm. 14:*141 (1992).
167. G. Bruche, A. Dietrich, and A. Mosandl, Stereoisomeric flavour compounds. LXXI: Determination of the origin of aroma-active dihydrofuranones, *Z. Lebensm. Unters. Forsch. 201:*249 (1995).
168. G. Bruche, A. Dietrich, and A. Mosandl, Stereoisomeric flavor compounds. Part LXI: Enantioselective analysis of aroma-relevant dihydrofuranones, *J. High Resolut. Chromatogr. 16:*101 (1993).
169. B. Maas, A. Dietrich, and A. Mosandl, Enantioselective capillary gas chromatography-olfactometry in essential oil analysis, *Naturwissenschaften 80:*470 (1993).
170. V. Karl, J. Gutser, A. Dietrich, B. Maas, and A. Mosandl, Stereoisomeric flavour compounds LXVIII. 2-, 3-, and 4-alkyl-branched acids, Part 2: Chirospecific analysis and sensory evaluation, *Chirality 6:*427 (1994).
171. D. Bartschat, D. Lehmann, A. Dietrich, and A. Mosandl, Chiral compounds of essential oils XIX. 4-Methyl-5-decanolide: chirospecific analysis, structure and properties of the stereoisomers, *Phytochem. Anal. 6:*130 (1995).

172. D. Lehmann, A. Dietrich, U. Hener, and A. Mosandl, Stereoisomeric flavour compounds. LXX: 1-p-Menthene-8-thiol: separation and sensory evaluation of the enantiomers by enantioselective gas chromatography-olfactometry, *Phytochem. Anal. 6:*255 (1995).
173. B. Koppenhoefer, Lin Bingcheng, V. Muschalek, U. Trettin, H. Willisch, and E. Bayer, Epimerization and enantiomer resolution of tripeptides by GC on L-Chirasil-Val, Proceedings 20th European Peptide Symposium 1988 Tuebingen (G. Jung and E. Bayer, eds.), de Gruyter, Berlin, 1988, p. 109.
174. B. Koppenhoefer, A. Nothdurft, J. Pierrot-Sanders, P. Piras, C. Popescu, C. Roussel, M. Stiebler, and U. Trettin, CHIRBASE, a graphical molecular database on the separation of enantiomers by liquid-, supercritical fluid-, and gas chromatography, *Chirality 5:*213 (1993).
175. C. Roussel and P. Piras, CHIRBASE: a molecular database for storage and retrieval of chromatographic chiral separations, *Pure Appl. Chem. 65:*235 (1993).
176. W. A. König, A. Krüger, D. Icheln, and T. Runge, Enantiomeric composition of chiral constituents in essential oils, *J. High Resolut. Chromatogr. 15:*184 (1992).
177. W. A. König, The direct resolution of enantiomeric drugs by chiral-phase gas chromatography, *Drug Stereochemistry. Analytical Methods and Pharmacology* (I. W. Wainer, ed.), Marcel Dekker, New York, 1993, p. 107.
178. M. Lindström, T. Norin, and J. Roeraade, Gas chromatographic separation of monoterpene hydrocarbon enantiomers on α-cyclodextrin, *J. Chromatogr. 513:*315 (1990).
179. F. Kobor, K. Angermund, and G. Schomburg, Molecular modelling experiments on chiral recognition in GC with specially derivatized cyclodextrins as selectors, *J. High Resolut. Chromatogr. 16:*299 (1993).
180. F. Kobor and G. Schomburg, 6-tert-Butyldimethylsilyl-2,3-dimethyl-α-, β-, and γ-cyclodextrins, desolved in polysiloxanes, as chiral selectors for gas chromatography. Influence of selector concentration and polysiloxane matrix polarity on enantioseparation, *J. High Resolut. Chromatogr. 16:*693 (1993).
181. A. Venema, H. Henderiks, and R. v. Geest, The enantioselectivity of modified cyclodextrins: studies on interaction mechanisms, *J. High Resolut. Chromatogr. 14:*676 (1991).
182. D. Icheln, B. Gehrcke, T. Runge, and W. A. König, Modified cyclodextrins—selective acylation and alkylation lead to specific selectivities for enantiomer separation in capillary gas chromatography, Proceedings 15th International Symposium Capillary Chromatography 1993 Riva del Garda (Italy) (P. Sandra, ed.), Hüthig, Heidelberg, 1993, p. 278.
183. C. Bicchi, G. Artuffo, A. D'Amato, V. Manzin, A. Galli, and M. Galli, Cyclodextrin derivatives in the GC separation of racemic mixtures of volatile compounds. Part V: Heptakis 2,6-dimethyl-3-pentyl-β-cyclodextrins, *J. High Resolut. Chromatogr. 15:*710 (1992).

7

Ion Trap Mass Spectrometry for Food Aroma Analysis

CHARLES K. HUSTON
Varian Chromatography Systems, Walnut Creek, California

I. INTRODUCTION

Each step of an analytical method provides some information that can be used for the overall characterization of a complex sample. Simple sample-preparation techniques (e.g., solvent extraction) provide the first qualitative information about an analyte's physicochemical characteristics. More selective sample-enrichment techniques (e.g., SPME) and chromatographic methods (e.g., capillary gas chromatography) provide further information that can allow the analyst to "build the case" for compound identification. Quantitation can be accomplished by analyzing the signal output of most chromatographic detectors because their response is proportional to the amount of analyte in the sample.

Much of the aforementioned information can be provided by a single system that combines chromatographic separation with a multichannel detector (e.g., mass spectrometer). Mass spectrometry (MS) simultaneously provides both qualitative and quantitative information and, thus, is extremely useful for analyses of food aroma samples containing many compounds of interest. Because of the volatile nature of food aromas, gas chromatography/mass spectrometry (GC/MS) is the most common method used for their MS analysis. Each data point of the complex chromatogram from a GC/MS analysis of beer headspace (Fig. 1), for example, contains a second dimension of data (a "mass spectrum"). Comparison of the mass spectrum (via computer searching) to known databases (Fig. 2) tentatively identified the compound at scan 435 in Figure 1 as phenylethyl alcohol. Closer examination of the spectrum (Fig. 3) showed the characteristic minor presence of the molecular ion (122 peak) as well as a major fragment ion (91 peak) resulting from the loss of CH_2OH. The combination of chromatographic retention time with a characteristic mass spectrum thus provides positive chemical identification for a large percentage of aroma analytes. GC/MS systems are becoming more widely used because of the increased availability of low-cost, high-speed computer hardware, which provides both instrument control and rapid data reduction (e.g., spectral library searching) capabilities.

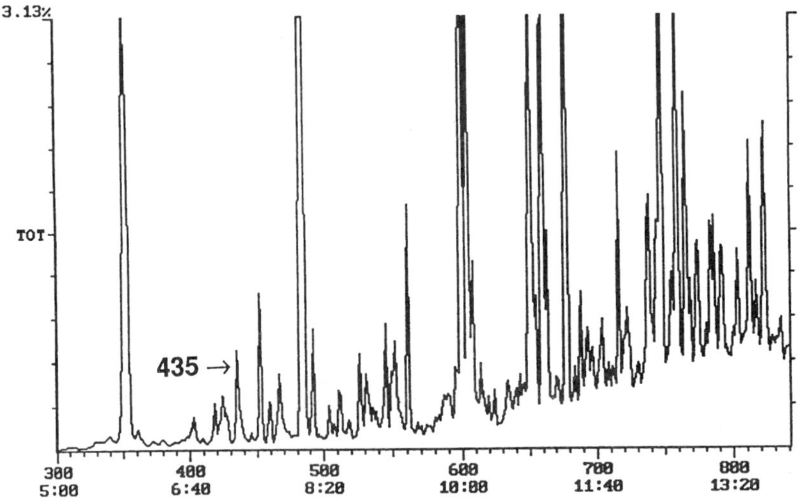

FIGURE 1 A total ion chromatogram (TIC) from ion trap GC/MS analysis of beer headspace. The TIC is characteristically presented in terms of time (x axis) versus relative signal intensity (y axis). Time is labeled in terms of both spectral scan number and hours:minutes.

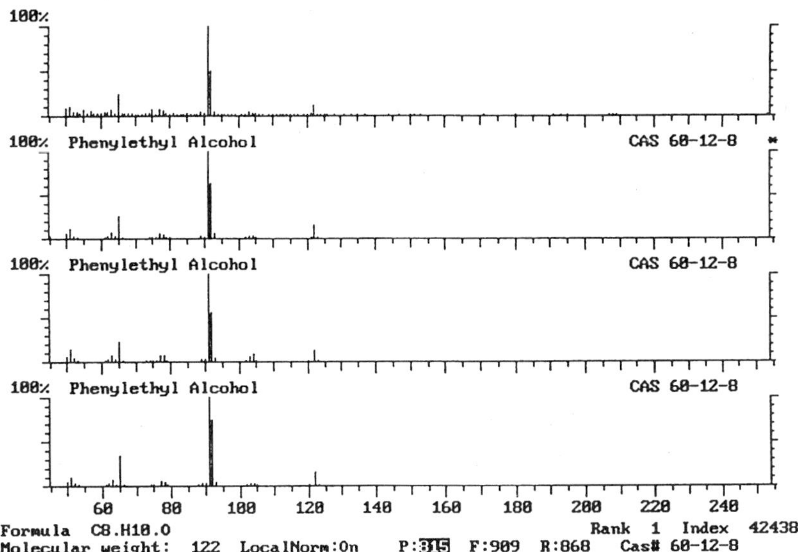

FIGURE 2 Spectral libraries often contain more than one example spectrum of a given compound; in this case, the library contained at least three "phenylethyl alcohol" spectra that closely matched spectrum 435 from Figure 1.

Quadrupole ion trap GC/MS systems are particularly applicable to the analytical challenges of food aromas because they provide capabilities ranging from sensitive, full-scan mass detection to multidimensional MS. This chapter will provide an overview of the operational aspects of ion trap GC/MS for the purpose of providing insight into its present and potential applications for food aroma analysis. The examples contained in this chapter were acquired via ion trap GC/MS; a number of references describing other mass spectral aroma analyses are also cited because of their immediate applicability to ion trap GC/MS.

II. THEORY AND INSTRUMENTATION

Mass spectrometry is an analytical technique where the sample (analyte) is first ionized to create a population of ion fragments with a distribution of mass-to-charge ratios (m/z). By separating this ion population on the basis of m/z and measuring (and integrating) the signal intensities, a mass spectrum is

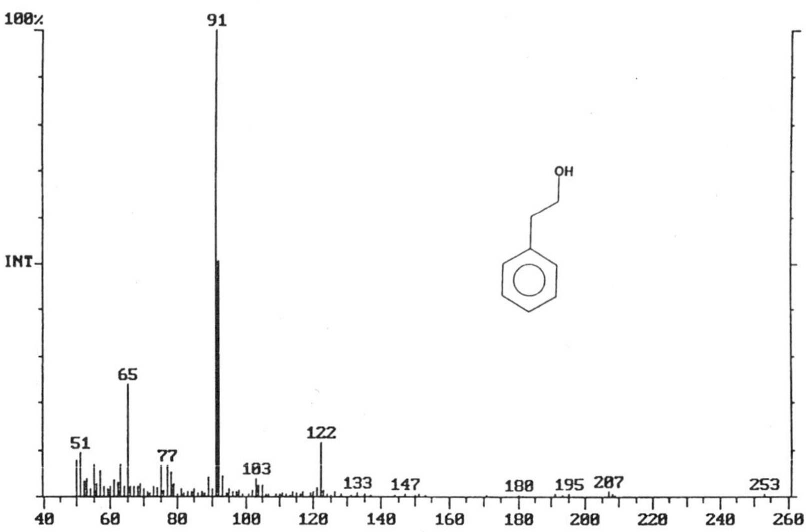

FIGURE 3 The mass spectrum from scan 435 of the TIC shown in Figure 1. The chemical structure of phenylethyl alcohol is also shown.

obtained that is characteristic of the analyte. MS instruments can differ in the ways that they create and/or separate and analyze ions. Most commonly, acquired MS data are analyzed via computer matching to spectral databases of known compounds ("library searching"). Large commercial libraries (e.g., NIST, Wiley, etc.) provide thousands of individual mass spectra, with multiple entries for selected compounds (e.g., the three library spectra for phenylethyl alcohol in Figure 2). Aroma analysts often additionally construct custom spectral libraries in the course of their work [e.g., volatile components in red wine (1)] and have also developed automated forms of computer data handling to deal with more complex aroma analyses (2). In the absence of library searching, successful interpretation of the MS information from unknown compounds (3) requires a basic knowledge of ion chemistry and a certain amount of experience.

A. Quadrupole Mass Spectrometry

Quadrupole MS instruments use various electrode configurations to establish conditions that affect the analyte ions in predetermined ways (4). The most common instrument, a transmission quadrupole, provides mass spectra by sequentially scanning through instrumental settings that selectively permit only ions with specific m/z to pass through the MS and into the detector. These mass filters are commonly able to analyze low nanogram quantities of compounds in the full-scan mode (the mode required to conduct library searches), while lower levels can often be detected using selected ion monitoring (SIM). For trace aroma analyses, special sample concentration methods are often required to overcome the sensitivity limitations of benchtop GC/MS systems based on transmission quadrupoles.

The same electrical fields used by transmission quadrupole instruments, however, can be established using electrodes with different geometries (5) to create an ion trap (Fig. 4). The ion trap stores and concentrates ions prior to mass analysis, and, thus, it is inherently more sensitive than a mass filter instrument. Typically, full-scan spectra (needed for successful library searches) can be obtained from picogram quantities of an analyte. The ion-storage capabilities of the ion trap are also very useful for advanced, MS ion-preparation techniques (e.g., MS/MS) that greatly increase the analytical power of the instrument.

B. Ion Trap Theory of Operation

As their name implies, quadrupole mass spectrometers utilize a quadrupole electrical field to affect the motion of ions. Ion motion can be determined from solutions to the Mathieu equation (6). For ion traps, the stable solutions to the

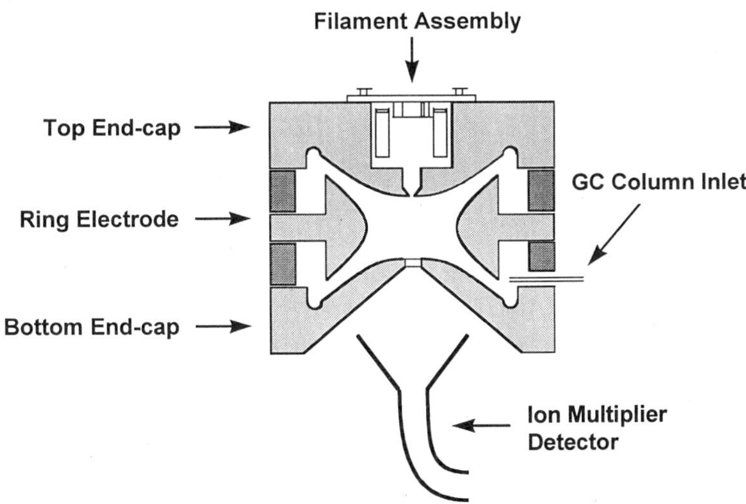

FIGURE 4 A schematic diagram of a quadrupole ion trap mass spectrometer.

equations are characterized by the dimensionless parameters, q_z and a_z, that define the conditions under which ions are trapped. These parameters are defined as (6):

$$q_z = -8eV/m(r_0^2 + 2z_0^2)/\Omega^2$$
$$a_z = -16eU/m(r_0^2 + 2z_0^2)/\Omega^2$$

Where V is the amplitude (0 to peak) of the RF potential applied to the ring electrode (Fig. 4), U is the DC potential applied to the end-cap electrodes, m is the m/z of the ion, r_0 is the radius of the ring electrode, z_0 is the separation between the end-caps, and Ω is the RF drive frequency. In most routine uses, no DC field is used, thus $a_z = 0$. The secular frequency of an ion, ω_z, can be determined from the value of β_z (6):

$$\omega_z = (\beta_z/2)\Omega$$

The value of β_z, and thus the secular frequency of a trapped ion, is a function of the operating conditions set for the ion trap. The practical message to be gained from examination of these equations is simply that ion trap operational conditions can be easily manipulated both to affect inherent ion characteristics (i.e., secular frequency) and to determine whether or not a population of ions (or portion of it) will be trapped. Quadrupole ion traps thus provide the analyst with both a sensitive mass analyzer (to obtain a mass spectrum) and the equivalent of a MS ion-preparation system in a single instrument (7).

C. Ion Trap GC/MS Instrumentation

In addition to the three electrodes discussed previously, the basic ion trap assembly (5) typically includes both a filament assembly and an ion multiplier detector (Fig. 4). The filament assembly is normally used to ionize the sample as it enters the trap (e.g., via the GC column inlet). After the ions are trapped and, subsequently, ejected by the electrodes, the ions are detected by the ion multiplier detector. This uses an electron multiplier tube (EMT) assembly to provide a signal that is related to the number of ions coming in contact with it. Ion traps designed for internal ion creation provide both maximum sensitivity and simplicity of maintenance (e.g., electrode cleaning) and thus are ideal for food aroma analysis.

Analyte ions can also be created outside of the trap; these systems include the hardware (lens assemblies, additional vacuum systems, etc.) necessary to transfer the externally created ions into the ion trap for analysis. External interface ion trap systems are most widely applied to nonvolatile (nonaroma) analyses (e.g., coupling to liquid chromatography, capillary electrophoresis). Due to their additional complexity and lower trace performance (resulting from inefficient transfer of the ions into the trap), these systems are infrequently used for GC/MS of food aromas.

The major mechanical parts of a typical ion trap GC/MS instrument are shown in Figure 5. In its simplest configuration, the GC consists of an injector and an analytical column (capillary column). The purpose of the injector is to vaporize the aroma sample so that its component parts can be resolved on the basis of both analyte volatility and its selective interaction with the stationary phase of the column. The injector is also often used as the interface between sample-handling techniques (e.g., supercritical fluid extraction) and the GC. For example, an on-column inlet gave optimal results for ion trap SFE/GC/MS of cloves (8). The entire GC system is thermally regulated (GC oven) to control selectivity and precision of the chromatography (discussed in more detail elsewhere in this book). Once resolved, the analytes elute from the end of the GC column and are transferred to the ion trap for MS analysis. A number of chromatographic interfaces (discussed below) can be used either prior to or in place of the transfer line shown in Figure 5. For successful ionization, trapping, and analysis of the transferred sample, the ion trap assembly must also be maintained under vacuum conditions (e.g., 10^{-5} Torr). The most reliable pumping system used to establish these low operational pressures

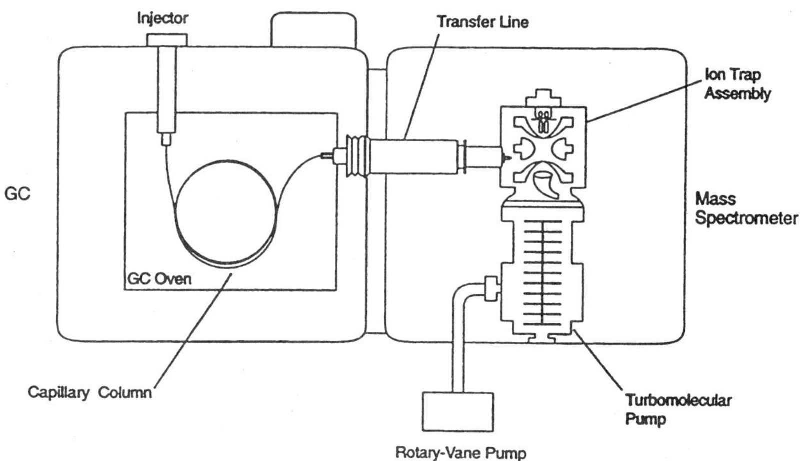

FIGURE 5 A schematic diagram of a direct interface ion trap capillary GC/MS system.

consists of a turbomolecular pump connected in series with a rotary vane pump (Fig. 5). Finally, although they are not shown, the control electronics and computer data system are also critical to both the performance and ease of use of any ion trap GC/MS system (9).

D. Chromatographic Interfaces

Because mass spectrometers operate at low pressures, an appropriate interface between the ion trap and the gas chromatograph is necessary for the system to operate properly. The objective of any interface is to transfer the analyte molecules from the inlet (e.g., the GC capillary column) to the MS while removing most of the carrier gas and maintaining inlet performance. With GC, the pressure reduction required by narrow-bore WCOT columns (typically used with low flow rates ranging from 1 to 3 ml/min) can be accommodated by the vacuum systems of most ion trap MS instruments. In these cases, a "direct interface" (i.e., the transfer line shown in Figure 5) can be used which transfers both the carrier gas and the sample molecules directly to the mass spectrometer. Direct interface hardware provides vacuum coupling between the two systems as well as thermal regulation (heating) to maintain the chromatographic separation. Once transferred, the carrier gas molecules (with smaller mass) are pumped away more rapidly than the sample. The direct interface is easy to use and provides complete sample transfer to the mass spectrometer (an important consideration for trace aroma analyses).

The higher flow rates used with large-bore capillary and packed columns are incompatible with direct interface approaches. For these applications, an effluent splitter can be used to handle the larger pressure differentials characteristic of higher-flow GC systems. The most common, an open split interface (Fig. 6), consists of a simple assembly that butts the column end against a restrictor line that is directly connected to the mass spectrometer (10). As its name implies, the GC sample stream is split before introduction into the mass spectrometer, and no sample enrichment occurs. A small flow of helium is passed around the low dead volume connection sleeve to assure a consistent split of the sample. GC column changes are relatively easy with the open split interface, because the restrictor (not the column) establishes a constant pressure differential between the gas chromatograph and the mass spectrometer (11). The open split interface provides the best chromatographic integrity of the nondirect MS interfaces (12). Additionally, the vent flow can be used for other analytical purposes ranging from the use of another type of GC detector to human sensory evaluation. Because much food aroma characterization includes sensory data, correlation of MS results with sensory evalu-

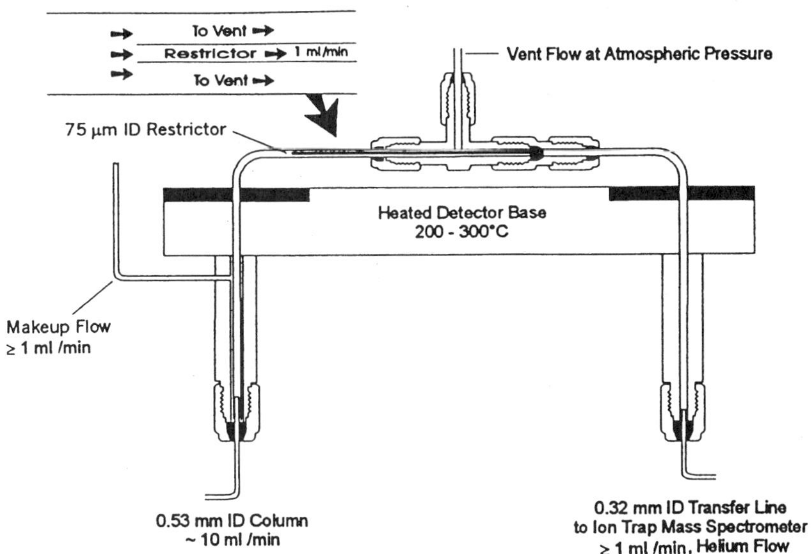

FIGURE 6 An open split interface.

ation of the vent flow (via a sniffer port) can be useful. For example, GC/MS/sniffing analysis has been successfully applied to cheddar cheese headspace (13) and fruit volatiles (14).

A jet separator can also be useful for higher-flow GC applications where sample enrichment is desired. The sample and carrier gas are passed through a small jet orifice where they increase in velocity and pass into a vacuum region. In the gap (ca. 0.5 mm) between the exit orifice and a collector orifice, the lighter carrier gas molecules are preferentially pumped away while the heavier sample molecules, having greater momentum, continue their path and enter the collector orifice for transfer to the MS. Generally, jet interfaces are made of inert glass to minimize sample interactions, and the orifice dimensions are designed to accommodate the intended flow rates of the GC.

III. OPERATION AND APPLICATIONS

A. Basic Ion Trap Operation

All mass spectrometers follow three basic steps to obtain a mass spectrum: (a) ion creation, (b) ion separation, and (c) ion detection. As mentioned previously, the ion trap accumulates and stores ions prior to analysis, thus, their ion creation step also includes establishing instrumental conditions that will cause the created ions to be trapped. The amplitude of the RF voltage applied to the ring electrode is primarily responsible for what ions will, or will not, be stable in the ion trap. At low RF levels, a wide range of m/z (e.g., 10–650 m/z) can be stored and, as the RF is increased (ramped), ions with increasingly larger m/z become unstable and are sequentially ejected from the trap. Ion separation results from this selective relationship between ion stability and RF level. As ions of increasing m/z are axially ejected from the trap in response to the RF ramp, the detector integrates the signal and collects a mass spectrum (containing m/z versus signal intensity information). The preceding scan sequence, the most basic in ion trap MS operation, is generally referred to as mass instability scanning (6).

The use of a buffer gas, axial modulation, and automatic gain control (AGC), in conjunction with the basic electron ionization (EI) scan sequence, allows the ion trap to effectively deal with the dynamics of a changing analyte ion population (i.e., real world analyses). A technique that affects ions with a particular characteristic (e.g., mass instability scanning) can only be maximally selective if the ion population is uniform. A partial pressure of buffer gas in the trap (normally 10^{-3} Torr He) serves to collisionally dampen the kinetic energy of the ions as they are trapped and improves spectral quality (resolution). At high sample concentrations, large numbers of ions in the trap may influence each other in the form of space charging, which adversely affects MS performance. An axial modulation technique (6) in combination with AGC is automatically used to eliminate space-charging problems. AGC also serves to maximize the sensitivity of ion trap MS. AGC is an automatic scan sequence conducted before the basic EI/MS scan sequence (or other scan sequences). Its primary purpose is to acquire a rough quantitative measurement of the ions formed and stored in the trap. When large numbers of ions are measured by AGC, the subsequent EI/MS scan will be modified to produce and analyze fewer ions (eliminating space charge problems). Conversely, when a very small ion signal is measured by the AGC scan sequence, the EI/MS scan will be modified to produce more ions for analysis. AGC thus maintains an optimal number of analytical ions in the trap for a wide range of scan techniques.

B. Electron Ionization

A compound must first be ionized before its mass spectrum can be obtained. As mentioned previously, the most common technique is EI. EI of a sample is accomplished using an electrically heated filament to produce high-energy electrons. The electrons are directed at the sample within the ion trap via a lens assembly (filament assembly in Figure 4) and, as they impact the neutral analyte molecules, analyte ions are produced, trapped, and mass analyzed (i.e., the basic ion trap EI/MS scan sequence). The extent of ionization and subsequent fragmentation is a characteristic of the compound itself (i.e., its characteristic mass spectrum). An ion trap EI/MS analysis of orange extract is shown in Figure 7. A number of trace flavor components can be seen in the total chromatogram (top), and an example EI/MS spectrum from the compound at scan 1196 is also shown (bottom). This trace spectrum shows the characteristic presence of numerous peaks, many of which may have been contributed by the matrix (orange) rather than the analyte itself. These contaminants were seen despite the fact that this was a background-substracted spectrum. The spectral axis notation SMP/BKG indicated that spectral data from a background region of the analysis were subtracted from the 1196 spectrum scan before presentation. In addition to library matching of spectrum 1196 with databases of known aroma/flavor spectra, molecular information may also be obtained via CI/MS analysis.

C. Chemical Ionization

Because of the energetics involved with EI, compounds with similar chemical structures may give similar spectra or may fragment to such an extent that little useful information can be obtained from EI/MS. For these cases, a less energetic ("softer") means of creating analyte ions is needed. Chemical ionization (CI) creates analyte ions by allowing neutral sample molecules to react with a population of reagent ions. The basic ion trap CI/MS scan sequence, then, includes (a) creation and storage of reagent ions, (b) a reaction period between the reagent ions and analyte molecules, (c) ejection of remaining reagent ions, and, finally, (d) mass analysis of the CI products. Although CI can be conducted with either positive or negative reagent ions, positive ion CI is most often used (15). CI reagent gas ions (R^+) can react with neutral sample molecules (M) in several ways:

Proton Transfer:	$(RH)^+ + M \rightarrow (MH)^+ + R$
Charge Transfer:	$R^+ + M \rightarrow M^+ + R$
Hydride Abstraction:	$R^+ + MH \rightarrow M^+ + RH$
Association:	$R^+ + M \rightarrow MR^+$

Proton transfer is the pathway most commonly associated with CI/MS, however, depending on the analyte and types of reagent ions used, products from any combination of the above pathways are possible. The typical goal for

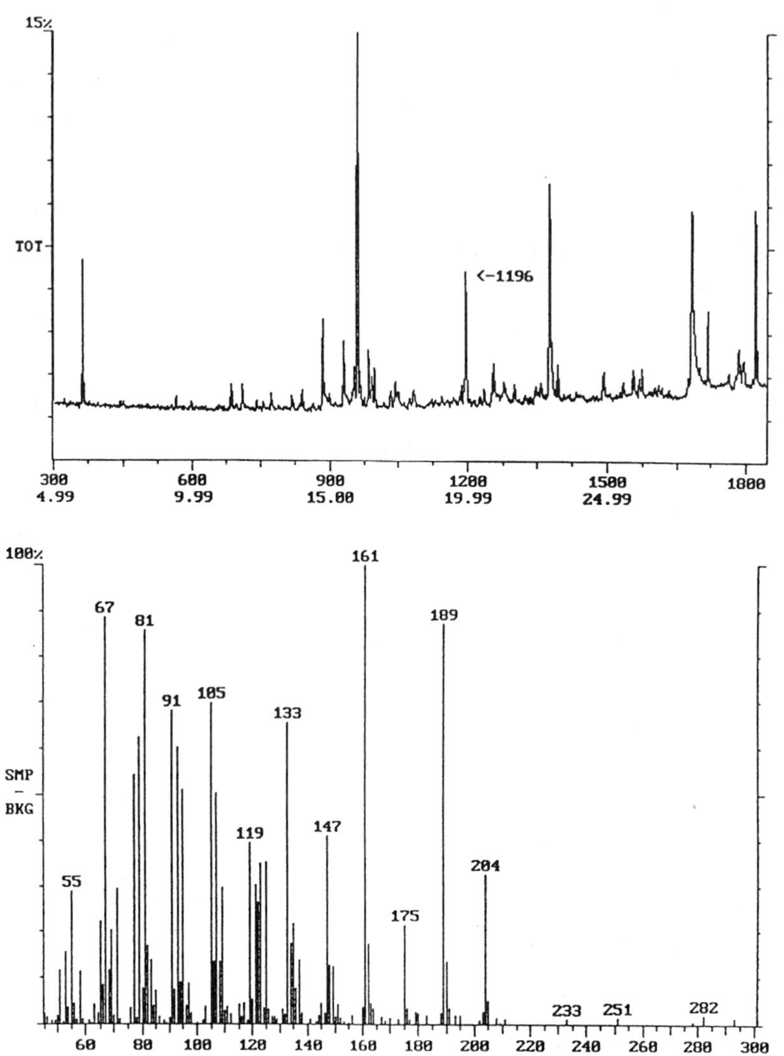

FIGURE 7 Ion trap GC/MS analysis of orange extract using EI. The EI mass spectrum shown (bottom) was taken at scan 1196 from the total ion chromatogram (top).

CI/MS, however, is the production of ions at a m/z equal to the molecular weight plus one (M + 1). Energetic proton transfer can cause subsequent charge transfer fragmentation.

Because of the sensitivity derived from internal ion creation, ion traps operate with low partial pressures of reagent ions and, thus, can utilize both gases and liquid vapors as CI reagents. Examples of common ion trap CI reagents include methane, methanol, acetonitrile, isobutane, and ammonia; these are listed in order from "hard" (creating much secondary framentation) to "soft" (creating little fragmentation) reagent type. In addition to the energetics of a particular CI reaction, multiple pathways may be possible because of the presence of more than one characteristic reagent. When methane, for example, is used as the reagent gas, four major reagent ions are created as follows:

Primary Ion Formation:

$CH_4 + e^- \rightarrow (CH_4^{\bullet})^+ + 2e^-$ (m/z = 16)

$CH_4 + e^- \rightarrow CH_3^+ + e^- + H^-$ (m/z = 15)

Secondary Ion Formation (Predominant):

$(CH_4^{\bullet})^+ + CH_4 \rightarrow CH_5^+ + CH_3^{\bullet}$ (m/z = 17)

$CH_3^+ + CH_4 \rightarrow C_2H_5^+ + H_2$ (m/z = 29)

Production of methane reagent ions results from both EI (primary ion formation) and CI (secondary ion formation) reaction pathways and, thus, a mixture of analyte ions from the various competing reaction pathways is also possible.

The orange extract component at scan 1196 in Figure 7 was also analyzed using ion trap CI/MS with two different reagent types (Fig. 8). Both CI analyses showed characteristic selectivity enhancement (relative to EI) in the form of fewer low m/z interferences. It was also possible, from either spectrum, to conclude that the 204 peak in the EI spectrum was the molecular ion because CI showed enhanced production of M + 1 (205 peak). Methane CI/MS (top) showed both a smaller M + 1 peak and more fragmentation because it was a harder reagent ion than acetonitrile (bottom). The acetonitrile spectrum (resulting from softer CI) gave enhanced production of M + 1, less secondary fragmentation, and a higher mass adduct ion. The characteristic adduct ion (M + 54 = 258) resulted from an association reaction between the neutral molecule and one of the acetonitrile reagent ions (CH_3CN reagent ions were seen at m/z = 42 and 54).

Finally, much higher reagent partial pressures are needed to conduct CI/MS with external ion sources. Because of this, the choice of reagents is limited (e.g., liquid reagents are less applicable) and a dedicated CI interface

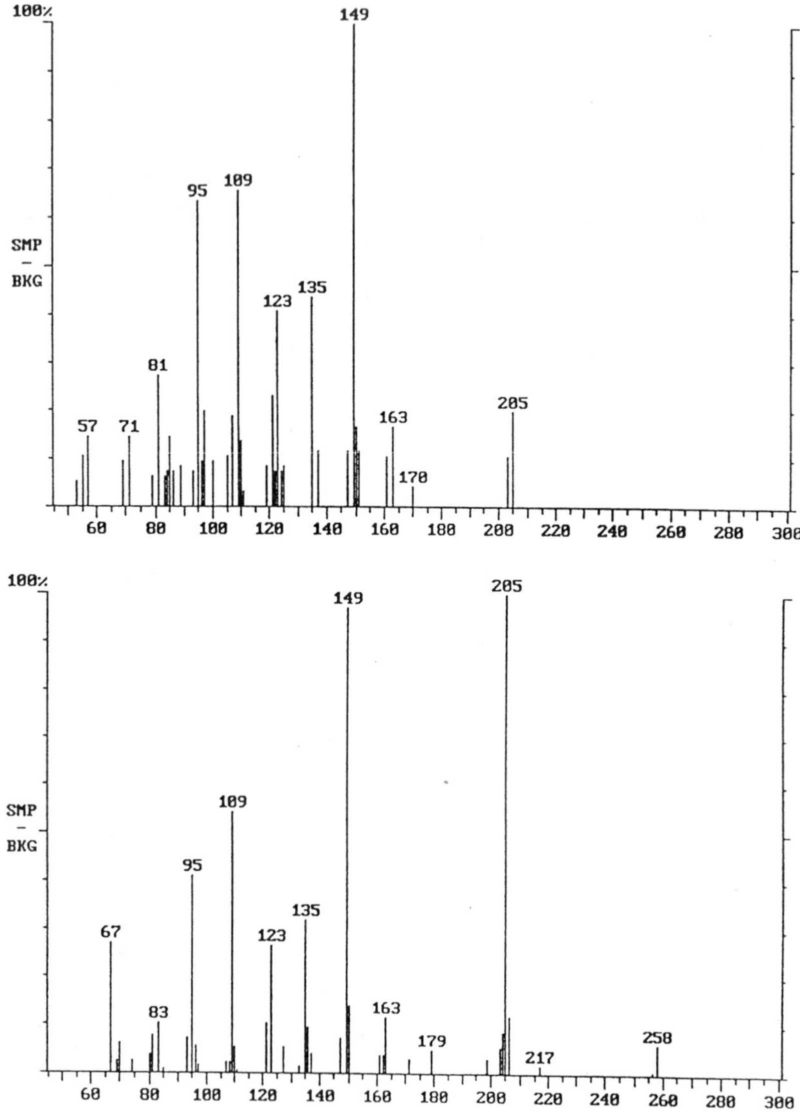

FIGURE 8 Ion trap GC/MS analyses of orange extract using two examples of CI (the spectra shown are representative of the same compound analyzed by EI in Figure 7). The CI reagent used for the top spectrum was methane (a gas), while acetonitrile (a liquid vapor) was used for the bottom CI/MS analysis.

must be used. This not only adversely affects CI performance (qualitative and quantitative), but it eliminates the ability of the analyst to easily switch from EI/MS to CI/MS during a chromatographic run.

D. Trapped Ion Chemistry

The ability of the ion trap to manipulate the time domain of an MS analysis (through its analysis sequences) provides a unique opportunity to capitalize on the inherent ion chemistries for some aroma compounds. For example, it is often difficult to identify saturated fatty acid methyl esters (FAMEs) with transmission quadrupole MS because they often give similar EI spectra that contain little molecular ion information. For this reason, CI techniques have often been applied to their analysis (16). FAME EI spectra, however, commonly show a base peak at m/z = 74, which is the product of a well-characterized ion rearrangement and dissociation pathway (Fig. 9). In ion traps, this fragment can protonate the neutral sample molecule (self-CI) to form an M + 1 ion. Ion trap instrumental parameters (17) can be manipulated to either minimize or enhance the production of M + 1 ions for these compounds. Other compounds of interest to aroma chemists found to produce proton-donating EI product ions include ketones, aldehydes, and amines (Fig. 10).

E. Selected GC/MS Aroma Applications

Industrial quality control (QC) is the most obvious application of simple GC/MS for food aromas. GC/MS data have been used to characterize such

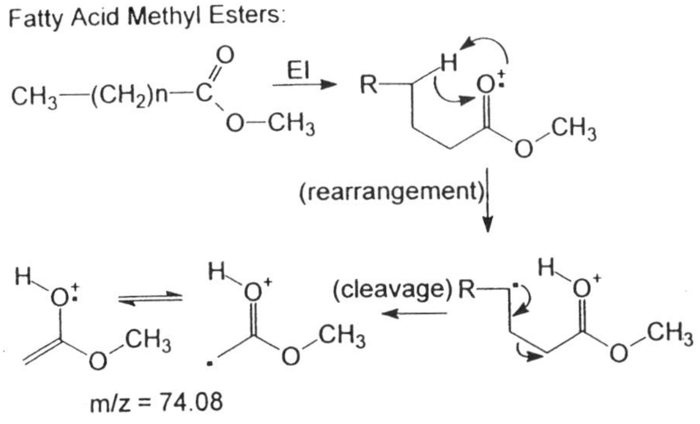

Fatty Acid Methyl Esters:

$CH_3-(CH_2)n-C(=O)-O-CH_3$ EI → (rearrangement) → (cleavage) → m/z = 74.08

FIGURE 9 Under EI conditions, FAMEs produce a major proton-donating ion at m/z = 74.08 via the pathway shown.

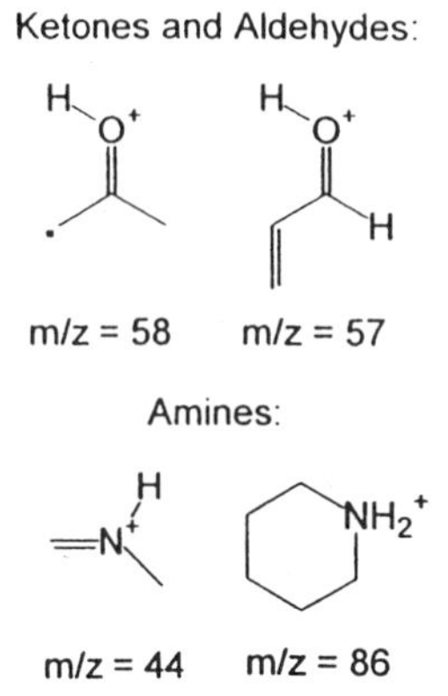

FIGURE 10 Characteristic proton donating ions resulting from EI of ketones, aldehydes, and amines.

QC concerns as the aromatic quality of ready-made tomato sauces (18), the organoleptics of olive oil (19), the flavor-active components in cooked commercial shrimp (20), and the aging process for Swiss Emmentaler cheese (21).

Sample preparation techniques can often be used to improve analytical results, and their effective development and application to GC/MS is an active research area for many analytical food chemists. Solid phase microextraction (SPME) was shown to complement ion trap GC/MS analyses of volatile components in wine (22,23). SPME is a very simple and robust technique that often provides analytical results that are equivalent to (or better than) traditional, static headspace sampling (SHS). Figure 11, for example, compares SHS and SPME for ion trap GC/MS analyses of terpene alcohols in a muscat wine. The SPME technique itself is described in more detail in another chapter in this book. The performance of four standard extraction, concentration, and injection techniques was evaluated for dynamic headspace GC/MS aroma profiling of unifloral honeys (24). Reversed carrier flow sampling was found to improve the analytical results from a headspace GC/MS system used for volatile constituent analyses of various foods (25), and direct interface ion trap GC/MS analyses were improved when purge and trap (P&T) was used to recover volatile organic compounds (VOC) from water (26). In addition to their use for P&T, porous polymer thermal desorption traps have been applied to analyses of VOCs in air (27), vegetable flavors (28), and the aroma profiles of nonalcoholic beers (29).

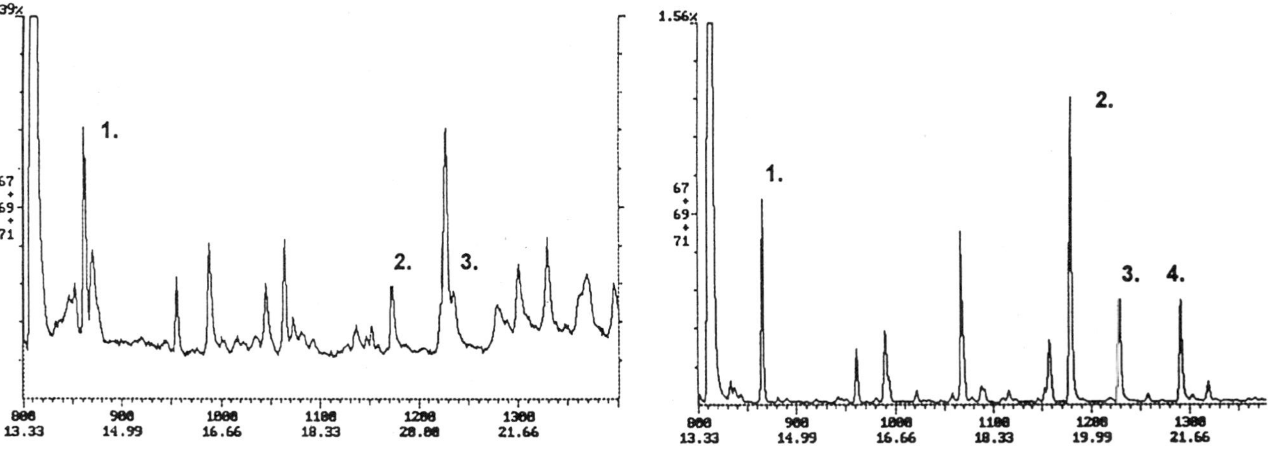

FIGURE 11 Ion trap GC/MS analysis of volatile terpene alcohols (150 ppb each alcohol) in a muscat wine. Static headspace sampling was used for the analysis shown on the left, while SPME was used prior to the GC/MS acquisition shown on the right. 1, Linalool; 2, citronellol; 3, nerol; 4, geraniol.

Advanced ion trap MS techniques (described below) can be effectively used when little or no separation of components is accomplished prior to the introduction of material into the ion trap. Their capabilities can minimize or eliminate the resolution requirements for GC. For aroma applications, systems have been developed with inlets that allow the ion trap to directly sample a gas or vapor stream. These "direct inlet" ion trap instruments use a simple restriction tube to provide a flow rate within the pumping capacity of the vacuum system (30).

Finally, other multidimensional detection techniques and novel separation methods (31) can be used to complement GC/MS analyses of food aromas. Fourier transform infrared spectrometry (FTIR), for example, has been applied to analyses of seed oil volatiles (32) and kiwi flavors (33), and an ion trap pyrolysis GC/MS system has been used to relate wood aging cask components with the aromatic compounds normally monitored in alcoholic beverages (34).

IV. ADVANCED MS ION-PREPARATION TECHNIQUES

Like any other separation method, mass spectrometry (essentially m/z chromatography) can be adversely affected by the presence of unwanted compounds (and their ions). Because of their use of ion accumulation prior to analysis, ion traps are particularly susceptible to these analytical challenges. Food chemists have become very familiar with the benefits of sample preparation techniques prior to GC. Regardless of whether "sample preparation" refers to selective sample enrichment (e.g., SPME) or the use of multiple chromatographic separations (e.g., GC column switching), it can generally be shown to dramatically improve the performance of complex GC aroma analyses. Until the development of the ion trap, mass spectral ion-preparation techniques involved the use of multiple, expensive MS instruments and hardware (35) to conduct a simple hyphenated MS analysis. For example, the hyphenated MS instrument called a "triple quad" actually consists of three transmission MS instruments. Each of the three parts conducts a single step of the MS/MS sequence (isolation, dissociation, and analysis), and thus MS/MS is conducted in space as analyte ions are transferred from one instrument to another. Because the ion trap conducts MS separations in time (using scan sequences) rather than in space, however, it possesses the unique ability to perform its own ion preparation prior to mass analysis. The advanced ion-preparation techniques implemented with the ion trap provide the aroma analyst with qualitative and quantitative benefits ranging from selective sample enrichment to multidimensional qualitative confirmations.

A. Selective CI/MS

As discussed previously, CI/MS is accomplished by creating reagent ions in the ion trap, allowing the reagent ions to react with neutral sample molecules, ejecting the reagent ions by raising the RF, and then analyzing the CI product ions. CI adds another dimension of selectivity to the MS analysis, however, the process of internally producing reagent ions via EI can also result in the production of a small number of EI analyte ions. While these ions do not normally interfere with the accuracy or precision of the MS analysis, they can be undesirable in some cases (e.g., qualitative spectral analyses or the use of certain CI libraries).

The technique known as SECI (simultaneous ejection CI) eliminates any interference from analyte EI products via the addition of another processing step to the ion trap CI/MS sequence (36). The use of SECI is analogous to a chromatographic sample clean-up, and thus it can be thought of as a simple ion-preparation method. Following reagent ion production, a waveform is applied (to the end-cap electrodes) which selectively ejects all ions with m/z greater than that for the largest reagent ion being used. This finite ejecton step does not affect the trap's subsequent ability to trap CI reaction products, but effectively ejects any analyte EI products that may have been formed. During the reaction portion of the CI sequence, thus, sample molecules only come into contact with CI reagents (or CI reaction products). The spectrum obtained from a SECI/MS analysis thus contains ion fragments that were solely produced by CI (primary and/or secondary) reaction pathways. The orange extract CI analyses using two different reagents (Fig. 8) were conducted using the SECI technique.

The ability of the ion trap to eject ions of particular m/z also allows for the selection of individual CI reagent ions prior to the reaction portion of the CI/MS sequence (37). This technique, reagent ion selected chemical ionization (RISCI), provides a means for very specific CI/MS characterization of aroma analytes and is also useful for gas phase ion chemistry research.

B. Selective Ion Storage

Like any chromatographic technique, an ion separation (MS) might not provide enough information for complete characterization of the analyte. This inadequacy might result from the unwanted presence of contaminants (high background) or might be due to the fact that a class of analytes provides similar spectra when a single ion creation method is used. Selective ion storage (SIS) (38) addresses the former situation by applying a selective ion-ejection technique both during ion creation and for a short time thereafter. In this way, the ion trap both creates and accumulates only the ions in the specified m/z range (or ranges) while all other ions are ejected from the trap. This selective sample-enrichment technique often allows detection limit performance to be maintained even in the presence of a significant background interference. Depending on the mass range requirements for the analysis, a further refinement of the SIS technique (39) (see Sec. IV.D.3) can also be used.

C. Multidimensional Mass Spectrometry

Tandem mass spectrometry can be used not only to overcome high background problems, but also to provide additional dimensions of spectral selectivity that are useful for differentiation between compounds with similar fragmentation patterns (35). Referred to as MS^n (most commonly MS/MS when $n = 2$), these approaches are analogous to GC column switching because they provide the means for adding further, selective MS-separation dimensions to the analysis. The basic MS/MS scan sequence (40) involves (a) ion creation, (b) ion selection, (c) ion dissociation, and (d) mass analysis. Ion creation can occur via either EI or CI. The selection step involves selective isolation (similar to SIS) of a user-specified ion that is characteristic of the target compound (the parent ion). After isolation, the parent ion is dissociated into product ions that are monitored during mass analysis. In order to account for variability in how target compounds may fragment, ion traps can utilize one of two different collision induced dissociation (CID) techniques: resonant excitation or dipole ion excitation. Although well characterized by simple GC/MS (41), an example of ion trap GC/MS/MS of a coffee sample is shown in Figure 12. In this case, the ion at m/z = 128 was chosen as the parent ion, and resonant CID was used. The parent ion was chosen to screen for 2[(methylthio)methyl]-Furan at m/z = 128 and the characteristic fragment ion in the inset spectrum (m/z = 81) is the result of a well-known fragmentation pathway (Fig. 13). The further dimensions implied by the term MS^n (with $n > 2$) are created by inserting additional isolation and dissociation sequences prior to mass analysis. Regardless of the dimension number used for MS^n, however, its analytical benefits include greater spectral selectivity, lower detection limits, and a reduction in both chromatographic requirements and the need for prior sample cleanup.

D. MS Acquisition Programming

For the ion trap to be a useful part of a GC/MS system, it must have some way of controlling not only how, but when its unique capabilities are applied. The following ion trap features make the advanced MS capabilities of commercial ion trap GC/MS instruments easily available for routine analyses.

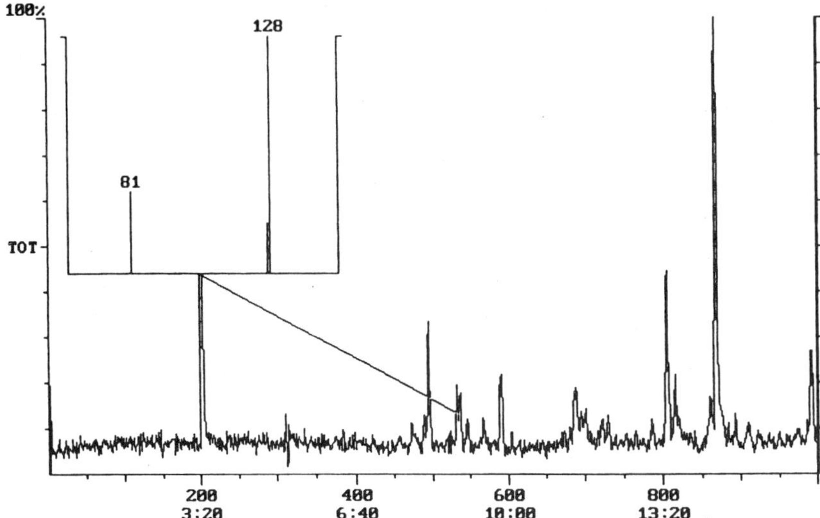

FIGURE 12 Ion trap GC/MS/MS of a coffee sample. The parent ion selected for MS/MS was at m/z = 128. Resonant CID was used to produce the product ion spectrum (inset).

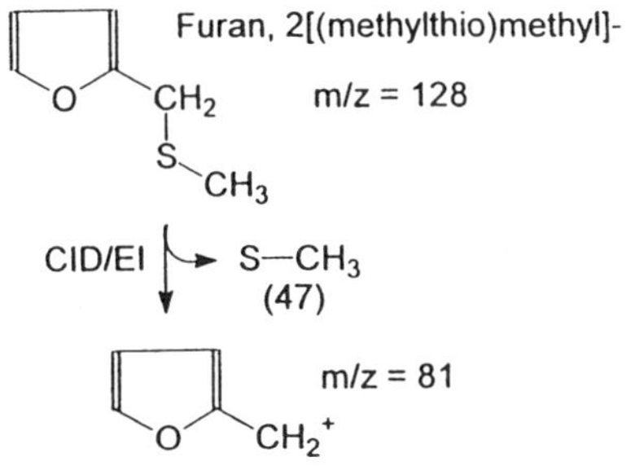

Furan, 2[(methylthio)methyl]-

CH_2 m/z = 128

S

CH_3

CID/EI → S—CH_3 (47)

m/z = 81

O CH_2^+

FIGURE 13 Reaction pathway for the ion trap GC/MS/MS spectrum shown (inset) in Figure 12.

1. Programmable Acquisition Segments

The fact that aroma samples can contain hundreds of compounds of interest, each one potentially requiring its own selective ion trap MS method, makes it essential to be able to operationally change between MS techniques during the course of the chromatographic run. Modern computer systems, combined with the use of direct interface ion trap GC/MS systems, allow the analyst to switch between ionization modes (EI and CI) and both standard and advanced scan sequences (42). MS method programming in chromatographic time is an essential part of most target compound screening methods.

2. Automated Methods Development

One of the most analyte-dependent, and thus variable, portions of an ion trap GC/MS method is the CID step of the MS/MS sequence. The CID voltage should be optimized to produce the desired amount of analyte fragmentation. The automated methods development (AMD) technique (43) allows the CID voltage to be changed on a scan-by-scan basis during compound elution. Examination of the spectra from a single AMD analysis can be used for MS/MS method optimization. AMD allowed for optimization of resonant CID for a MS/MS method in Figure 14. The parent ion (m/z = 173) in this example could be seen in the upper left spectrum, where no resonant CID (voltage = 0) was applied (MS/MS isolation only). For each successive MS/MS scan, the CID voltage was increased by an increment of 0.2 V (results shown in the inset spectra) up to a maximum of 1.6 V. As the voltage was increased, the parent ion fragmented into characteristic product ions (e.g., 127 and 99). Different AMD methods can be applied throughout the chromatographic run, greatly simplifying MS/MS methods development for complex target screening analyses.

3. Unit Mass Selective Ion Storage

Because of the relationships between mass and frequency, the SIS technique (based solely on waveform ejection using resonant frequencies) cannot provide unit mass isolation across the operational mass range of the ion trap. In the majority of cases, the small number of unwanted additional ions stored does not affect the storage efficiency and, thus, the analytical performance of SIS. In cases where a major contaminant ion exists near the m/z of an analyte ion, however, unit mass isolation may be desirable. In these cases, the two-step isolation technique used for MS/MS (40) can be used for selective ion storage (39). Unit mass selective ion storage (uSIS) provides the capability to isolate ions of a single m/z regardless of the m/z of interest. The technique can be se-

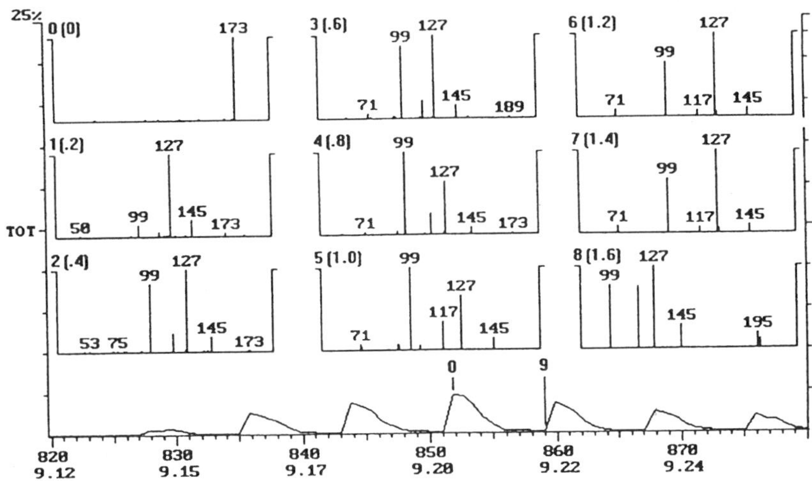

FIGURE 14 An example AMD application allowing the optimum MS/MS CID voltage to be determined. The parent ion (m/z = 173) in this example is shown in the upper left spectrum, where no resonant CID (voltage = 0) was applied. The voltage was increased in increments of 0.2 V (results shown in the spectra inset).

quentially applied (i.e., AMD) to provide the capability of monitoring multiple ions; the current commercial maximum is 10 m/z (or 10 ranges of m/z), and the spectral data can be easily merged for reduction and quantitation.

4. Multiple Reaction Monitoring

The same sequential (scan-to-scan) application of MS methods used by AMD and uSIS can be implemented for ion trap MS/MS methods. While programmable acquisition segments allow MS/MS methods to be applied in chromatographic time (i.e., for the duration of a GC peak), peak co-elution requires a higher degree of MS/MS method variability. MRM provides the capability to conduct sequential MS/MS scans for up to 10 different parent ions. Because high-resolution capillary GC is often used for food aroma analyses, however, the ability to scan for 10 different compounds is rarely required. The most frequent use of multiple reaction monitoring consists of an application known as isotopically labeled internal standards (ILIS). In this application, the sample is spiked with a known amount of an isotopically labeled internal standard, which coelutes with the compound of interest. The analysis in Figure 15 con-

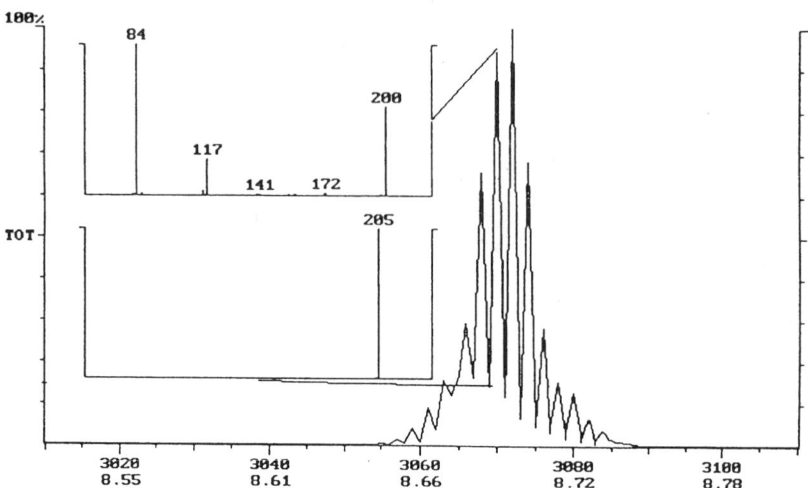

FIGURE 15 MRM analysis consisting of two alternating scans: MS/MS analysis where the parent ion at m/z = 200 was isolated and dissociated (top spectrum), and MS/MS isolation of a deuterated form (D5) of the paren tion (m/z = 205, bottom spectrum).

sisted of two alternating MS scans that were applied during the elution of the peak shown: (a) MS/MS analysis, where the parent ion at m/z = 200 was isolated and dissociated (top spectrum), and (b) MS/MS isolation of a deuterated form (D5) of the parent ion (m/z = 205, bottom spectrum). These types of techniques, when used to sequentially analyze for both the target compound and an internal standard, provide excellent qualitative and quantitative data.

ACKNOWLEDGMENTS

The advanced MS "ion-preparation" techniques of the quadrupole ion trap described in this chapter are the result of more than 6 years of collaborative instrumental research and development that involved the expertise of a number of key chemists, engineers, and programmers. It has been a pleasure to be associated with these individuals and to be a part of these technological developments.

Data illustrating various ion trap GC/MS analyses of orange extract were acquired using a *Saturn 2000 GC/MS System* (Varian Chromatography Systems, Walnut Creek, CA) by Dr. Robert D. Brittain. Analyses of beer and coffee samples were conducted by Dr. John R. Berg and Dr. Charles K. Huston. Dr. Zelda Penton provided the analyses of wine.

REFERENCES

1. G. Vernin, C. Boniface, J. Metzger, D. Fraisse, D. Doan, and S. Alamercery, Aromas of Syrah wines: identification of volatile compounds by GC-MS-spectral data bank and classification by statistical methods, *Dev. Food Sci. 17:*655 (1988).
2. A. Rozenblum and P. Brunerie, Automatic processing of GC-MS analysis using a two-dimensional search system, *Dev. Food Sci. 35:*133 (1994).
3. F. W. McLafferty, *Interpretation of Mass Spectra*, University Science Books, Mill Valley, CA, 1980.
4. R. E. March and R. J. Hughes, *Quadrupole Storage Mass Spectrometry*, John Wiley & Sons, New York, 1989.
5. R. E. March and J. F. J. Todd, *Practical Aspects of Ion Trap Mass Spectrometry—Volume II: Ion Trap Instrumentation*, CRC Press, Inc., Boca Raton, FL, 1995.
6. R. E. March and J. F. J. Todd, *Practical Aspects of Ion Trap Mass Spectrometry—Volume I: Fundamentals of Ion Trap Mass Spectrometry*, CRC Press, Inc., Boca Raton, FL, 1995.
7. R. E. March and J. F. J. Todd, *Practical Aspects of Ion Trap Mass Spectrometry—Volume III: Chemical, Environmental, and Biomedical Applications of Ion Trap Mass Spectrometry*, CRC Press, Inc., Boca Raton, FL, 1995.
8. C. K. Huston and H. Ji, Optimization of the Analytical Supercritical Extraction of Cloves via an On-Column Interface to an Ion Trap GC/MS System, *J. Agric. Food Chem. 39(7):*1229 (1991).
9. F. W. Karasek and R. E. Clement, *Basic Gas Chromatography—Mass Spectrometry, Principles and Techniques*, Elsevier, Amsterdam, 1988.
10. R. F. Severson and O. T. Chortyk, Open split interface for capillary GC/MS, *Anal. Chem. 56:*1533 (1984).
11. C. Feigel and W. Holmes, Direct split interface for analysis of volatile organic compounds, *GC/MS Application Note #19*, Varian Chromatography Systems, Walnut Creek, CA, 1992.
12. R. D. Brittain, Determination of EPA methods 524.2, 624, and 8260 analytes with an open split interface to the Saturn GC/MS, *GC/MS Application Note #16*, Varian Chromatography Systems, Walnut Creek, CA, 1991.
13. G. Arora, F. Cormier, and B. Lee, Analysis of odor-active volatiles in cheddar cheese headspace by multidimensional GC/MS/sniffing, *J. Agric. Food Chem. 43(3):*748 (1995).
14. E. J. Brunke, P. Mair, and F. J. Hammerschmidt, Volatiles form naranjilla fruit (Solanum quitoense Lam.). GC/MS analysis and sensory evaluation using sniffing GC, *J. Agric. Food Chem. 37(3):*746 (1989).
15. A. G. Harrison, *Chemical Ionization Mass Spectrometry*, CRC Press, Inc., Boca Raton, FL, 1992.

16. C. P. R. Jennison and J. Jennison, The Determination of Trace Level FAMES Using CI Mode GC/MS, *GC/MS Application Note #37*, Varian Chromatography Systems, Walnut Creek, CA, 1993.
17. C. K. Huston, Manipulation of ion trap parameters to maximize compound-specific information in gas chromatographic-mass spectrometric analyses, *J. Chromatogr. 606:*203 (1992).
18. F. Tateo, A. Ferrillo, and A. Orlandi, Correlation between aromatic qualities and GC-MS composition of ready-made tomato sauces, *Dev. Food Sci. 35:*107 (1994).
19. F. Tateo, N. Brunelli, S. Cucurachi, and A. Ferrillo, New trends in the study of the merits and shortcomings of olive oil in organoleptic terms, in correlation with the GC/MS analysis of the aromas, *Dev. Food Sci. 32:*301 (1993).
20. S. Mandeville, V. Yaylayan, and B. Simpson, GC/MS analysis of flavor-active compounds in cooked commercial shrimp, *J. Agric. Food Chem. 40(7):*1275 (1992).
21. B. Klein, Comparison of four extraction, concentration and injection techniques for volatile compounds analysis by GC-MS: an application to the study of the volatile flavor of Swiss Emmentaler cheese, Proceedings, 6th Weurman Symposium on Flavour Science Technology (A. F. Thomas, ed.), J. Wiley & Sons, 1990, p. 205.
22. Z. Penton, Characterization of flavor components in wines with solid phase microextraction (SPME), GC and GC/MS, *SPME Application Note #3*, Varian Chromatography Systems, Walnut Creek, CA, 1995.
23. Z. Penton, Characterization of flavor components in wines with solid phase microextraction (SPME), GC and GC/MS, *SPME Application Note #6*, Varian Chromatography Systems, Walnut Creek, CA, 1995.
24. A. Bouseta, S. Collin, and J. P. Dufour, Characteristic aroma profiles of unifloral honeys obtained with a dynamic headspace GC-MS System, *J. Apic. Res. 31:*96 (1992).
25. R. Barcarolo, P. Casson, and C. Tutta, Analysis of the volatile constituents of food by headspace GC-MS with reversal of the carrier flow during sampling, *J. High Resol. Chromatogr. 15(5):*307 (1992).
26. R. D. Brittain and N. A. Kirchen, Determination of volatile organic compounds in water with the Saturn GC/MS, *GC/MS Appliction Note #8*, Varian Chromatography Systems, Walnut Creek, CA, 1992.
27. E. Almasi and N. Kirshen, The determination of volatile organic compounds (VOC's) in air by the TO-14 method using the Saturn II GC/MS system, *GC/MS Application Note #18*, Varian Chromatography Systems, Walnut Creek, CA, 1992.
28. A. L. Boyko, M. E. Morgan, and L. M. Libbey, Porous polymer trapping for GC/MS analysis of vegetable flavors, Proceedings, Anal. Foods Beverages (George Charalambous, ed.), Academic Press, 1978, p. 57.
29. A. Kaipainen, A study of the aroma profiles of non-alcoholic beer by thermal

desorption and GC-MS, *J. High Resol. Chromatogr. 15(11):*751 (1992).

30. M. B. Wise, C. V. Thompson, and M. R. Guerin, Real-time determination of volatile organic compounds in air and water using direct sampling ion trap mass spectrometry, Proceedings—42nd ASMS Conference, Chicago, IL, 1994.
31. M. Woerner and P. Schreier, Multidimensional gas chromatography/mass spectrometry (MDGC/MS): a powerful tool for the direct chiral evaluation of aroma compounds in plant tissues. III. (1S)-(-)-2-endo-Acetyxy-3-exo-hydroxybornane (vulgarole) in mugwort (Artemisia vulgaris L.) herb, Pytochem. Anal. 2(6):260 (1991).
32. L. Jirovetz, W. Jaeger, and G. Remberg, Analysis of the volatiles in the seed oil of Hibiscus sabdariffa (Malvaceae) by means of GC-MS and GC-FTIR, *J. Agric. Food Chem. 40(7):*1186 (1992).
33. W. Pfannhauser, R. Kellner, and G. Fischboek, GC/FTIR and GC/MS analysis of kiwi flavors, *Dev. Food Sci., 24:*357 (1990).
34. G. C. Galletti, A. Carnacini, P. Bocchini, and A. Antonelli, Chemical composition of wood casks for wine ageing as determined by pyrolysis/GC/MS, *Rapid Commun. Mass Spectrom. 9:*1331 (1995).
35. K. L. Busch and G. L. Glish, *Mass Spectrometry/Mass Spectrometry: Techniques and Applictions of Tandem Mass Spectrometry*, VCH Publishers, New York, 1988.
36. C. K. Huston, B. Bolton, M. Wang, and G. Wells, Chemical ionization in ion trap GC-MS using selective ion ejection techniques, Proceedings—41st ASMS Conference, San Francisco, CA, 1993.
37. C. Huston and G. Wells, Reagent ion selected chemical ionization in ion trap GC-MS, Proceedings—42nd ASMS Conference, Chicago, IL, 1994.
38. G. Wells and C. Huston, Field-modulated selective ion storage in a quadrupole ion trap, *J. Am. Soc. Mass Spectrom. 6:*928 (1995).
39. G. Wells and C. Huston, High resolution selected ion monitoring in a quadrupole ion trap mass spectrometer, *Anal. Chem. 67(20):*3650 (1995).
40. S. Schachterle, R. D. Brittain, and J. D. Mills, Analysis of pesticide residues in food using gas chromatograph-tandem mass spectrometry with a benchtop ion trap mass spectrometer, *J. Chromatogr. 683:*185 (1994).
41. M. Shimoda and T. Shibamoto, Isolation and identification of headspace volatiles from brewed coffee with an on-column GC/MS method, *J. Agric. Food Chem. 38(3):*802 (1990).
42. O. D. Sparkman and R. D. Brittain, Programmable acquisition of tune events in ion trap gas chromatography/mass spectrometry, Proceedings—42nd ASMS Conference, Chicago, IL, 1994.
43. G. Wells and C. Huston, High speed method optimization for routine GC/MS/MS in an ion trap, Proceedings—43rd ASMS Conference, Atlanta, GA, 1995.

8

Off-Flavors and Malodors in Foods: Mechanisms of Formation and Analytical Techniques

RAY MARSILI
Dean Foods Company, Rockford, Illinois

I. INTRODUCTION

The chemicals responsible for off-flavors and malodors in foods and beverages can originate from incidental contamination from environmental (outside) sources (e.g., air, water, or packaging material) and from chemical reactions occurring within the food material itself (e.g., lipid oxidation, enzymatic action, microbial metabolic reactions). In addition, "imbalance" off-flavors can occur when certain ingredient components that are normally present and often essential to the product are present in abnormally high or low concentrations.

No type of food or beverage product is immune to off-flavor development. When the problem does occur, several questions should be answered as quickly as possible: What is the mechanism of formation? Is it an isolated problem caused by a single case of product abuse by one customer, or is it the result of processing, ingredient, packaging, or microbiological problems involving an entire production run and requiring significant product recalls? Does the off-flavor signal a problem that is a potential threat to public health? Has the same type of malodor occurred in the past? What is the likelihood that the problem will reoccur in the future, and can it be prevented? Answers to these questions can avoid expensive product recalls and minimize damage to a food processor's reputation.

The purpose of this chapter is to illustrate a few examples of the types of food taints and to show how the analytical techniques presented earlier in this book can be used to elucidate their mechanism of formation.

II. PACKAGING

A. Residual Packaging Solvents

Ironically, packaging materials, which are designed to preserve the freshness and flavor of foods and beverages, can actually be directly responsible for causing flavor defects. Although plastic packaging material consists primarily of nonvolatile high molecular weight polymers, volatile low molecular weight compounds are often added to improve functional properties of the materials: plastizers to improve flexibility, antioxidants to prevent oxidation of the plastic polymers or the food inside the packaging, and UV blockers to prevent "yellowing" of polymeric material when it is exposed to light. Additional additives include polymerization accelerators, cross-linking agents, antistatic chemicals, and lubricants (1).

Occasionally packaging materials are not adequately cured before they are used, and a small amount of solvent associated with the manufacturing of the packaging materials remains. Residual solvents in packaging materials can migrate into food products, imparting malodors and off-flavors (2). For example, Goldenberg and Matheson (3) reported that residual styrene monomer from polystyrene trays was responsible for imparting "plastic" off-flavors to chocolate and lemon cookies and frozen TV dinners.

1. Solvents from Inks and Dyes

Several examples of food malodors caused by solvents from packaging material have been reported. In one example, cardboard boxes (46 cm × 25 cm × 25 cm) filled with several dozen 3-g packets of nondairy coffee creamer were contaminated with a highly objectionable odor. The packets were a paper polyfoil material (flexible web). No contamination of the actual nondairy creamer was observed.

To determine the chemical responsible for the musty odor, the atmosphere in the box was sampled at four different locations with a gas-tight syringe. Four 5-ml injections were piggy-backed to give a total injection volume of 20 ml. Each of the 5-ml gas samples was injected onto a gas chromatography (GC) column (DB-5, 30 m × 0.25 mm, 1 μm film thickness). Volatiles were cryofocused in a narrow band by cooling a small portion of the front end of the capillary column to –100°C with liquid nitrogen. Cryofocusing permitted large-volume injections of air samples and provided sharp, well-defined chromatographic peaks. Three minutes after the last air samples were injected, the cryofocusing device was heated to 200°C to initiate injection into the analytical column.

The effluent from the capillary column was split (50:50) between an ion trap (mass spectrometry) detector and an olfactory detector (sniff port). Peaks were identified by mass spectrometry, and their aromas were determined by olfactometry. Several solvent peaks were observed in the air from the boxes with the malodor but not in control samples (previous lots of boxes of samples with no malodor). The largest peak in the chromatogram of the boxes with the malodor was 1,3,5-trimethylbenzene (mesitylene). The odor of the peak was determined by sniffing the effluent of the olfactory detector and proved to be identical to the malodor of the complaint samples.

According to the packaging supplier, the ink used for packaging graphics had been changed recently. Analysis of the new ink showed it contained high levels of trimethylbenzenes. The original ink was used in subsequent production runs, and the malodor problem never reoccurred.

GC/mass spectroscopy (MS) static headspace analysis with a gas-tight syringe is rapid and useful for the qualitative identification of chemicals responsible for off-flavors and malodors. However, the technique using gas-tight syringes is not recommended for quantitative work because volatiles may condense in the syringe body or needle. Specifically designed commercially available GC injection systems for static headspace analysis allow for accurate reproductibility and quantitation and have been previously described (4–7).

2. Solvents from Packaging Films

Another example of a food off-flavor from solvent packaging material occurred with half-and-half packaged in 13-ml polystyrene cups. Normal-tasting control samples and samples with a "chemical, solventlike" off-flavor were analyzed by purge-and-trap GC/MS. Five-gram samples were purged at room temperature for 20 minutes; volatiles were trapped on a Tenax TA column, desorbed at 180°C, and cryofocused at −100°C prior to injection onto a DB-5 capillary column (30 m × 0.25 mm. 1 μm film thickness) using the same olfactometry/MS detection configuration described above.

As shown in Figure 1, the most significant differences in the chromatograms of control and tainted samples were an increase in the acetone levels and the presence of a significant propylacetate peak in the tainted samples. The odor of the propylacetate peak was characterized with the sniff port and judged to be similar to the sample's odor defect.

The packaging lidstock consisted of three layers: an outer paper layer impregnated with water-based inks, a middle metal-foil layer and an inner plastic film used for heat sealing. The inner heat-seal film, which is actuated by heat and pressure to seal the lid to the cup, is applied to the foil as slurry and dried. The solvent used by the packaging supplier to form the slurry was propylacetate. After application of the plastic film to the foil, sheets of the lidstock material pass through drying ovens to remove all residual propylacetate solvent. According to the packaging supplier's specifications, the lidstock should contain less than 1000 mg propylacetate per 3000 sq. ft. of material. After the problem was reported to the packaging supplier, quality control specifications were more closely monitored and no further off-flavors occurred.

B. Absorption of Flavor Chemicals by Packaging Materials (Scalping)

Another problem that can occur when inappropriate packaging is selected for specific food applications is a phenomenon referred to as scalping—the absorption of flavor-important chemicals from the food product into the packaging material. This problem has been observed, for example, in orange juice. Weak flavor in orange juice can result from many sources, including poor quality and perhaps even adulterated frozen concentrate, overheating of juice during processing, and scalping of flavorful orange oil components by carton packaging material.

Numerous chemicals, including monoterpenes, sesquiterpenes, aldehydes, and other oxygenated compounds, contribute to the distinctive flavor of fresh orange juice. These chemicals possess a wide range of volatility—from acetaldehyde and ethylbutyrate, two chemicals associated with the fresh-squeezed flavor of orange juice, to tetradecyl aldehyde and valencene, a sesquiterpene. Analyzing chemicals with such a wide range of boiling points and concentrations is challenging. Numerous isolation and concentration tech-

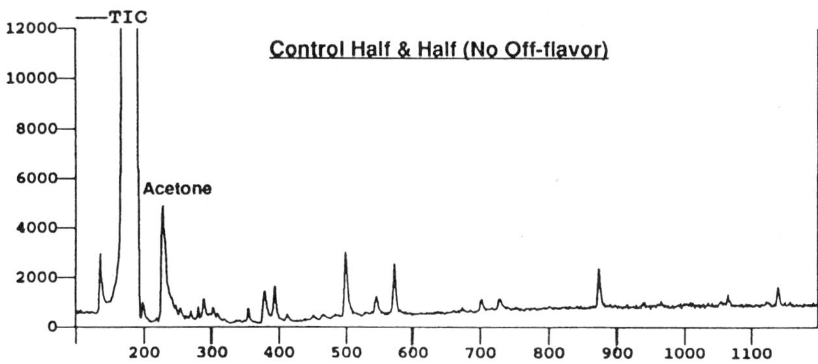

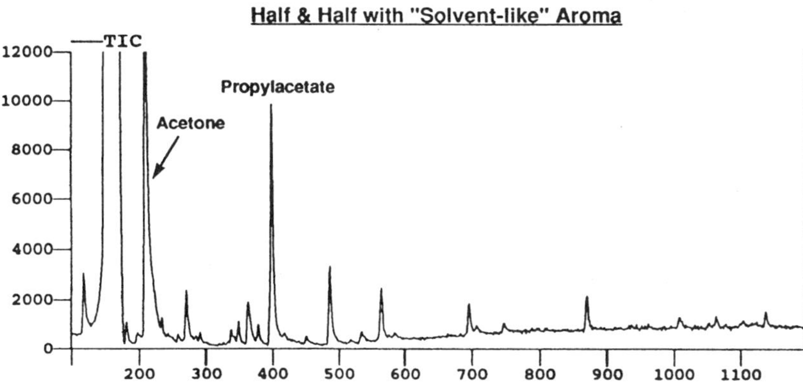

FIGURE 1 Chromatograms of control (normal tasting) and complaint half-and-half samples analyzed by purge-and-trap GC/MS. Five-gram samples were purged at room temperature for 20 minutes. Propyl acetate, a solvent contaminant from packaging material, is the primary chemical responsible for the complaint sample's malodor/off-flavor.

niques prior to GC analysis have been used to analyze flavor-contributing chemicals in orange juice, including purge and trap, vacuum distillation, simultaneous distillation–solvent extraction (SDE) and solvent extraction.

Purge-and-trap methods with Tenax traps do not work well because the extremely volatile polar components are difficult to trap at high recovery rates, and the highest boilers are not volatile enough to be purged from the juice in sufficient quantities for detection. Applying distillation-based methods to the analysis of volatiles in high-sugar samples can lead to artifact formation and alterations in the quantitative relationships of volatiles.

Bicchi et al. (8) were among the first researchers to emphasize the importance of preextracting flavor volatiles from sugars prior to heating. For quantitating organic volatiles in honey, Bousita and Collin more recently proposed a two-step protocol, including preliminary dichloromethane extraction in an inert atmosphere followed by simultaneous steam distillation of the dichloromethane extract (9).

Another strategy that is well suited to the analysis of volatiles in high-sugar samples like orange juice is to use solvent extraction for higher–boiling point components (i.e., limonene and higher boilers) and static headspace at room temperature for extremely volatile components (e.g., acetaldehyde, ethanol, ethyl acetate, ethyl butyrate, *trans*-2-hexenal, and hexanal).

A chromatogram of an ethanol/pentane extract of orange juice is shown in Figure 2 (10). Orange oil components in the extract were concentrated by evaporating the volume of pentane solvent from 3 ml to approximately 75 μl. 1,2,4-Trimethyl benzene was used as an internal standard. Analysis of orange juice spiked with various levels of orange oil components showed the method was quantitative, with percent recoveries of 93% or higher for all 13 components tested. (α-Pinene was the most volatile compound tested by solvent extraction.)

Solvent-extraction methods have been used to optimize packaging choices for orange juice. For example, shelf-life experiments with various types of cartons revealed that flavor-important aldehydes were readily absorbed by "juice board" (paper board sandwiched between two layers of low-density polyethylene) but were absorbed to a lesser extent and at a slower rate by "barrier board" (paper board sandwiched between two layers of low-density polyethylene with an inner layer of ethylene vinyl alcohol copolymer). Also, compared to storage in glass and barrier board, samples stored in the more permeable juice board allowed higher levels of atmospheric oxygen to penetrate, and they developed higher concentrations of carvone, carveol, and α-terpineol—oxidation/degradation products of limonene known to contribute off-flavors to orange juice.

This type of analytical testing allows food manufacturers to judiciously select appropriate packaging materials for their products. In general, the more effective the barrier, the higher the cost of the packaging material. Food processors can use analytical studies in combination with organoleptic taste panels to objectively determine how much product deterioration or scalping has occurred, how much can be tolerated, and how much barrier protection will be re-

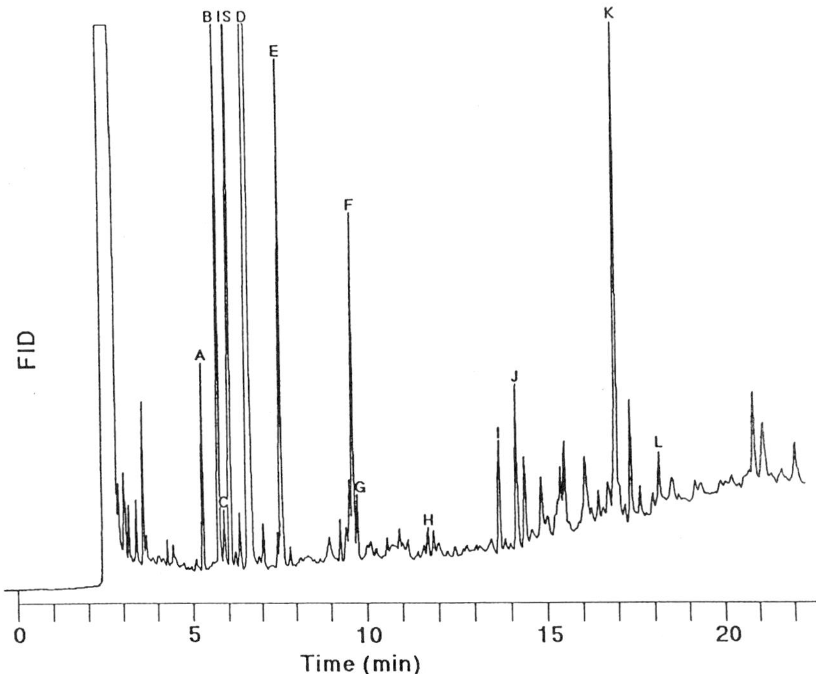

Figure 2 Chromatogram of an ethanol/pentane extract of orange juice (after concentration with nitrogen stream). Solvent extraction is a simple and rapid sample preparation technique for studying scalping of desirable flavor chemicals by packaging materials. Peak identities are as follows: A = α-pinene (0.31 ppm); B = myrcene (2.33 ppm); C = octanal (0.12 ppm); IS = internal standard (6.00 ppm 1,2,4-trimethylbenzene); D = limonene (109.5 ppm); E = linalool (1.12 ppm); F = decanal (1.69 ppm); G = α-terpineol (0.15 ppm); H = carvone (0.13 ppm); I = dodecanal (0.48 ppm); J = caryophellene (0.53 ppm); K = valencene (1.85 ppm); L = tetradecyl aldehyde (0.22 ppm).

quired. Investing in insufficient barrier protection can cause off-flavors, but spending more than is necessary for barrier protection is a waste of money.

Static headspace GC techniques have been used to monitor chemical changes in orange juice stored in glass containers for various time periods in the dark and when exposed to fluorescent light (4). Although loss of flavor chemicals through scalping would not occur in glass containers, flavor loss was still noted in the light-exposed samples. The most significant trend observed in the chemical data was the loss of acetaldehyde, an important aroma chemical, in samples exposed to light.

Like all analytical techniques, static headspace methods have their biases, shortcomings, and limitations. Analyzing limonene in orange juice by static headspace methods seems like a good idea. Limonene, which accounts for approximately 90–95% of the composition of orange oil, appears to be a good candidate for static headspace analysis since it has a relatively low boiling point and is present in relatively high concentrations. In practice, however, obtaining accurate, reproducible quantitative results for limonene in orange juice by headspace techniques is difficult (11).

For accurate quantitation with static headspace, the analyte should be an ideal dilute solution (7). Under these conditions, gas phase equilibrium can be attained, the activity coefficient of the analyte is constant, and a linear detector response results when standards of increasing concentration are analyzed. (The method-of-additions calibration technique is the preferred calibration method for headspace analysis of food systems.) In orange juice, limonene is present as an emulsion at concentration levels that exceed the solubility limit in the liquid phase. As a result, the vapor concentration is independent of the liquid concentration, and the peak area are in a vapor sample is no longer sensitive to the concentration in the liquid. For this reason, quantitative analysis of limonene by static headspace is inadvisable.

III. LIGHT-INDUCED OFF-FLAVORS

Milk is highly susceptible to formation of off-flavors and malodors. One reason for this is that milk's bland taste does a poor job masking off-flavors. Another reason is that the primary components of milk—lactose, casein, whey proteins, and milkfat—are not only good substrates for microorganism growth, which can generate off-flavor metabolites, but are also subject to degradation by exogenous enzymes, heat, and/or light. Shipe et al. (12) have listed seven descriptors of off-flavors in milk based on causes: heated, lipolyzed, microbial, transmitted (from feed and weeds), light-induced, oxidized, and miscellaneous.

Light-induced off-flavors, undoubtedly the most common flavor defect in milk, have two distinct components. Initially a burnt, activated sunlight flavor develops and predominates for about 2 or 3 days. Degradation of sulfur-containing amino acids of the serum (whey) proteins has been blamed for this reaction. The second component is attributed to lipid oxidation. This off-flavor, often characterized as metallic or cardboardy, usually develops after 2 days and does not dissipate.

The increasing use of high-density polyethylene (HDPE) milk jugs has promoted the occurrence of light-induced off-flavors. Exposure of milk in blow-mold plastic containers to the fluorescent lights of supermarket dairy cases is responsible for the development of light-induced off-flavors in some 80% of store samples (13).

As illustrated in Figure 3, autoxidation of unsaturated fatty acids involves a free radical reaction, forming fat hydroperoxides and various malodorous ketones and aldehydes (6)—e.g., hexanal in the case of linoleic acid (14). Singlet oxygen, metal catalysts, heat, and light are all possible initiators of the chain reaction.

A. Oxidation of Milkfat

In resolving off-flavor problems in foods, it is important to consider not only agents that may be initiating off-flavor chemical reactions, but also subtle compositional changes that may have occurred in the food product (i.e., the substrate) to enhance off-flavor development.

In one study, for example, several milk samples from one geographical

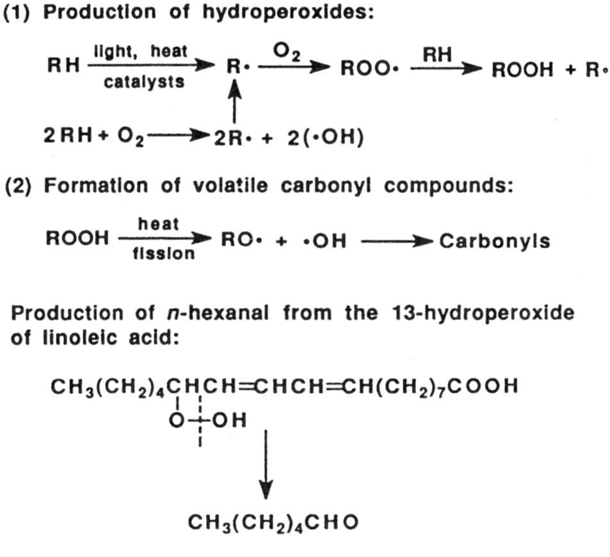

(1) Production of hydroperoxides:

$$RH \xrightarrow[\text{catalysts}]{\text{light, heat}} R\cdot \xrightarrow{O_2} ROO\cdot \xrightarrow{RH} ROOH + R\cdot$$

$$2RH + O_2 \longrightarrow 2R\cdot + 2(\cdot OH)$$

(2) Formation of volatile carbonyl compounds:

$$ROOH \xrightarrow[\text{fission}]{\text{heat}} RO\cdot + \cdot OH \longrightarrow \text{Carbonyls}$$

Production of *n*-hexanal from the 13-hydroperoxide of linoleic acid:

$$CH_3(CH_2)_4\underset{\substack{|\\O-OH}}{C}HCH{=}CHCH{=}CH(CH_2)_7COOH$$

$$\downarrow$$

$$CH_3(CH_2)_4CHO$$

Figure 3 Production of malodorous carbonyl compounds from the reaction of light and oxygen with unsaturated fatty acids.

region were analyzed by purge-and-trap GC/MS to determine the source of the severe off-flavor characterized as "oxidized" by dairy technologists. Purge-and-trap analysis revealed unusually high concentrations of hexanal, suggesting autoxidation of linoleic acid in milkfat. The off-flavor problem had occurred during winter months for the previous 4 years but was getting progressively worse each successive year. Because the level of hexanal was so high, copper contamination from processing lines or from diet supplements was initially suspected as the source of activation/catalysis. Previous studies of milk samples intentionally abused by UV light exposure and contact with copper revealed that hexanal levels tend to be significantly higher when prooxidant metals are involved than when milk is light-abused without added prooxidant metals.

Further testing of "bad" milk samples by atomic absorption spectrometry ruled out contamination by copper, nickel, or iron. Another suspected contributing factor was lack of naturally occurring antioxidants (e.g., α-tocopheral) due to changes in winter feed regimens. However, high-performance liquid chromatography (HPLC) analysis showed samples contained normal levels of α-tocopherol.

When fatty acid profiles of complaint and normal milk samples were compared, samples with the intense oxidized off-flavor consistently contained 200–300% more linoleic acid than normal-tasting milk from different geographical areas. Linoleic acid (C18:2) is highly susceptible to photooxidation.

The high linoleic acid content was traced to the cows' diet. Dairy farmers in this region had been feeding cows increasingly high levels of soybeans each year. Feeding high levels of soybeans has been shown to increase milkfat's linoleic acid content and make milk more susceptible to oxidation than usual (14). This problem can be corrected by regulating levels of unsaturated lipids in feed to decrease the proportion of unsaturated fat in milkfat. Resolution of this important off-flavor problem involved not only protecting milk from UV light sources, but also modifying the food substrate by altering the feeding regimen of the cows.

B. Degradation of Proteins

Milk isn't the only dairy product that can develop light-induced off-flavors. Figure 4 shows chromatograms of a normal-tasting control sample of vanilla ice cream and one that had a strong "putrid, burnt-feather" odor. For this analysis, 10 g of sample plus 20 ml of distilled water were purged at room temperature. Volatiles were trapped on Tenax TA and analyzed by GC/MS after desorption onto a 30 m × 0.25 mm DB-5 capillary column.

A large peak identified by mass spectrometry as dimethyl disulfide was

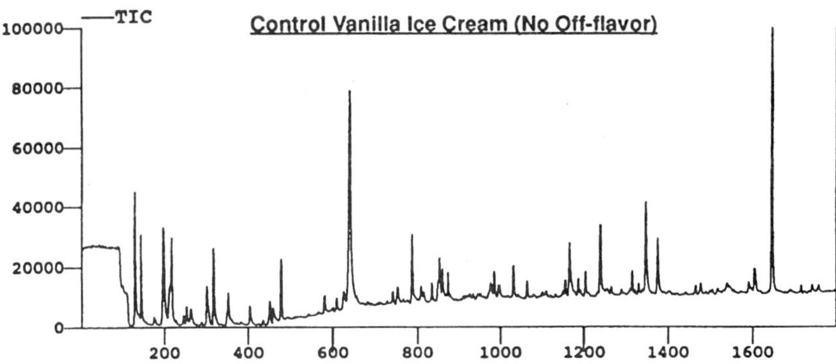

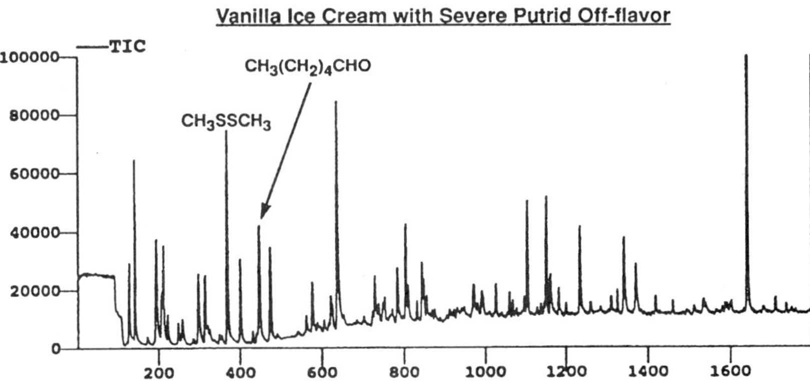

FIGURE 4 Chromatograms of control (no off-flavor) and complaint (putrid) vanilla ice cream samples, showing hexanal (from reaction of light with linoleic acid) and dimethyl disulfide (from reaction of light with dairy protein components). The dimethyl disulfide is the major contributor to the complaint sample's off flavor. Samples were analyzed by purge-and-trap GC/MS. Ten grams of sample were diluted with 20 ml of water and purged for 20 minutes at room temperature.

detected in the foul sample. Olfactometry revealed the peak had an intense cabbage, burnt-feather aroma. UV radiation exposure of methionine in the presence of riboflavin and oxygen generates methional (potato odor), which further degrades to methanethiol, dimethyl sulfide, and dimethyl disulfide—all of which can contribute a cabbage or burnt-feather–type aroma. Free radicals derived from methionine, methional, and cysteine can combine to form the three odiferous sulfur compounds shown in Figure 5 (15). A significant increase in the level of hexanal in complaint samples compared to control samples provided further evidence that complaint samples had been light-abused.

Careful inspection of the warehouse storage conditions revealed that samples were stored in close proximity to high intensity lights. Lighting adjustments were made, and the problem was easily and quickly remedied.

Light-induced off-flavors have been reported in numerous nondairy food systems. For example, Tressl et al. (16) demonstrated that the "skunky" off-flavor sometimes observed in beer is attributed to light-catalyzed degradation of the isohumulones.

IV. MICROBIOLOGICAL OFF-FLAVORS

A. Metabolites from Growth of Bacteria and Molds

Microorganisms can cause off-flavors in foods in numerous ways. The most common way is by contributing malodorous chemicals produced as metabolites during their growth phase in food materials.

Fish and milk are highly susceptible to microbial-induced off-flavors. The "fishy" off-flavor associated with stale fish is the result of trimethylamine production via a bacterial enzymatic reduction reaction with trimethylamine oxide, a naturally occurring constituent of fish muscle (17). Intense malodors that occur during later stages of spoilage are caused by a variety of nitrogen- and sulfur-containing compounds associated with putrefaction reactions.

Postpasteurization contamination of milk with psychotrophic bacteria—bacteria that can grow at refrigerated temperatures—is a common cause of off-flavors in milk. Raw milk contaminated with psychrotrophic bacteria prior to pasteurization can even cause malodor problems. While pasteurization destroys the bacteria, their heat-stable lipases and proteases sometimes survive, and the action of these extracellular enzymes on milk components can also generate off-flavors.

Some characteristic off-flavor notes in milk are associated with specific psychotrophic bacteria. For example, contamination by *Pseudomonas fragi*, a psychotrophic gram-negative organism, often causes "fruity" off-notes in milk. Initially a lipase from this bacteria hydrolyzes short-chain fatty acids from milkfat; other *Pseudomonas fragi* enzymes then convert the acids to ethyl esters (ethyl butyrate and ethyl hexanoate) (18). A malty off-flavor in milk can occur when 3-methyl butanal is produced from the conversion of leucine by *Streptococcus lactis* subsp. *maltigenes* or *Lactobacillus malaromicus* (19).

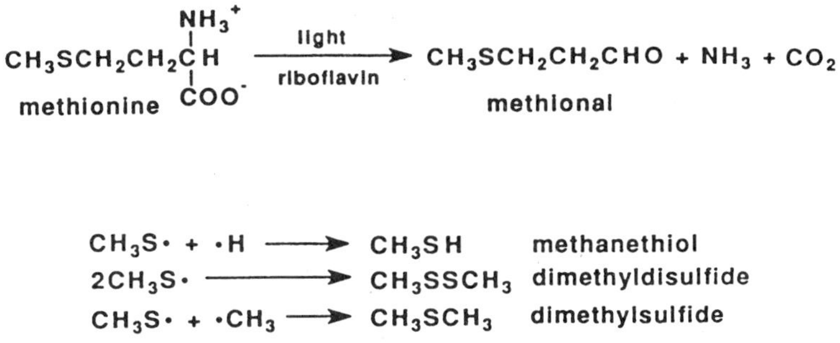

$$CH_3SCH_2CH_2\underset{COO^-}{\overset{NH_3^+}{C}}H \xrightarrow[\text{riboflavin}]{\text{light}} CH_3SCH_2CH_2CHO + NH_3 + CO_2$$

methionine → methional

$$CH_3S\cdot + \cdot H \longrightarrow CH_3SH \quad \text{methanethiol}$$
$$2CH_3S\cdot \longrightarrow CH_3SSCH_3 \quad \text{dimethyldisulfide}$$
$$CH_3S\cdot + \cdot CH_3 \longrightarrow CH_3SCH_3 \quad \text{dimethylsulfide}$$

FIGURE 5 Reaction of light with methionine in the presence of riboflavin catalyst to produce methional, which further degrades by free radical reactions to three highly malodorous sulfur-containing chemicals: methanethiol, dimethyl disulfide, and dimethyl sulfide.

Microorganisms can generate malodorous chemicals in unexpected and interesting ways. Potassium sorbate is often used as a fungistatic agent for cultured dairy products, cheeses, and fruit drinks. In 1966, Marth et al. demonstrated that a large number of molds in the genus *Penicillium* could grow in the presence of up to 7100 ppm potassium sorbate (20). The occurrence of a plastic, paint, or kerosene off-flavor in feta cheese, a geranium off-flavor in wine, and a strong hydrocarbon off-note in grape drink have all been attributed to the presence of *trans*-1,3-pentadiene, a strong odorant produced from the enzymatic decarboxylation reaction of sorbic acid (*trans,trans*-2,4-hexadienoic acid).

B. Example: Malodors in Beet Sugar

One significant quality problem with white beet sugar is a characteristic earthy, musty, barny, silagelike odor, which is frequently perceived in samples. The cause of this malodor has only recently been elucidated (21). While the characteristic aroma defect is usually not detectable once the sugar is solubilized, it can be extremely strong and objectionable when sealed canisters of the granulated sugar are initially opened by consumers.

Parliment and coworkers (22) used atmospheric steam distillation, extraction with ether, and concentration by distillation prior to GC/MS and infrared analysis to identify the volatile constituents of cooked beets and assess their importance in beet aroma. Of the 17 compounds identified, the major component to the odor of cooked beets was 4-methylpyridine. The presence of geosmin [*trans*-1,10-dimethyl-*trans*-(9)-decalol] and 2-methoxy-3-*sec*-butylpyrazine was also confirmed. In earlier work, Murray et al. (23) reported the presence of geosmin in beetroot. The low flavor/odor thresholds for pyrazines and geosmin and their musty/earthy notes make them good candidates for study with respect to the beet sugar odor problem.

1. Closed-Loop Stripping and Direct Thermal Desorption

In the author's lab, several beet sugar samples with various intensities of the characteristic beet sugar malodor were tested using two different GC purge-and-trap techniques: closed-loop stripping analysis (CLSA) and direct thermal desorption (DTD). Identification and quanitatation of GC peaks was accomplished with an ion trap detector (ITD), and odor characterization of chemicals eluting from the GC column was done with an olfactory detector (OD). Our sample preparation techniques prior to GC injection avoid the high-heat treatments associated with distillation techniques (e.g., Likens-Nickerson extraction) and do not require extraction solvents.

CLSA has been shown to be an effective sample-preparation technique prior to GC/MS for determining ultra-trace levels of geosmin, 2-methylisoborneol, and other malodorous/musty chemicals in drinking water. Using salted CLSA at 25°C, Hwang and coworkers (24) analyzed 48 water samples spiked with 4–20 ng/liter of geosmin and obtained an average recovery value of 105%, with a relative standard deviation of ±15%. This technique was approved in 1988 as an official method by the Standard Methods Committee for testing geosmin in water. The closed-loop stripping apparatus used to analyze the malodorous beet sugar samples was a modified version of the one described by Krasner and coworkers (25).

A second purge-and-trap technique was employed to study potential odorants that were poorly recovered by CLSA. With the technique, approximately 0.8 g of beet sugar was accurately weighed and placed into a glass thermal desorption cartridge. The cartridge was then placed in the desorber interface chamber of the thermal desorption device of the concentrator (PeakMaster™, CDS Analytical, Inc.). Volatiles were desorbed from the sugar in the cartridge by heating the desorption chamber to 75°C and purging with helium at a rate of 30 ml/min for 15 minutes. CLSA/GC/MS analyses provided clues, which indicated that several smaller, poorly resolved, non–Gaussian-shaped peaks might be carboxylic acids. Therefore, an FFAP fused-silica column with a film thickness of 0.25 μm was used for DTD analysis.

Our analytical strategy for determining the cause of the characteristic odor defect in beet sugar was based on analytical testing and organoleptic sensory analysis. First, malodorous sugar samples were analyzed by GC (CLSA and DTD) using the OD ("sniff port") to smell eluting peaks to determine which chemicals were potential contributors to the odor problem. Using a capillary column outlet splitter, half of the column effluent was directed to the ITD for identification and quantitation of peaks. Once suspect chemical contributors to the odor problem were identified and quantitated (or at least their maximum levels estimated), odorless cane sugar samples were spiked with these chemicals at concentration levels similar to those found in the beet sugar to determine which chemicals were responsible for the malodor. Using this approach, we were able to identify the primary chemicals responsible for the characteristic malodor of beet sugar and propose a mechanism for their formation.

2. Olfactometry

For both CLSA and DTD, effluent from the capillary was split 1:1, with half of the effluent routed to an ITD and half directed to an OD/sniff port. Olfactometry is an excellent detection technique for studying the aromas of food products. In fact, the nose is by far the most valuable detector for flavor chemists.

The OD allows chemists to incorporate the sense of smell into analytical investigations of off-flavors and malodors in foods. With the OD, the outlet stream from a GC capillary column (or, as in our work, a portion of it) is transferred to a nose cone, where it is mixed with a humidified air stream. A diagram of an olfactory detector is shown in Figure 6.

3. Aromagrams

By continuously sniffing column effluent at the nose cone and assigning descriptors to the aromas detected, the chemist can generate an "aromagram"—a documentation of sensory responses to odors that elute during a chromatographic run. Aromas can be detected even when no observable peaks occur in the chromatogram because, for some chemicals, the sense of small is a far more sensitive detector than any available GC detector. Aromagrams are valuable for studying off-flavors because they can indicate which chemicals are the most likely contributors to the odor or flavor defect being studied.

The beet sugar aromagrams obtained with the aid of the OD were important tools in identifying which chemicals were possible contributors to the characteristic beet odor problem. Figure 7 shows an example of a typical beet sugar aromagram obtained with CLSA. Chemicals that had intense aromas and were judged to be possible contributors to the characteristic odor defect were 2,5-dimethylpyrazine, furfural, butyric acid, isovaleric acid, and geosmin. While none of the chemicals detected with the OD exactly matched

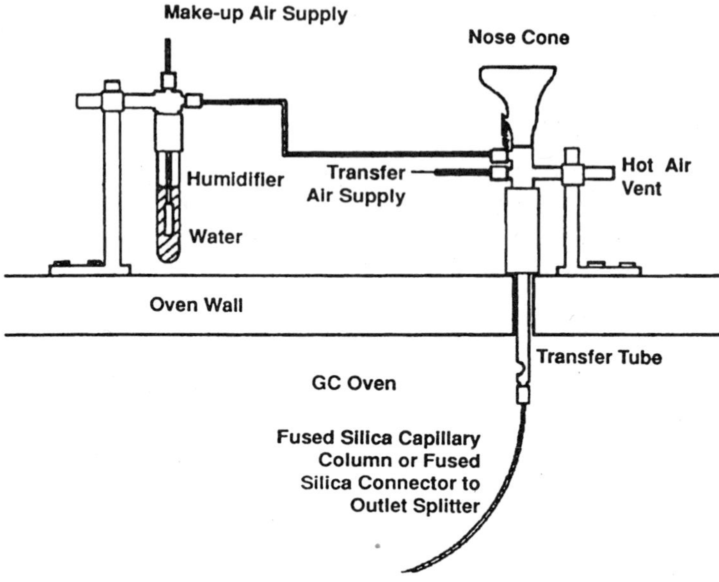

FIGURE 6 The olfactory detector (from SGE, Inc., Austin, TX) is designed to transfer the outlet stream (or a portion of the outlet stream) from a gas chromatograph to a nose cone in which it is mixed with a humidified air stream, allowing the operator to use the nose to characterize aroma attributes of individual components as they elute from the column.

the characteristic beet odor defect, the single chemical that most closely matched the odor defect was isovaleric acid.

Although CLSA generated numerous odors that were detectable with the OD, the technique did not offer satisfactory quantitative reproducibility or sensitivity for 2,-5-dimethyl pyrazine and volatile organic acids. CLSA was, however, a sensitive and quantitative sample-preparation technique for geosmin.

To obtain more accurate quantitation of organic acids and other polar peaks, an FFAP fused-silica capillary column was used in conjunction with DTD. A typical beet sugar aromagram is presented in Figure 8.

4. Recombination and Sensory Panel Studies

Using qualitative and quantitative data from the CLSA and DTD of sugar samples, odor-free cane sugar of the same granulation size as the beet sugar was spiked with various amounts of 2,5-dimethylpyrazine, furfural, acetic

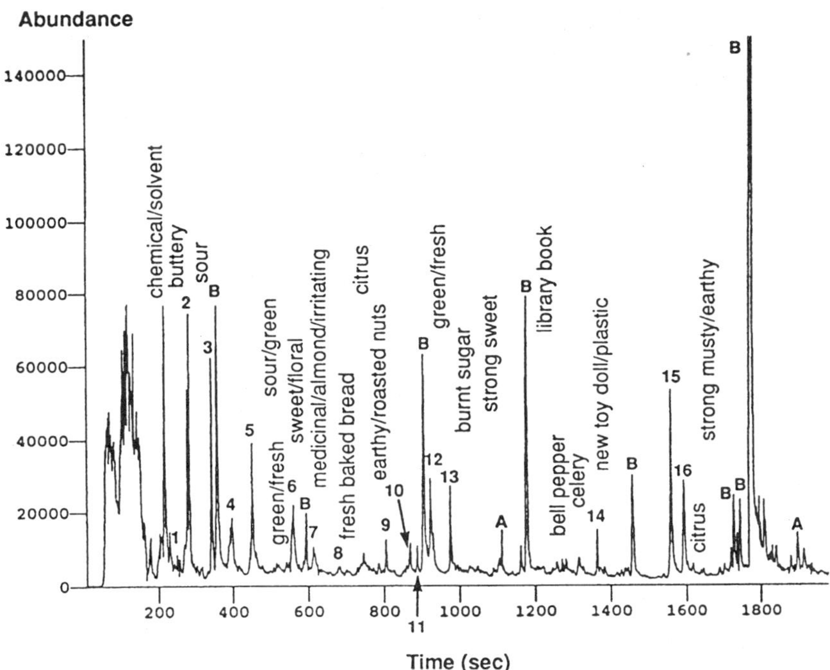

FIGURE 7 Closed-loop stripping aromagram of a malodorous (musty) beet sugar sample (50 g of sugar, 1 drop of antifoam, 2 g sodium chloride, and 70 ml water). Peak identities are as follows: A = unknown alkane; B = chemical contributed by blank (i.e., chemical originating from Tenax traps, antifoam, GC septa, etc.); 1 = chloroform; 2 = pentane, 3 = methylbutanal; 4 = acetic acid; 5 = tetrahydro-2,3-dimethyl-2-furanol*; 6 = butyl acetate; 7 = furfural; 8 = furfuryl alcohol; 9 = 5-methyl-2(3H)furanone; 10 = benzaldehyde; 11 = 1-octene-3-ol; 12 = 2-octanol; 13 = 2-ethylhexan-1-ol; 14 = carvone; 15 = 2-methylhexylpropanoate*; 16 = 2-methyl-2-ethyl-3-hydroxyhexylpropanoate*. (* = Tentative identification by mass spectrometry.)

acid, butyric acid, isovaleric acid, and geosmin. Chemicals were mixed individually with odorless cane sugar to determine approximate sensory threshold levels and also in combinations to determine resulting aromas.

Based on sensory threshold data for individual components, none of the suspect odorant chemicals would be expected to contribute odor to the sugar

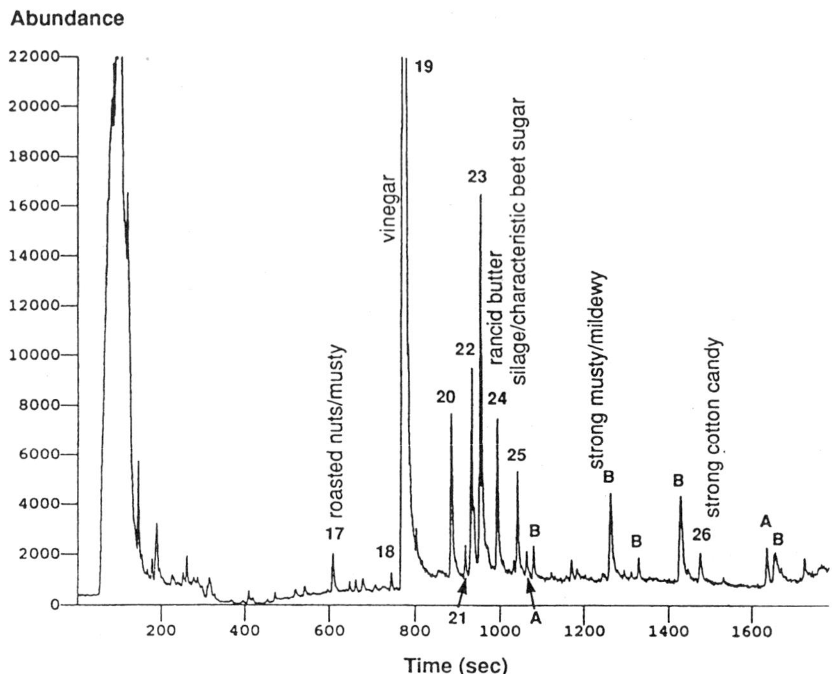

FIGURE 8 Direct thermal desorption aromagram of a malodorous (musty) beet sugar sample (0.8000 g desorbed at 75°C for 15 min). Peak identities are as follows: A = unknown alkane; B = chemical contributed by blank (i.e., chemical originating from Tenax traps, antifoam, GC septa, etc.); 17 = 2,5-dimethylpyrazine; 18 = dichlorobenzene; 19 = acetic acid; 20 = 3-methyl-2-butanol; 21 = propanoic acid; 22 = 2-pentanol; 23 = 2-butanol; 24 = butyric acid; 25 = isovaleric; 26 = 2-pyrrolidinone.

samples since all were present at concentrations below the threshold limits. Geosmin is perhaps the only exception to this since the sensory threshold detection level and the detection limit of geosmin by the CLSA method with the ITD are approximately the same.

However, when sugar samples were spiked with various combinations of suspect odorants and sniffed by sensory panelists, an important observation was made: mixtures of volatile acids in combination with geosmin produced an aroma identical to the typical odor defect of beet sugar. Furthermore, a synergistic effect was observed—i.e., the concentrations of acids and geosmin that would produce discernible odors were considerably less than the concentration required when each chemical was added by itself to the sugar. Mixing each acid separately with geosmin produced the characteristic beet sugar odor defect, no matter which specific volatile acid was used. However, slight nuances in aromas were observed depending on the type of acid and its concentration. For example, an acetic acid/geosmin combination provided earthy notes, while an isovaleric/geosmin combination had an odor more reminiscent of musty silage. A mixture of 25 ppt geosmin, 500 ppb acetic acid, 60 ppb isovaleric acid, and 200 ppb butyric acid provided an excellent match to the typical beet sugar odor defect.

The chemicals responsible for the characteristic odor defect of beet sugar originate from the action of soil microorganisms on sucrose in sugarbeets. Geosmin is produced by numerous actinomycetes and other types of soil molds (26). Butyric and isovaleric acids are metabolites of soil bacteria (e.g., *Clostridium butyricum* and other species of clostridia). Cleary (27) reports that fructose, glucose, and organic acids tend to increase in concentration in beets stored for prolonged periods prior to processing.

This beet sugar example illustrates the usefulness of olfactory detectors and the importance of using various types of concentration/isolation techniques as well as how different polarity GC capillary columns can be used to achieve resolution of critical malodorous chemicals. Also, it demonstrates the shortcoming of relying too heavily on CharmAnalysis and aroma dilution analysis methods for solving malodor problems. Recombination studies (e.g., spiking odorless substrate with mixtures of potential odor-causing chemicals) are sometimes essential for understanding possible critical synergistic effects between odorants.

V. TOOLS AND TECHNIQUES FOR EVALUATING GC AND OLFACTOMETRY RESULTS

Resolving off-flavor and malodor problems in foods using gas chromatography–olfactometry (GCO) techniques can be extremely difficult when samples contain complicated aroma volatile profiles. Even with complex samples, however, it is possible to determine the cause of off-flavors with the aid of various tools and techniques.

A. Dilution Analysis Techniques: CharmAnalysis and Aroma Extraction Dilution Anaysis

One popular technique that provides quantitative estimates of the potency levels of the various volatiles eluting from the GC capillary column is dilution analysis. The primary goal of dilution analysis studies is to identify the chemical components that contribute to the aroma of the food and to assess the relative potency of each odorant. Two types of dilution analysis are CharmAnalysis™ (28) and aroma extraction dilution analysis (AEDA) (29).

With dilution analysis techniques, a series of increasing dilutions of food sample extracts is prepared and analyzed by GCO. Each successive dilution is sniffed until no significant odor is detected. With AEDA, the number of dilutions necessary to eliminate the presence of an odor at a particular retention time (referred to as the flavor dilution value) is used to estimate odor potency of chromatographic peaks.

With the CharmAnalysis technique, times of the individual sniffs are combined and graphed. The resulting graph resembles a chromatogram and consists of peaks that can be integrated to provide peak areas ("charm values"). The greater the charm value, the more potent the odor contribution of the peak. The mathematics involved in CharmAnalysis have been described elsewhere (28).

Dilution analysis has been used to study a variety of food aromas. A few examples include apples (30), milk (31), mushrooms (32), packaging materials (33), breadcrust (34), honey (35), cherries (36), and beer (37).

A major disadvantage of both dilution analysis techniques is that they can be extremely time consuming, since often several dilutions must be sniffed until no odor is detected. Another problem is that humans have different abilities to detect aromas. Therefore, several different sniffers should be used to verify results, and this could extend the evaluation process over a period of several weeks or even several months. Another shortcoming of dilution analysis is that, unlike recombination studies like the one described above for beet sugar, it provides no insights into important synergistic effects of odiferous chemicals and how odors from more than one chemical may be combining to cause off-flavors.

B. Multivariate Statistical Analysis

While dilution analysis methods focus on the olfactory part of GCO, multivariate analysis emphasizes the quantitative relationships between GC peak area data.

Capillary GC methods incorporating modern GC detectors provide resolution and sensitivity unimagined a few years ago. A single analysis of a food product can easily generate more than 100 chemical peaks that may be potential malodor contributors in a particular food sample. Unfortunately, more data does not always easily translate into more useful information.

Frequently, the real challenge confronting aroma researchers is how to identify a few aroma-influencing chemical peaks (or perhaps just one peak) among a forest of dozens of peaks that have no significance to the malodor problem under study. Univariate data analysis methods, while useful for a wide array of applications, can easily overlook meaningful information in complex data sets. In contrast to univariate methods, multivariate statistical methods, which are based on the mathematics of matrix algebra and include the use of vectors, eigenvectors, and eigenvalues, examine many variables simultaneously and are capable of revealing measurements that are intercorrelated. The mathematics principles and techniques of multivariate analysis have been described elsewhere (38–40).

Easy-to-use, sophisticated computer programs are now available to perform multivariate analysis (41). Initially, exploratory data analysis is performed on the data set. This step involves the computation and graphical display of patterns of association in multivariate data sets. Often the exploratory phase is accomplished with two techniques: hierarchical cluster analysis (HCA) and principal component analysis (PCA). HCA and PCA can be used to show clustering and to reveal outliers.

Classification modeling can be conducted and involves the computation and graphical display of class assignments based on the multivariate similarity of one sample to others. One example of this technique is identification of bacteria based on the fatty acid profiles of lipid extracts from the bacterial cell walls. Two different classification models that are commonly used are K-Nearest Neighbors (KNN) and Soft Independent Modeling of Class Analogy (SIMCA).

In addition, regression techniques such as principal component regression (PCR) and partial least squares (PLS) can be used to measure the degree of predictability. With regression models, the analyst is interested in predicting some value (rather than assigning a class designation) for an unknown sample.

Multivariate analysis has been applied to the study of a wide variety of food and beverage problems. A few examples include milk shelf-life prediction (42), chemotyping of essential oils (43), discriminating aromas of coffee samples (44), classifying wine samples (45), and characterizing peppermint oils (46).

In the author's lab, a chemometrics study is currently being conducted to allow classification of milk samples as to the cause of off-flavor development. For this work, control samples of normal, good-tasting milk are analyzed by dynamic headspace GC/MS techniques. The samples are then subjected to various abuse conditions (e.g., exposure to light, high-heat treatment, contamination with sanitizers, addition of copper salts, contamination with various known types of psychotrophic bacteria, etc.) and reanalyzed. The abused samples provide the basis for SIMCA classification modeling.

Once the appropriate classification model has been developed and validated, chemists will be able to rapidly and accurately classify complaint milk samples as to the cause of off-flavor. This type of testing will (a) identify the specific mechanism of off-flavor development, (b) provide clues as to specific processing, packaging, distribution, and warehouse problems responsible for causing off-flavors, and (c) hopefully lead to improved milk quality in the long term.

C. Computer Databases and Expert Systems

The likelihood of resolving off-flavor and malodor problems based on GCO experiments is highly dependent on researcher experience. There are numerous reference books and technical journal articles dealing with off-flavors in foods and beverages, and the amount of new information in the field is increasing at an overwhelming rate. One approach that is helpful in organizing and retrieving facts and information is a computer database/expert system.

Databases can be set up to provide rapid retrieval of specific kinds of off-flavor information, including type of chemicals observed in GC profiles, type of food or beverage product associated with off-flavor development, descriptors to characterize the aroma of observed peaks, etc. The major advantage of an expert system is that it allows relatively untrained researchers to benefit from the knowledge base of more experienced researchers.

Ney (47) has described a database approach for studying off-flavors in foods. Ney's database fields include name (descriptor) of off-flavor, name of food or beverage, name of off-component, formula of off-component, off-flavor type, off-flavor formation, and off-flavor avoidance.

In the author's lab, a similar database of off-flavor facts has been developed and is constantly being upgraded and enlarged. One record of the database is shown in Figure 9. Chemical structures and diagrams of chemical reaction mechanisms are inputted into picture fields in the database using a chemistry drawing program. One field that is particularly useful is the "References" field, which lists the pertinent journal articles used in compiling the information in the database record.

A researcher studying, for example, a catty off-flavor note in beer by dynamic headspace GC/MS/olfactometry might observe a peak with a cat urine–like odor and identify it as 4-methyl-4-mercapto-2-pentanone based on MS matching of peak spectrum with library spectra. The analyst could use this information in a variety of ways to improve understanding of the problem. He

Chemical Name, General

mesityl oxide
isopropylideneacetone
thioketone

Chemical Name, Specific

4-methyl-3-penten-2-one
4-methyl-4-mercapto-2-pentanone

Chemical Structure(s)

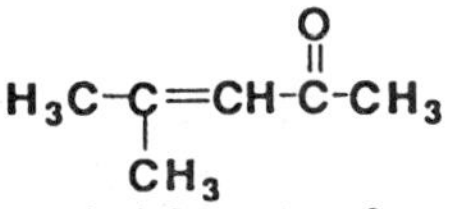

$$H_3C-C(CH_3)=CH-C(=O)-CH_3$$

4-methyl-3-penten-2-one
(mesityl oxide)

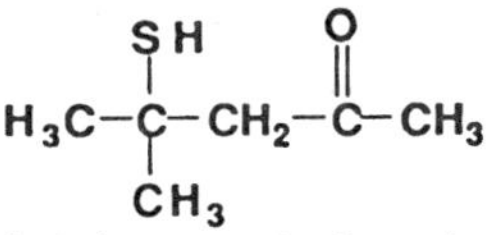

$$H_3C-C(SH)(CH_3)-CH_2-C(=O)-CH_3$$

4-methyl-4-mercapto-2-pentanone
("thioketone")

Off Flavor/Aroma

Mesityl oxide (also called isopropylideneacetone or 4-methyl-3-penten-2-one) has a honey-like odor. Thioketone (also called 4-methyl-4-mercapto-2-pentanone) has ribes or catty taint (cat-urine odor).

Mechanism of Formation

Two acetone molecules can condense to form 4-methyl-4-ol-penten-2-one. Dehydration of this compound yields mesityl oxide. Hydrogen sulfide -- from (microbial) degradation of proteins containing cysteine, cystine, and/or methionine amino acids in cheese, sausage, and other processed meat products -- adds to the carbon-carbon double bond of mesityl oxide to generate thioketone. The thioketone has a strong cat-urine-like odor at extremely low concentration thresholds (<0.1 ppb). Thioketone, however, is partially responsible for the pleasant flavor of black currants.

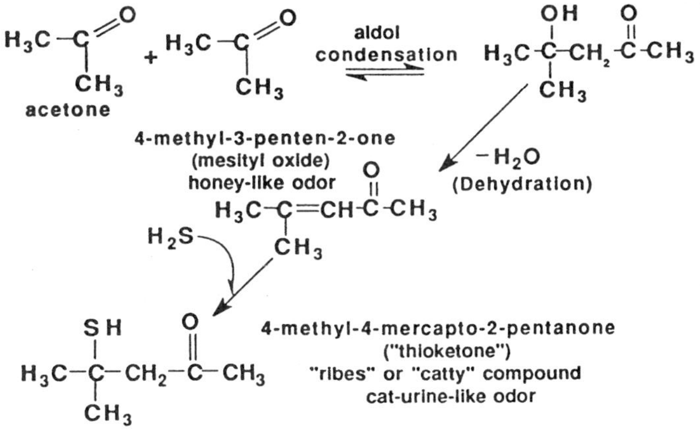

$$H_3C-C(=O)CH_3 + H_3C-C(=O)CH_3 \xrightleftharpoons{\text{aldol condensation}} H_3C-C(OH)(CH_3)-CH_2-C(=O)-CH_3$$

acetone

$$\xrightarrow{-H_2O \text{ (Dehydration)}} H_3C-C(CH_3)=CH-C(=O)-CH_3$$

4-methyl-3-penten-2-one
(mesityl oxide)
honey-like odor

$$\xrightarrow{H_2S} H_3C-C(SH)(CH_3)-CH_2-C(=O)-CH_3$$

4-methyl-4-mercapto-2-pentanone
("thioketone")
"ribes" or "catty" compound
cat-urine-like odor

FIGURE 9 Computer databases are an efficient tool for storing, searching for, and retrieving information about off-flavors in foods and beverages. This is an example of one record from an off-flavor database.

Occurrence/Comments

Acetone vapors can occur in numerous ways in food systems. Bovine ketosis, for example, is responsible for ppm levels of acetone in milk. Dyes and inks on packaging graphics sometimes use acetone as a solvent. Acetone solvent is sometimes used in extracting spices.

While dehydration of 4-methyl-4-ol-pentan-2-one is one way to generate mesityl oxide in foods, mesityl oxide can also occur in foods because of environmental contamination. Mesityl oxide is used as a solvent for nitrocellulose, many gums and resins, particularly vinyl resins. It is also used in lacquers, varnishes and enamels and in making methyl isobutyl ketone.

One of the staling off flavors of beer is described as ribes flavor. This flavor develops rapidly in some beers when packaged with a high air content in head space (1). The off flavor reaches a peak after 4-8 weeks and thereafter becomes gradually less noticeable (2) .

Tressl et al. reported that 4-methyl-4-mercapto-2-pentanone was formed by addition of hydrogen sulfide to the corresponding α, β–unsaturated ketone, and this mercaptoketone was responsible for the ribes flavor (3).

In a catty off-flavored beer, Cosser et al. also found 4-methyl-4-mercapto-2-pentanone which was transformed from mesityl oxide, an impurity in a paint used for the malting plant (4).

References

1. Clapperton, J.F. J. Inst. Brew., 82 (1976), 175-176.

2. Dalgliesh, C.E. Euro. Brew. Conv., Proc. 16th Congr., Amsterdam (1977), 623-659.

3. Tressl R., D. Bahri, and M. Kossa. In: Charalambous, G. (Ed.), *The Analysis and Control of Less Desirable Flavors in Foods and Beverages*, Academic Press, New York, 1980, p. 315.

4. Cosser, K.B., J.P. Murray, and C.W. Hazapfel. Tech. Quart., Master Brewers Assoc. Am. (1980), 53-59.

FIGURE 9 Continued

or she could, for example, enter "4-methyl-4-mercapto-2-pentanone" into the chemical name field, retrieving all records that list this chemical. The analyst could then inspect the known reaction mechanisms for this compound and decide if one or more are reasonable for the particular food or beverage system being studied. Or perhaps, even prior to analyzing samples, the analyst could enter the word "ribes" (see Fig. 9) or "catty" in the "Off-Flavor/Aroma" field and the word "beer" in the "Occurrence/Comments" field and obtain all records discussing a ribes, catty off-flavor in beer.

Although developing and maintaining computer databases of this type is a monumental task, properly designed databases can make an invaluable contribution to understanding and resolving off-flavor problems and to passing along research experience gained to future analysts.

VI. CONCLUSION

As the few examples presented in this chapter illustrate, numerous mechanisms exist for off-flavor formation in foods and beverages. In some ways, discovering the chemical or chemicals responsible for a particular food malodor is like looking for a needle in a haystack. However, recent advances in chemical instrumentation, olfactometry, new techniques for introducing volatiles into GC capillary columns, statistical techniques like multivariate analysis, and other tools for interpreting GCO results now make the chance of finding that needle more likely than ever before.

REFERENCES

1. T. G. Hartman, J. Lech, K. Karmas, J. Salinas, R. T. Rosen, and C.-T. Ho, Flavor characterization using adsorbent trapping-thermal desorption or direct thermal desorption GC and GC-MS, *Flavor Measurement* (C.-T. Ho and C. H. Manley, eds.), Marcel Dekker, Inc., New York, 1993, p. 55.
2. H. Kim-Kang, Volatiles in packaging materials, *Crit. Rev. Food Sci. Nutri. 29:*255 (1990).
3. N. Goldenberg and H. R. Matheson, Off-flavors in foods, a summary of experiences: 1948–1974, *Chem. Industry 5:*551 (1975).
4. R. T. Marsili, Measuring volatiles and limonene oxidation products in orange juice by capillary GC, *LC.GC 4:*359 (1986).
5. R. T. Marsili, Monitoring bacterial metabolites in cultured buttermilk by HPLC and headspace GC, *J. Chromatogr. Sci. 19:*451 (1981).
6. R. T. Marsili, Measuring light-induced chemical changes in soybean oil by capillary headspace GC, *J. Chromatogr. Sci. 22:*61 (1984).
7. H. Hachenberg and A. P. Schmidt, *Gas Chromatographic Headspace Analysis*, Heyden & Son Ltd., London, 1977, p. 32.
8. C. Bicchi, F. Belliardo, and C. Frattini, Identification of the volatile components of some piedmontese honeys, *J. Apic. Res. 22:*130 (1983).
9. A. Bousita and S. Collin, Optimized Likens-Nickerson methodology for quantifying honey flavors, *J. Agric. Food Chem. 43:*1890 (1995).
10. R. T. Marsili, G. J. Kilmer, and N. Miller, Quantitative analysis of orange-oil components in orange juice by a simple solvent extraction-GC procedure, *LC GC 7:*778 (1989).
11. H. A. Massaldi and C. J. King, Determination of volatiles by vapor headspace

analysis in a multi-phase system: d-limonene in orange juice, *J. Food Sci. 39:*434 (1974).
12. W. F. Shipe, R. Bassette, D. D. Deane, W. L. Dunkley, E. G. Hammond, W. J. Harper, D. H. Kleyn, M. E. Morgan, J. H. Nelson, and R. A. Scanlan. Off-flavors of milk: nomenclature, stanards and bibliography, *J. Dairy Sci. 61:*855 (1978).
13. S. E. Barnard, Importance of shelf life for consumers of milk, *J. Dairy Sci. 55:*134 (1973).
14. C. D. Azzra and L. B. Campbell, Off-flavors of dairy products, *Off-Flavors in Foods and Beverages* (G. Charalambous, ed.), Elsevier, Amsterdam, 1992, p. 345.
15. G. D. Forss, Review of the progress of dairy science: mechanisms of formation of aroma compounds in milk and milk products, *J. Dairy Res. 46:*691 (1979).
16. R. Tressl, D. Bahri, and M. Kossa, Formation of off-flavor components in beer, *The Analysis and Control of Less Desirable Flavors in Food and Beverages* (G. Charalambous, ed.), Academic Press, New York, 1980, p. 293.
17. M. E. Stansby, Speculation on fishy odors and flavors, *Food Technol. 16:*28 (1962).
18. M. E. Morgan, The chemistry of some microbially induced flavor defects in milk and dairy foods, *Biotechnol. Bioeng. 18:*953 (1976).
19. A. Miller, M. E. Morgan, and L. M. Libbey, *Lactobacillus maltaromicus*, a new species producing a malty aroma, *Int. J. Syst. Bacteriol. 24:*346 (1974).
20. E. H. Marth, C. M. Capp, L. Hasenzahl, H. W. Jackson, and R. V. Hussong, Degradation of potassium sorbate by *Penicillum* species, *J. Dairy Sci. 49:*1197 (1966).
21. R. T. Marsili, N. Miller, G. J. Kilmer, and R. E. Simmons, Identification of the primary chemicals responsible for the characteristic malodor of beet sugar by purge and trap GC-MS-OD techniques, *J. Chromatogr. Sci. 32:*165 (1994).
22. T. H. Parliment, M. G. Kolor, I. Y. Maing, Identification of the major volatile components of cooked beets, *J. Food Sci. 42:*1592 (1977).
23. D. E. Murray, P. A. Bannister, and R. G. Buttery, Geosmin: an important volatile constituent of beetroot, *Chem. Ind. 973:*457 (1975).
24. C. J. Hwang, S. W. Krasner, M. J. McGuire, M. S. Moylan, and M. S. Dale, Determination of subnanogram per liter levels of earthy-musty odorants in water by the salted closed-loop stripping method, *Environ. Sci. Technol. 18:*535 (1984).
25. S. W. Krasner, C. J. Hwant, and M. J. McGuire, A standard method for quantification of earthy-musty odorants in water, *Water Sci. Technol. 15:*127 (1983).
26. Y. S. Abo Gnah and N. D. Harris, Determination of musty odor compounds produced by *Streptomyces griseus* and *Streptomyces odorifer*, *J. Food Sci. 50:*132 (1985).
27. M. Cleary, Carbonation process in beet sugar manufacture, *Chemistry and Processing of Sugarbeet and Sugarcane* (M. A. Clarke and M. A. Godshall, eds.), Elsevier, Amsterdam, 1988, p. 20.
28. T. A. Acree, J. Barnard, and D. Cunningham, A procedure for the sensory analysis of gas chromatographic effluents, *Food Chem. 14:*273 (1984).

29. F. Ullrich and W. Grosch, Identification of the most intense odor compounds formed during autoxidation of linoleic acid, *Z. Lebensm. Unters. Forsch. 184:*277 (1987).
30. D. G. Cunningham, T. A. Acree, J. Barnard, R. Butts, and P. Braell, Charm analysis of apple volatiles, *Food Chem. 19:*137 (1986).
31. L. Moio, D. Langlois, P. Etievant, and F. Addeo, Powerful odorants in bovine, ovine, caprine and water buffalo milk determined by gas chromatography-olfactometry, *J. Dairy Res. 60:*215 (1993).
32. K. H. Fischer and W. Grosch, Volatile compounds of importance in the aroma of mushrooms (*Psalliota bispora*), *Lebensm. Wiss. Technol. 20:*233 (1987).
33. A. B. Marin, T. E. Acree, J. H. Hotchkiss, and S. Nagy, Gas chromatography-olfactometry of orange juice to assess the effects of plastic polymers on aroma character, *J. Agric. Food Chem. 40:*650 (1992).
34. P. Schieberle and W. Grosch, Evaluation of the flavor of wheat and rye bread crusts by aroma extraction dilution analysis, *Z. Lebensm. Unters. Forsch. 185:*111 (1987).
35. I. Blank, K. H. Fischer, and W. Grosch, Intensive neutral odorants of linden honey. Differences from honeys of other botanical origin, *Z. Lebensm. Unters. Forsch. 189:*426 (1989).
36. W. Schmid and W. Grosch. Identification of highly aromatic volatile flavor compounds from Morello cherries (*Prunus cerasus*), *Z. Lebensm. Unters. Forsch. 182:*407 (1986).
37. N. B. Sanchez, C. L. Lederer, G. B. Nickerson, L. M. Libbey, and M. R. McDaniel, Sensory and analytical evaluation of beers brewed with three varieties of hops and an unhopped beer, *Proceedings of the 6th Int. Flavor Conf., Rethymnon, Crete* (G. Charalambous, ed.), Elsevier, Amsterdam, 1992, p. 403.
38. M. Chien and T. Peppard, Use of statistical methods to better understand gas chromatographic data obtained from complex flavor systems, *Flavor Measurement* (Chi-Tang Ho and C. H. Manley, eds.), Marcel Dekker, Inc., New York, 1993, p. 1.
39. C. Zervos and R. H. Albert, Chemometrics: the use of multivariate methods for the determination and characterization of off-flavors, *Off-flavors in Foods and Beverages* (G. Charalambous, ed.), Elsevier, Amsterdam, 1992, p. 669.
40. M. A. Sharaf, D. L. Illman, and B. R. Kowalski, *Chemometrics*, John Wiley & Sons, New York, NY, 1986, p. 180.
41. *Pirouette: Multivariate Data Analysis for IBM PC Systems*, Version 1.2, Infometrix, Inc., Woodinville, WA, 1990.
42. B. Vallejo-Cordoba and S. Nakai, Keeping quality assessment of pasteurized milk by multivariate analysis of dynamic headspace gas chromatographic data: shelf-life prediction by principal component regression, *J. Agric. Food Chem. 42:*989 (1994).
43. P. Ramanoelina, J. Viano, J. Bianchini, and E. M. Gaydou, Occurrence of various chemotypes in Niaouli (*Melaleuca quinquenervia*) essential oils from

Madagascar using multivariate statistical analysis, *J. Agric. Food Chem. 42:* 1177 (1994).

44. T. Aishima, Aroma discrimination by pattern recognition analysis of responses from semiconductor gas sensor array, *J. Agric. Food Chem. 39:*753 (1991).
45. I. Moret, G. Scarponi, and P. Cescon, Chemometric characterization and classifiction of five Venetian white wines, *J. Agric. Food Chem. 42:*1143 (1994).
46. F. Chialva, A. Ariozzi, D. Decastri, P. Manitto, S. Clementi, and D. Bonelli, Chemometric investigation on Italian peppermint oils, *J. Agric. Food Chem. 41:*2028 (1993).
47. K. H. Ney, Specification of a computer program for off-flavors, *Off-Flavors in Foods and Beverges* (G. Charalambous, ed.), Elsevier, Amsterdam, 1992, p. 665.

9

Gas Chromatography–Olfactometry for the Determination of Key Odorants in Foods

BEHROZE S. MISTRY, TERRY REINECCIUS, AND
LINDA K. OLSON
Aspen Research Corporation, St. Paul, Minnesota

I. INTRODUCTION

The early nineteenth century saw the beginnings of analytical work on food flavors. Benzaldehyde was the first flavoring material isolated from bitter almonds by Vogel in 1818 and by Martres in 1819 (1), but it was not identified until 1832. Fifty years later, Tiemann and Haarmann (2), and later Reimer (3), isolated, identified, and synthesized vanillin. This was the first flavor compound to be synthesized (1), and it heralded the era of the flavor industry.

Initial studies in flavor research were hampered by the inadequate separation provided by packed column gas chromatography (GC), and thus flavor chemists were the pioneers of capillary column chromatography. The evolution of capillary column GC and the interfacing of GC with mass spectrometry (MS) resulted in the separation and identification of numerous volatile compounds existing in different foods. Today, more than 6900 volatile compounds have been identified in foods and beverages (4). However, of all these volatile compounds, only a few determine the characteristic odor of a specific food. Sometimes only one compound is responsible for the characteristic odor of a particular food—this type of compound is known as a "character impact compound." Great strides have been made in flavor research, which is being directed towards combining olfactometry and sensory techniques with instrumental methods to gain insight into better characterization of food flavors.

In this chapter, we will take the reader through different phases—past and present—of odor and flavor characterization by several pioneers in the field of flavor chemistry. Here we will talk about the development of gas chromatography–olfactometry (GCO), followed by the development of extract dilution methods and Osme. The existing new area of aroma recombination, which is the last piece of the puzzle, will also be mentioned. We will also critically review each method, presenting its strengths and limitations, and provide insight into work needed to further strengthen this aspect of flavor chemistry.

II. HISTORY AND CURRENT DEVELOPMENTS IN THE CHARACTERIZATION OF KEY ODORANTS IN FOODS

In 1997, the concept of odor activity value (also known as OAV, unit flavor base, odor unit, odor value, or aroma value) will celebrate its fortieth year in the field of gas chromatography–olfactometry. The concept of OAV was first proposed by Patton and Josephson (5) shortly after the introduction of gas chromatography by James and Martin in 1952. In this early work, GCO simply referred to smelling the GC effluent after its separation. This was an exciting period for flavor chemists, who were now able to assign odor descriptions to GC peaks and to separate odor active chemicals from volatile chemicals with no or minimal odor response. There were great expectations of GCO being able to unlock flavor secrets; however, when GCO was used, most food systems failed to produce distinct character impact compounds (6,7). The challenge then was to determine the relative importance of a flavor compound to the overall flavor of the food, giving rise to the idea of aroma effectiveness. A value to express aroma effectiveness was originated by Patton and Josephson (5), who proposed relating the concentration of a compound to its sensory threshold. The concept was first termed "aroma value" by Rothe and Thomas in 1963 (8). Other authors used the terms "odor unit" (6), "unit flavor base" (9), and "odor value" (7). "Aroma value" is the ratio of the concentration of an aroma compound to its threshold, thereby indicating how much the actual concentration of a compound exceeds its sensory threshold.

Since the concept of "aroma value" was proposed, GCO and OAV have been extensively applied in the area of flavor chemistry. These techniques have clearly demonstrated that the most abundant volatiles may have little if any odor significance in a food. These techniques have been invaluable in determining undesirable or foreign off-odors in foods or in determining differences between a control and variant of the control (e.g., aged product, different source, process effect). Unfortunately, the original vision of using GCO and OAV for flavor duplication work has met with very limited success. With the exception of works by Buttery et al. on tomato flavor (10,11), Blank and Grosch on dill herb flavor (12), Schieberle et al. on butter flavor (13), and Grosch on cheese flavor (14), no sensory confirmations of OAVs of compounds or their contribution to the original flavor have been published.

The last forty years have served as a long incubation time for the evolution of GCO methods. During this time, three methods have emerged: Aroma Extract Dilution Analysis (AEDA) (15), CharmAnalysis (16), and Osme (17). Their emergence as academic and commercial GCO methods and a divergence in theory, technique, and interpretation has only occurred within the last 12 years.

III. IMPORTANCE OF ISOLATION TECHNIQUES

The importance of selecting the appropriate isolation technique for GCO work should not be overlooked. The success of flavor characterization of foods by GCO depends largely on the isolation technique employed to isolate the flavor compounds from the food matrix. The number of odorants detected by GCO depends on the method used to isolate the flavor volatiles from the food. Due to large numbers of volatile compounds found in foods, their differences in physical and chemical properties, and their low threshold levels, isolation of volatiles from foods becomes very challenging. There are innumerable methods of flavor isolation from a food matrix; however, each method will introduce biases into an aroma profile. Therefore, different methods may provide different aroma profiles. Other variables that influence GCO results include the amount of food sampled, dilution of the volatile fraction by the solvent, and aliquot of extract injected into the gas chromatograph. The interested reader can refer to an in-depth article by Reineccius (18) on the biases in flavor profiles introduced by isolation techniques.

The importance of aroma isolation method in aroma recovery is illustrated by Guth and Grosch (19). Known amounts of odorants were dissolved in ethyl ether, added to sunflower oil, and then isolated by sublimation in vacuo. The yields of odorants obtained by this isolation method ranged from 1% (for 4,5-epoxy-(*E*)-2-decenal) to 78% (for 1-octen-3-one). In another example, Leahy and Reineccius (20) compared 10 different methods for the recovery of a flavor model system from dilute aqueous solutions. The percent recoveries of the compounds were unique for each method evaluated (recoveries ranged from 0 to 100% depending upon aroma compound and isolation method). By direct solvent extraction of an aqueous solution containing methyl anthranilate, only 10% was recovered using pentane as the solvent compared to approximately 80% recovery using dichloromethane (20). In investigating "foxy" character in wines made from Concord grapes, the contribution of methyl anthranilate to this "foxy" note (21) may be missed if pentane is chosen as an extraction solvent.

Since any subsequent work by GCO is dependent on how well an extract represents the aroma in question, substantial time must be invested in this phase of the study. Each isolation method has its unique weaknesses; hence, more than one isolation method may have to be used to accurately view the true aroma of the food (e.g., headspace and vacuum distillation). Numerous aroma isolation methods should first be investigated and the aroma extracts evaluated by formal sensory evaluation techniques. The isolation methods selected should be based on sensory confirmation of the best representation.

IV. GAS CHROMATOGRAPHY–OLFACTOMETRY

GCO, sometimes referred to as "GC sniffing," is an important analytical tool in flavor research because it characterizes the odors of single compounds or complex mixtures of volatiles emerging from the sniffing port. Here, the human nose is the detector used for evaluating the effluent of the GC column. The nose has a theoretical odor detection limit of about 10^{-19} moles (22), making GCO a very valuable and sensitive tool for the detection of odor active volatiles like 2-methoxy-3-hexyl pyrazine (odor threshold of 1 part in 10^{12} parts of water) (22). Acree (23) indicated that a person would be able to detect 50–500 fg (10^{-15}) of β-damascenone by GCO. Volatile compounds with different odors, even those with very small differences in retention index, will be differentiated from one another by GCO (23).

GCO has often been used to detect trace amounts of character impact compounds or off-odors in foods. For example, when the effluent of a pineapple extract was sniffed by GCO, a typical pineapple odor was recognized in a certain region of the GC profile (24). However, the sensitivity of the FID (flame ionization detector of a GC) was too low to detect a peak. Upon subsequent enrichment of the extract, the peak was identified as allyl hexanoate (24). We saw a similar problem related to an off-odor in beet-sugar. A musty odor, similar to that of the original beet-sugar sample, was identified by GCO in a particular region of the GC profile. Once again, there were no peaks detected by the FID in that region. Upon further enrichment of the extract, geosmin was identified as the compound producing the musty odor. Since many flavor volatiles have extremely low odor thresholds, detection of these compounds by GC-FID becomes very difficult and one may have to rely on GCO to elucidate the odor of the GC peak of interest.

A. Limitations of GCO

To accurately perform the analysis and evaluate data, one should be aware of the limitations of GCO. Sensory perception of a food (good vs. bad, banana or coffee, etc.) is arrived at by the simultaneous integration of all of the taste and olfactory signals arising from the taste and aroma compounds in a food. In GCO, however, we are attempting to determine the contribution of a given aroma compound separately as it elutes as an individual peak on the gas chromatograph. This compound is being evaluated out of context, so to speak. This may make evaluation of its contribution to a food difficult or impossible to assess accurately. An alternative method might use GC effluent trapping of peak fractions and subsequent sensory evaluation of these collected fractions to simulate the original flavor of the food. Here, one could trap what is considered to be the most characteristic aroma compound and compare its odor to that of the entire food aroma complex. Assuming it fails to reproduce the food aroma, one could then add additional compounds until the reconstructed aroma fraction is judged to be indistinguishable from the entire food aroma. This would permit the evaluation of odors in combination as is done in normal tasting. Furthermore, the compounds needed in these fractions would be readily available in the aroma isolate and in the correct proportions as well. This approach would potentially compensate for attempting to evaluate an aroma compound out of context as is typically done by GCO methods.

The elution order, odor character, and perceived intensity of one compound will directly influence the perceived intensity of the compound eluting after it. This is referred to as the "contrast effect" and can be corrected for by balancing the presentation order (25). Manipulation of elution time and order of the compounds can be accomplished by column selection and chromatographic parameters (temperature, pressure, carrier gas). Manipulation of elution order, however, is limited by column selection (polar vs. nonpolar phases). A balanced presentation of elution order is not possible by GCO; however, evaluating the perceived intensities of eluting compounds on a minimum of two column phases (e.g., DB-1 and DB-Wax) would provide validity to the data.

Another limitation of GCO is that fatigue, sensory saturation, and adaption on the part of the human subject will negatively influence intensity measures and must, therefore, be minimized (26,27). There is no scientific evidence to show whether the perceived intensity of a compound detected at the fortieth minute of continuous sniffing would be similar to the intensity of the same compound if it were evaluated after 5 minutes of sniffing. These factors could be addressed by dividing the sniffing time into shorter intervals. The order in which a subject evaluated these shortened runs could be randomized and balanced in design among subjects; this would further reduce contrast effects.

The condition or physical environment under which GCO is conducted has a significant influence on the validity of the data. Noise, distractions, extraneous odors, and uncomfortable test conditions may introduce error. Ideally, GCO should be conducted in an isolated, quiet room with a positive pressure air-handling system to prevent and eliminate odors. The subject should be able to perform the test in a comfortable position, preferably seated versus standing over a warm gas chromatograph. The hot, dry carrier gas carrying the GC effluent to the nose may be irritating and uncomfortable. To correct this problem, a gentle stream (20–30 ml/min) of humidified air may be used. This prevents drying of olfactory mucosa and condensation of components on the walls of the olfactometer mask, if used.

GCO should not be conducted on substances of unknown composition. The health and safety of subjects evaluating samples by GCO should be the primary concern. Subjects conducting GCO should be aware of the nature of the material they will be exposed to during the analysis. Laboratories should have their own regulations and safety standards in this matter (e.g., GCO should be applied only to food extracts, not to industrial waste effluents). Currently, there are no OSHA regulations or university guidelines in place regarding this application of human subjects.

Selection, screening, and training of human subjects as "sniffers" during a GCO run should be carried out in an objective manner (25). Unfortunately, in GCO studies the researchers involved with the project may have a biased opinion when conducting GCO.

V. EXTRACT DILUTION TECHNIQUES

GCO has evolved over time to include dilution techniques (AEDA and CharmAnalysis), cross-modal matching (Osme), and maximum perceived intensity. Of these three GCO modifications, extract dilution techniques, and cross-modal matching have become the most common techniques used in analytical work on food flavors. A discussion of these methods follows.

Two extract dilution techniques were developed to overcome some of the limitations of a single run by GCO: the AEDA method by Grosch and coworkers (Deutsche Forschungsanstalt für Lebensmittelchemie, Garching, Germany) (15,28) and CharmAnalysis by Acree and coworkers (Cornell University, Ithaca, NY) (16). To date, these are the only two methods that have the goal of identifying the key odorants in food systems. These methods also attempt to rank key odorants in order of potency based on evaluation of individual GC peaks by GCO. The dilution value of a compound is assumed to be proportional to its OAV in air. Hence, the higher the dilution at which the compound can be detected by GCO, the greater the contribution of that compound to the odor of the food. While using these methods one must keep in mind the limitation of assessing one compound at a time by GCO (as discussed in the previous section).

The extract dilution technique involves stepwise dilution (typically 1:2 or 1:3) of the prepared extract with a solvent and evaluation of each dilution by GCO. GCO is conducted up to the dilution at which the odorant(s) of interest cannot be perceived in the GC effluent. The dilution value is equivalent to the magnitude required to reduce the concentration of a compound in the original extract to a level below its threshold. For example, if 1 part of extract is diluted into 2 parts of solvent, the dilution factor is 3. During GCO, if an odor active compound is then detected in the fifth dilution, the dilution value becomes $3^5 = 243$.

A. Limitations of Extract Dilution Techniques

Extract dilution techniques are very time consuming. It can take several days to conduct a dilution study by GCO since several dilutions have to be analyzed. It is, therefore, difficult to perform duplicate or triplicate analyses or to check reproducibility among different GCO users. Human fatigue also becomes a major concern.

Time requirements are further expanded since GCO of extract dilutions should be conducted on two different GC columns. Two different columns are needed since some odor compounds are better resolved by one of the GC columns and the GC elution order will be varied (29). To reduce this time problem, Schieberle (30) suggested that the original extract and two dilutions, 1:20 and 1:200, be analyzed by GCO on two GC columns of different polarities. He further stated that three panelists should conduct these studies. Then the column on which most of the odor active compounds are detected is the column of choice for further dilution studies. This approach will help reduce concerns for compound resolution but will not address the issue of compound elution order.

Both AEDA and CharmAnalysis are screening methods. They do not absolutely indicate which compounds make the greatest contribution to the aroma of food. This is partly because during GCO of the dilution extracts, the odor compounds are volatilized and then evaluated; in foods, the volatility of the aroma compounds depends on their solubility in the food matrix as well as their interactions with nonvolatile constituents. The FD factors or Charm values (dilution values during GCO) do not consider the physical factors of a food matrix or the physiological impressions of odor character that influence aroma perception. One should be aware that the dilution values do not represent the sensory thresholds of the odor active compounds in the food matrix; therefore, care must be taken in assigning any ranking of relative importance to these odor active compounds.

Abbott et al. (31) have observed gaps in coincident responses for a series of dilutions analyzed by GCO. An individual may not detect an odor at a certain Kovats Index in a particular dilution but will detect this odor at this same Kovats Index at a higher dilution. Abbott et al. (31) stated that there may be cross-adaptation between two compounds causing a gap in coincident response. For example, at one dilution, compound x may not be detected due to cross-adaptation from a prior-eluting compound y; however, in a more dilute sample, cross-adaptation has no effect and compound x can be detected. Schieberle (30) provided a solution to this phenomenon. He mentioned only AEDA, but this modification can be applied to any GCO dilution technique. Schieberle (30) stated that to avoid gaps, GCO should be conducted within 2 days. This, he said, can be done by sniffing the original extract and the dilutions 1:4, 1:16, 1:64, 1:256, and 1:1024 on the first day and the dilutions 1:2, 1:8, 1:32, 1:128, and 1:512 on the second day. He also recommended that the entire GC run be sniffed for each dilution.

While there are advantages to having one individual complete an entire sniffing run at one time, there are also concerns with this approach. Several researchers, among them McDaniel et al. (17) and Abbott et al. (31), have stated that an individual does not have the same GCO response at different times of the day or over longer time periods. For an individual concentrating only on one region of the chromatogram during GCO, a 3% coefficient of variance was found (32). This low coefficient of variance may be due to less fatigue on the part of the researcher concentrating on only one region as opposed to the entire GC profile.

B. AEDA and FD Factors

The volatiles in the initial extract can be sniffed by GCO in conjunction with FID detection or separately. Figure 1 is a GC profile of the initial extract of roasted beef (33) sniffed by GCO in conjunction with FID detection. Stepwise dilution of the extract and subsequent analysis of each dilution by GCO will yield a dilution where no more odorants are perceivable by GCO. The ratio of the concentration of the compound in the initial extract to its concentration in the most dilute extract in which the odor was detected by GCO is the FD factor of that compound. The FD factor by AEDA is identical to the peak maximum of a Charm value. The FD factor is a relative measure and is proportional to the OAV of that compound in air. Once the FD factors for the compounds are determined, an FD chromatogram is plotted. The FD chromatogram consists of the Kovats Index on the x-axis and the FD factors on the y-axis. An FD chromatogram for the odor active components of roasted beef (from Fig. 1) is shown in Figure 2 (33).

The AEDA technique has proven to be a valuable screening tool for determining key odorants in various foods. Some examples of foods investigated by AEDA include beef (33–35), beer (36), butter (13), butter oil (37), Emmentaler cheese (38), roasted coffee (39), cucumber (40), dill herb (12), honey (41), lemon oil (42), lovage (43), melon (40), mushroom (44), oat meal (45), olive oils (46), parsley (47), popcorn (48), puff pastry (49), rye bread crumb and crust (50), roasted sesame (51), strawberry (52), green and black tea (53), trout (54), and wheat bread crust (55) and crumb (56).

FD factors have found application in our laboratory for estimating the concentrations of compounds present at levels below their instrumental detection limits, e.g., differences in geosmin concentrations in extracts prepared from mold-infested grain. During a GCO run, the subject only smells at the specified retention time geosmin elutes. Dilutions are presented in a randomized order, and blanks are included in the analysis. We first prepare a standard solution of geosmin at an initial concentration that is easily detectable by all the subjects performing GCO. This concentration and subsequent dilutions of the standard are sniffed by GCO. The dilution (concentration) at which there is no perceptible odor by GCO for the geosmin standard (e.g., 0.03 ppb) is recorded as the odor threshold detection level for the subject. This threshold concentration (0.03 ppb) will be the same for geosmin in the standard and in

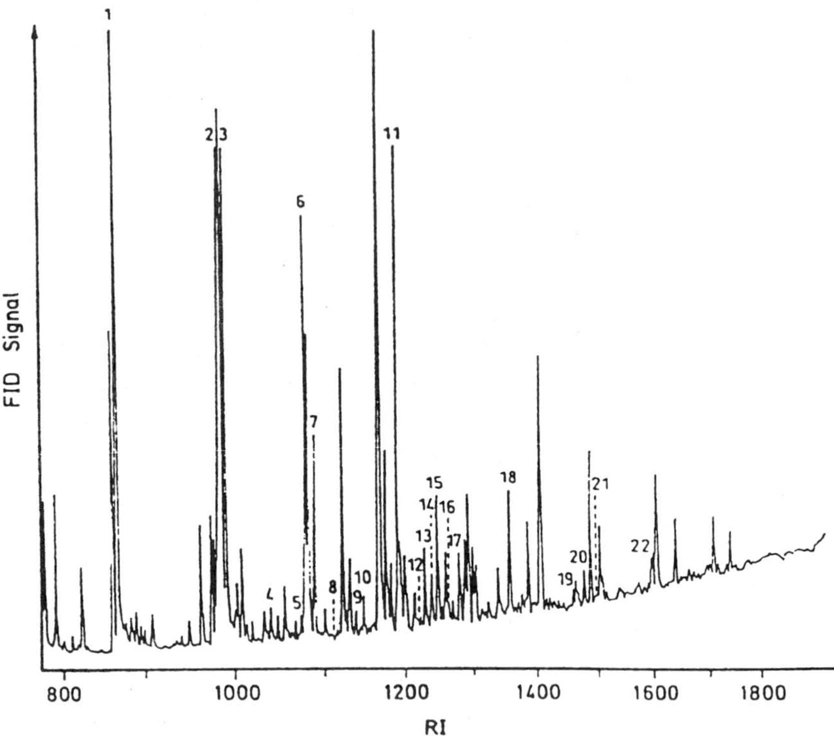

FIGURE 1 Gas chromatogram (GC-FID) of volatiles in roasted beef. Numbers 1–22 show the positions where an odor was detected by GCO. RI is the retention index on an OV-1701 capillary column. (From Ref. 33.)

the sample extracts for that particular subject. Next, the initial solvent extract of the sample and subsequent dilutions of the extract are also sniffed by GCO. The dilution at which there is no perceptible odor for geosmin in the sample extract is noted and the dilution factor determined (e.g., 3^6). The concentration of geosmin in the sample extract can be estimated by multiplying the dilution factor of geosmin at which no perceptible odor is detected (3^6) by its odor threshold (0.03 ppb).

1. Comparative AEDA

AEDA can also be used to identify flavor differences between two samples, e.g., a control and a sample containing an off-flavor. Once the odorant(s) caus-

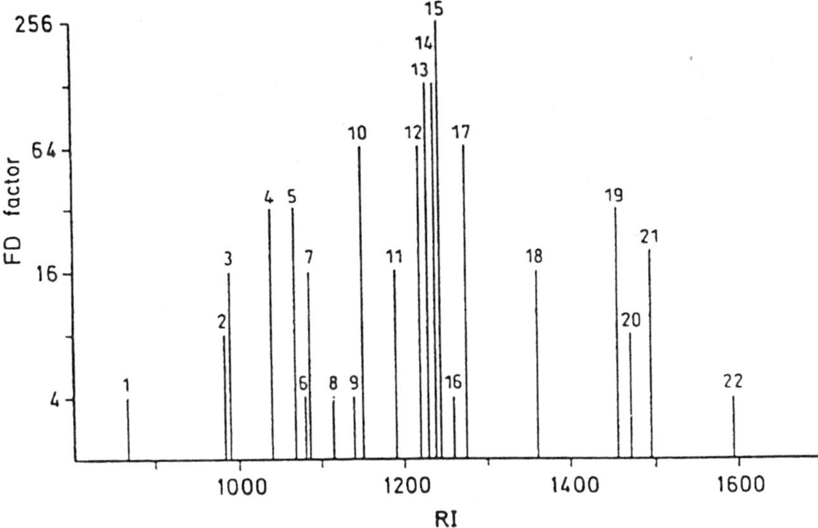

FIGURE 2 FD chromatogram of odor active compounds (1–22 in Fig. 1) of roasted beef. RI is the retention index on an OV-1701 capillary column. (From Ref. 33.)

ing the off-flavor has been identified, the odorant can be used as an indicator substance for an off-flavor. In comparative AEDA, the volatile compounds from the two samples (control and off-flavor) are isolated using exactly the same procedure. The flavor extracts then have to be concentrated to the same extent and the same amounts injected into the gas chromatograph for GCO work. Comparative AEDA assumes that if flavor extracts of both samples are prepared identically, AEDA and FD factors can be used to characterize differences between them (30).

Comparative AEDA has been used to identify off-flavors in soybean oil (57), butter oil (37), beer (36), extruded oatmeal (45), and trout (54). This technique has also been used to study the effects of processing on white sesame seeds (51) and strawberries (52).

2. Combined Headspace/AEDA

Most studies using AEDA are done with solvent extracts of volatiles isolated from foods. Unfortunately, highly volatile compounds may be lost during concentration of the solvent extract or they may cochromatograph with the solvent. In either case, AEDA would not be able to identify these compounds, leading to erroneous results. To overcome this limitation, a combined headspace/AEDA technique has been developed.

Both dynamic headspace (58) and static headspace (53,59–61) techniques have been used in conjunction with AEDA. Both dynamic and static headspace techniques offer the advantages of providing a solvent-free aroma isolate and potentially a more accurate view of the more volatile aroma constituents. However, static headspace methods provide too little material for identification by mass spectrometry. Dynamic headspace methods have a weakness in that they depend upon some method of aroma trapping (e.g., porous polymers or cryotrapping) to provide an aroma concentrate for analysis. Thus, dynamic headspace trapping also provides a biased view of the aroma isolate. Further, compounds that are difficult to isolate by vacuum distillation, solvent extraction, etc., may also be difficult to isolate by dynamic headspace methods. Combined headspace/AEDA potentially offers a view of the more volatile compounds and should always be used in conjunction with AEDA (using solvent extracts) where the key odorants have already been identified.

C. CharmAnalysis

The term "Charm" is an acronym for Combined Hedonic Aroma Response Measurements. The terms "charm" and "colors" are used to define peak areas and odor descriptors, respectively (16). CharmAnalysis is presented as a quantitative and qualitative tool for the analysis of gas chromatographic effluent. The method combines the use of GC-FID/GCO with a computer-assisted data-collection system (16,23,62). This method has developed into a commercially available system called CharmAnalysis™, which is assisted by the use of Charmware™ software.

The following procedure used in CharmAnalysis is summarized from Acree et al. (16) and Acree (23,62). The procedure first requires preparation of a representative extract of the aroma compound(s) of interest. This extract must be amenable to gas chromatographic analysis and suitable for the preparation of a series of dilutions. The extract is stepwise diluted by a constant factor, typically one part extract plus two parts diluent, until the last dilution results in no odor detection by GCO. An internal standard may be added to each dilution as a means of later monitoring the consistency of instrumental analysis over time. Gas chromatographic columns and operating conditions are selected based on composition of the extracts. CharmAnalysis recommends the use of shorter-length nonpolar columns (DB-1, OV-101, or SE-30) whenever possible to minimize the time required for complete elution of odor active compounds (23). A splitter is usually installed at the end of the column to divide the effluent for simultaneous detection by FID and GCO.

Before GCO of an aroma extract is performed, a standard of *n*-paraffins is chromatographed using the same conditions as those to be used for GCO, but with an FID detector. The retention times of the *n*-paraffins are used to determine retention indices of the eluting odors detected by GCO. Acree (62) makes use of *n*-paraffins to monitor chromatographic changes experienced over the time frame required to complete the CharmAnalysis. The extract dilution series is analyzed in a randomized order, the dilutions are coded, and subjects are not informed as to which sample they are evaluating. A single GCO run consists of first injecting an aliquot of a sample into the gas chromatograph. Following separation of the components by GC, the effluent exits the GC column into an olfactometer. The olfactometer delivers a stream of purified moist air (50–75% RH) at a linear velocity equal to or greater than the carrier gas in the chromatographic column (30–50 cm/sec). The flow design helps preserve chromatographic resolution. The olfactometer delivers the effluent to a subject seated comfortably away from the GC. The subject responds to the detection of an odor by depressing a button and holding it down till the odor changes in character or disappears. Depending on the software version, the subject can select a descriptive term on the screen to characterize the odor, or alternatively, the odor description is verbalized and recorded.

A computer data-handling system (Charmware) records the response time interval. For each CharmAnalysis, the retention time intervals of each odor are plotted to produce a square peak at a fixed height. Charm chromatograms are constructed by summing the square peaks produced at a given retention index from all the samples in a dilution series and then plotting peak areas at a specified retention index vs. dilution value (Fig. 3) (62). The added square waves are transformed to peak areas proportional to the concentration of the odor compound by use of an algorithm (62).

The areas under the curve are referred to as "charm values," and these areas are said to be proportional to the amount of odor active compound in the most concentrated sample (16,63). One of the purposes of integrating the area under the curve is an attempt to correct for the chromatographic properties of an aroma compound. For example, butyric acid will chromatograph poorly on a DB-5 column resulting in an irregular, lower, and broad peak; however, on a DB-wax column, butyric acid will exhibit the desired Gaussian peak shape and will be higher with narrow peak width. Hence, for the same concentration of butyric acid, the charm value (integrated area) determined using a DB-5 column should be approximately equal to that using a DB-wax column. The concept of including elution time range is unique to CharmAnalysis. The sig-

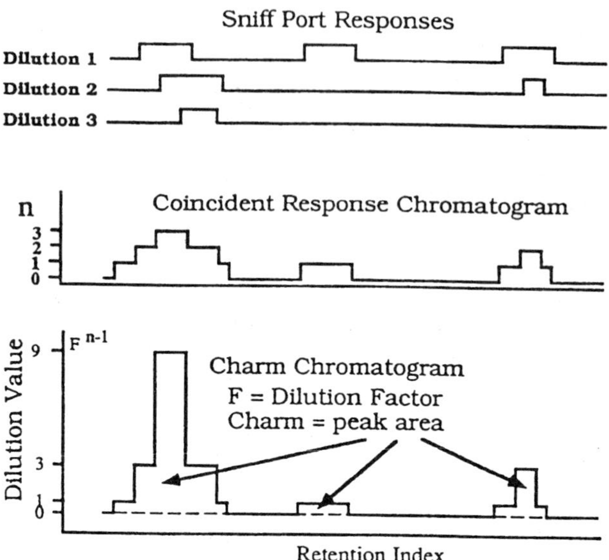

FIGURE 3 Stages in the development of a Charm chromatogram. (From Ref. 62.)

nificance of including time as a variable influencing the validity of the data is discussed in the following sections.

Although CharmAnalysis has limitations with respect to the validity of interpretations derived from Charm values, CharmAnalysis has proven useful as a comparative tool for evaluating differences in aroma extracts. CharmAnalysis also enables identification of odor active compounds within an aroma extract and determination of the odor characteristics of these compounds as a function of decreasing concentration. Perhaps of great interest would be the combination of extract dilution techniques and Osme. By incorporating these two methodologies, odor intensity–concentration curves for compounds of interest could be determined by GCO.

D. AEDA vs. CharmAnalysis

The main difference in interpretation of results between CharmAnalysis and AEDA methods is that in CharmAnalysis, the duration of the odor by GCO is taken into account while in AEDA, only the maximum dilution value detected is noted. The FD factor determined by AEDA has the same significance as the apex of the peak in CharmAnalysis. A study on beer conducted by Abbott et al. (31) is the only one we have found that compares the data from AEDA and CharmAnalysis. Abbott et al. (31) indicated that the method by which the data are treated (AEDA vs. CharmAnalysis) can lead to very different results. The order of potency of the key odorants was different for most of the six panelists when the data were presented as log FD factors vs. Kovats Index (AEDA) compared to log surface area vs. Kovats Index (CharmAnalysis). Abbott et al. (31) indicated that it was difficult for the panelists to detect the end of the odor active peak during a GCO run. This would lead to errors in determining surface areas of the odor active peaks using CharmAnalysis but have no influence on the FD factors. Therefore, the values for log surface areas showed greater errors compared to log FD factors. More work needs to be done to understand the differences in results and validity of AEDA and CharmAnalysis.

VI. OSME METHOD

Osme, a cross-modal method of GCO, was developed by McDaniel and coworkers at Oregon State University (17,64,65). Osme, derived from a Greek word meaning smell, is a quantitative bioassay that can be used to measure the perceived odor intensity of a compound eluting from a gas chromatograph olfactometer (64). Osme has been used to determine aroma differences in wines, hops and beers influenced by harvest time, hop variety, and added hop fraction (17,64–66).

Osme first involves preparation of a representative extract of the aroma being studied. The aroma extract is then analyzed by traditional GC methodology using a chemical detector to obtain an analytical profile. Subsequently, the detector end of the column is moved to a sensory detector port. The delivery of GC effluent to a subject is accomplished using a 1 cm i.d. × 60 cm length of silicon-coated glass venturi tube. The GC effluent is mixed with humidifed air (60% RH) and passed through the glass tubing at a rate of 11 liters/min to a subject seated away from the gas chromatograph. The subject rates the intensity of an eluting compound using an electronic time-intensity scaling device (15-cm scale) and at the same time describes the odor of the eluting compound, which is also recorded. The 15-cm scale is labeled as 0 = none, 7 = moderate, and 15 = extreme.

A subject's response is registered directly into a computer data-handling system (software program) developed for Osme. Data obtained by Osme are odor retention times, time intensity ranges, and corresponding odor descriptors. Times and intensities of peaks detected at least 50% of the time for a given sample by a subject are averaged and these averages used to construct individual Osmegrams. Next, a consensus Osmegram based on the individual subject's averages of times and intensities of peaks detected by at least three of the four subjects (4 replications × 4 trained subjects) is constructed. As with other GCO methods (AEDA and CharmAnalysis), the retention times are converted to retention indices. The resulting consensus Osmegram looks very much like a traditional chromatogram; however, the coordinates represent perceived average intensity (y-axis) vs. retention index (x-axis) (Fig. 4).

Osme differs from AEDA and CharmAnalysis in that only one concentration of the extract is evaluated. No dilution series is prepared; hence, results obtained by Osme are not based on odor detection thresholds. Osme is founded on principles consistent with current psychophysical theories. For example, the use of a trained sensory panel and the 15-cm scale is consistent with descriptive analysis techniques. The perceived intensity scores collected by Osme could be analyzed by common statistical methods such as *t*-test and analysis of variance to determine differences between compounds within a sample or between samples (25). It is unfortunate that statistics have not been applied to Osme because statistical analysis of the data would lend a credibility not yet attained by other GCO methods.

The formal application of intensity measurement of compounds detected by GCO is late in arriving, and consequently Osme competes with two traditional research methods (AEDA and CharmAnalysis). To its researcher's credit, Osme does not attempt to assign relative importance of a compound to an aroma based on its perceived intensity. To do so would perpetuate an error made by flavor chemists who use extract dilution methods (AEDA and CharmAnalysis) to rate compounds with the highest flavor dilution values as being most important to the aroma of the food (discussed in section on OAV). Osme stands by itself since the method is based on valid sensory relationships and the intensity data collected are quantitative, permitting statistical comparisons between compounds and samples.

Guichard et al. (67) compared the results of intensity response measurements of a model aroma extract (Osmelike) with those obtained by CharmAnalysis. No significant differences were observed between the two techniques. A close evaluation of the work suggests a reason for these results. First, in evaluating the two techniques, large coefficients of variation were found between judges. (Ten trained judges were used for intensity response, while three were used for CharmAnalysis.) Second, Steven's slope (n) and the threshold values for the compounds investigated were similar. For three of the six compounds investigated, n ranged from 0.40 to 0.52, and for the other three compounds, n ranged from 0.26 to 0.35. With regard to threshold, for

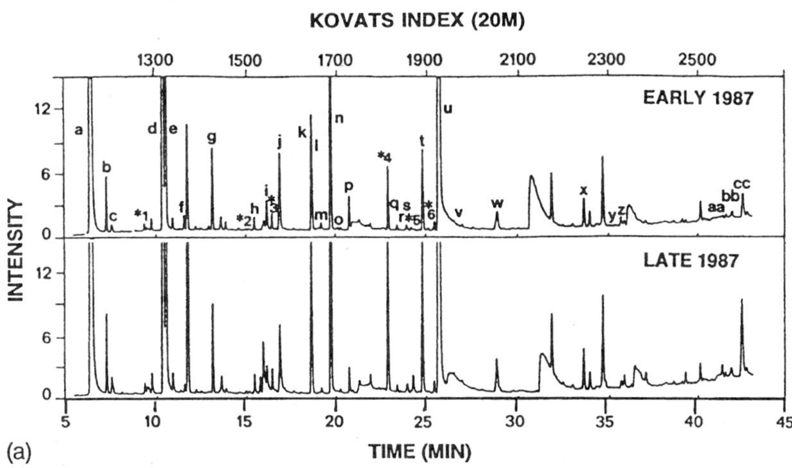

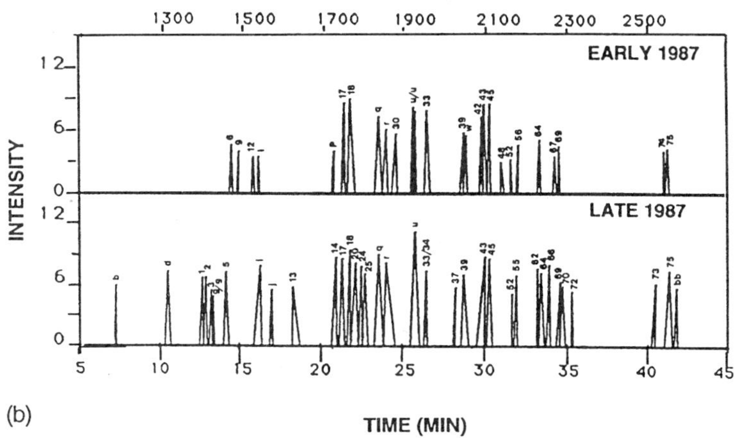

FIGURE 4 (a) Gas chromatograms of early 1987 and late 1987 wines. (b) Osmegrams of early 1987 and late 198 wines. (From Ref. 66.)

five of the six compounds, thresholds differed only by a factor of approximately 10; for the sixth compound, the threshold differed by a factor of approximately 100. The narrow differences between the power function slopes (n) within the two sets and corresponding narrow threshold range may not have been great enough to be detected by the judges (given the large coefficients of variation). Consistent results would be expected by both response methods if the values of n and the threshold values were within the variability range of the judges. However, one would not expect consistent results to prevail for compounds having a broader range in sensory thresholds and power function slopes (n).

VII. ODOR ACTIVITY VALUES

As mentioned in the previous section, AEDA and CharmAnalysis should be considered screening tools for ranking odor active compounds in foods. AEDA and CharmAnalysis are both based on the odor thresholds of compounds in air; in real life, the odor properties of these compounds are influenced by the food matrix. To overcome this and other limitations of the extract dilution techniques (which have been discussed), Grosch and coworkers took AEDA one step further by determining the OAVs of the odorants.

After AEDA is carried out to aid in the selection of key odorants of a food, OAVs of these volatiles are determined. In the OAV approach, the concentration of the selected odor active compound is first accurately determined by stable isotope dilution assay (see next section). Next, the nasal or retronasal threshold of the compound is determined in the matrix that most closely resembles the food being analyzed. For example, in their work on determining key odorants of butter, Schieberle et al. (13) used sunflower oil to determine odor thresholds of the odorants. Having determined the absolute concentrations and sensory threshold, the OAVs of all the key odorants are calculated.

Table 1 (33) shows the concentrations and OAVs of six key odor active compounds (out of the 22 compounds in Figure 2) responsible for the roasted aroma of beef.

A. Stable Isotope Dilution Assay

When determining OAV, it is imperative that the concentration of the odor active compound be accurately determined. In typical GC quantitation work, an internal standard with a chemical structure similar to that of the compound is used if the compound is present at concentrations of 0.1 ppm or higher (30).

TABLE 1 Concentrations and OAVs of Six Key Odor Active Compounds in Roasted Beef[a]

Compound	Concentration (μg/kg)	OAV[b]
4-Hydroxy-2,5-dimethyl-3(2H)-furanone	928	9
2-Acetyl-2-thiazoline	28	28
2-Ethyl-3,5-dimethylpyrazine	5.4	3
2,3-Diethyl-5-methylpyrazine	27	27
Guaiacol	2.1	1
Methional	12.5	7

[a]The beef was roasted for 7 min at temperatures increasing from 200 to 210°C.
[b]For OAV, a nasally estimated odor threshold in water was determined.
Source: Ref. 33.

However, when quantifying trace levels of volatile compounds or compounds that are labile or polar, the use of related chemicals as standards is not a choice. Typical examples of such compounds are 4-hydroxy-2,5-dimethyl-3(2H)-furanone and 3-hydroxy-4,5-dimethyl-2(5H)-furanone (68). For compounds such as these, the internal standard used for quantification is a stable isotope (typically m + 2) of the particular compound being analyzed. This technique has been applied to flavor work by Grosch and coworkers and is called stable isotope dilution assay. This labeled internal standard has the same chemical and physical properties as the analyte. Isolation losses experienced by the analyte will be experienced in a similar fashion by the stable isotope.

Grosch (68) has given a good overview of stable isotope dilution assay. Briefly, the food sample is spiked with a known amount of labeled isotope(s) of the odor active compound(s) previously screened by AEDA. The volatile fraction is then isolated and the extract containing the labeled isotope standard and the analyte(s) is analyzed by gas chromatography/selected ion mass spectrometry (SIM) in the chemical ionization mode. The SIM peak areas for the labeled isotope and the analyte give their relative concentrations. Knowing the exact amount of labeled isotope in the extract and using the peak areas, the concentration of the analyte can be calculated. One assumes that both the labeled isotope and the analyte suffer the same losses during isolation, GC analysis, and mass spectrometry.

It is very costly and time-consuming to synthesize stable isotopes for the 10–20 compounds previously selected by AEDA. The stable isotopes are not always commercially available, and they can be very expensive. Synthesis of stable isotopes requires expertise on the part of the researcher. Schieberle (30) has listed the 60 stable isotopes prepared for determining key odorants in foods in their laboratories.

Most of the stable isotopes used as internal standards are labeled with deuterium because their synthesis is less expensive (68). There are some deuterated odor active components that during quantification will undergo deuterium-protium exchange, producing erroneous results. Such compounds have to be labeled with ^{13}C instead. Examples of these components are 3-hydroxy-4,5-dimethyl-2(5H)-furanone and 4-hydroxy-2,5-dimethyl-3(2H)-furanone (69,70).

B. Determination of Threshold Values

Once absolute concentrations of the key aroma components have been determined, researchers must determine the sensory threshold of each of these compounds. When determining sensory thresholds, it is very important to use the same matrix (or a comparable one) as the food system containing the key aroma compounds. Threshold values of aroma compounds determined in air or in a simple solution will not be the same as those in a food matrix due to flavor/food interactions, which in turn will affect the release of these aroma compounds during eating (71).

Different components of the food matrix such as fats, carbohydrates, proteins, and macromolecules interact with the flavor compounds in the food. Most flavor compounds are hydrophobic and will interact with fat (72). Changing the fat content will affect the odor threshold of odor active compounds in the food. For example, the flavor thresholds of octanoic acid and γ-decalactone are 60 times higher in oil than in water (73). Bakker (71) indicated that carbohydrates influence the flavor thresholds of compounds; however, there is very little published data on carbohydrate/flavor interactions. Volatiles are selectively bound to proteins by hydrophobic interactions with discrete binding zones (74). Pangborn and Szczesniak (75) showed that hydrocolloids (hydroxypropylcellulose, sodium alginate, xanthan, and sodium carboxymethylcellulose) suppressed the odor intensities of select flavor compounds (acetaldehyde, acetophenone, butyric acid, and dimethyl sulfide).

Threshold values are determined by Grosch and coworkers in two ways: by GCO and by triangle testing in a medium prevailing in the food being tested (C. Milo, personal communication). In the first method, a standard compound, 2(E)-decenal, with a known odor threshold (2.7 ng/liter) (76) was chosen. A known concentration of this compound is added to a solution containing a known concentration of the odor active compound, y. This mixture and subsequent dilutions of it are then analyzed by GCO until there are no perceivable odors of the standard or compound y. Knowing the concentrations of the standard and compound y and the odor threshold of the standard, the odor threshold of compound y can be calculated.

Odor thresholds of key odor compounds are also determined by performing triangle tests nasally or retronasally (C. Milo, personal communication). Samples of known concentrations of the odor active compound are prepared in a medium (e.g., water, sunflower oil, cellulose, etc.) that predominates in the food. Then, two blanks and one sample containing known concentration of the odor active compound are presented as a set to a trained panel of at least five judges. These sets of samples are evaluated in decreasing order of concentration and the recognition threshold is determined.

The usefulness of odor thresholds has been summarized by Teranishi et al. (77). They indicated that their flavor research group (U.S.D.A., Agricultural Research Service, Western Research Center, Albany, CA) has been using the concept of odor threshold in foods for the past 30 years. They have used the concept to determine odor purity of compounds. The concept is also used by Teranishi et al. (77) to determine the amounts of starting materials, serve as a reference point in describing odor intensity and quality (odor quality changes with concentration) and evaluate the importance of key aroma compounds.

C. Limitations of OAV

As was noted earlier, the concept of odor activity value proposed by Grosch and coworkers is not new. However, OAV has been taken one step further by Grosch and coworkers in that it is not used as a stand-alone method but is used in conjunction with AEDA to determine key odorants in foods.

The main limitation of OAV is the lack of correlation between odor thresholds of compounds determined in air and in a medium that predominates in the food. Threshold values of odor active compounds in foods have traditionally been determined in air. This disregards the fact that the compound will interact with the water, carbohydrates, proteins, and fat present in the food, thus influencing its odor perception (71). The odor thresholds of compounds in air are lower than in oil (30). The threshold values of *trans*-2-decadienal and hexanal are approximately 0.03 and 14 ppb in air (78) and 135 and 120 ppb in oil, respectively (6). If equal concentrations of these compounds are present in the solvent extract obtained from potato chips, and the threshold values are determined in air, the OAV for hexanal would be lower (OAV is the ratio of concentration to threshold, and hexanal has a higher threshold in air than *trans*-2-decadienal). However, in potato chips, the thresholds of these two compounds are influenced by the presence of oil and will have about the same OAV if their concentrations are similar (here, the thresholds for *trans*-2-decadienal and hexanal in oil are 135 and 120 ppb, respectively). Researchers as early as Mulders (7) understood this limitation of determining odor and flavor thresholds in air or water and trying to correlate them to the food matrix. To overcome this limitation, Mulders (7) in his work on flavor of white bread, compared threshold values of compounds in the headspace of a synthetic aqueous solution to those in the headspace of bread.

There is also a lack of correlation between threshold values of compounds evaluated nasally (by smelling) or retronasally (by tasting). The method by which threshold values are determined will influence OAVs of odor active compounds. This in turn will influence the relative aroma rating given to these compounds in food. Table 2 (79) shows differences in threshold values of some odor active compounds in fresh cod determined both nasally and retronasally. The table also shows differences in OAVs of these compounds (79).

The chemical and physical properties of odor active compounds will in-

TABLE 2 Nasal and Retronasal Thresholds and OAVs of Some Odor Active Compounds in Fresh Cod

Compound	Threshold in water (μg/kg)		OAVs (conc./threshold)	
	Nasal	Retronasal	Nasal	Retronasal
Dimethyltrisulfide	0.006	0.008	25	19
(E,E)-2,4-Nonadienal	0.1	0.06	32	53
Methanethiol	0.2	2	500	50
Methional	0.2	0.04	55	275
(Z)-4-Heptenal	0.2	0.06	8	27
Dimethylsulfide	0.3	2	260	39
3-Methylbutanal	0.35	0.25	145	204
Hexanal	4.5	10.5	26	11
Diacetyl	15	5	13	40
1-Octen-3-one	0.05	0.01	14	70
2,3-Pentanedione	30	5	3	17

Source: Ref. 79.

fluence flavor/food interactions. One should keep in mind that odor threshold values of isomers of some compounds will be different. For example, α-ionone has a threshold of 0.5 ppb (w/v); its isomer, β-ionone, has a threshold of 20 ppb (w/v) (80).

Koster and Wouters (81) and Frijters (82) have severely criticized the meaningfulness of conclusions drawn from OAV (odor unit, aroma value, etc.). Frijters (82) stated that OAV is not a number of absolute physical concentration, but only an arbitrary scale defining the number of times by which the threshold concentration is exceeded.

Frijters (82) further stated that since OAV does not have physical and perceptual measurements, it is not a psychophysical measure for perceived odor intensity. Yet OAV makes erroneous assumptions based on psychophysical theories. These assumptions are that (82) (a) two odor active compounds with the same OAV will exhibit an equal perceived intensity and (b) a linear relationship exists between the concentration of the compound and its perceived intensity. Koster and Wouters (81) indicated that two compounds with the same OAV may not demonstrate the same odor intensity. Also, the compounds will most likely exhibit different concentration/perceived intensity behavior. This statement (81) was corroborated by Frijters (82) and Sauvageot (83), who stated that assumption (b) is invalid by both Fechner's and Stevens's laws (84), which indicate that a logarithmic or power relationship exists between perceived intensity and concentration of the odorant.

The odor character of the food will strongly influence the relative importance of an odor compound to the overall aroma. For example, if the concentrations of a foul-smelling substance like skatole and a pleasant-smelling substance such as vanillin in food are the same, the perceived intensities of these two compounds will not be the same: the perceived intensity of skatole will be higher than that of vanillin. For these reasons, ranking odor active components on the basis of their OAV values may not be a good indicator of their relative importance in a food system.

Frijters (82) also stated that the odor intensity of a mixture is not necessarily equal to the summed intensities of the individual components. It has been proven (with some exceptions) that the perceived intensity of a two-compound mixture is less than the sum of intensities of the single components but more than their arithmetic mean.

Despite the limitations of OAV, Frijters (82) states that "although this concept does not have precise validity, it can give some guidance in particular investigations." We need to expand our knowledge base in sensory perception, structure-activity relationships of compounds, and food matrix influences in order to correct some of the limitations of OAV. For now, the OAV method gives a good indication of contributions of key aroma compounds in foods. The OAV method is further strengthened when combined with aroma-recombination studies.

VIII. AROMA-RECOMBINATION STUDIES

Aroma-recombination studies take all the analytical information obtained in determining key odorants in foods and correlate it with sensory studies. The key odorants determined in foods are combined in specific concentrations, as determined by stable isotope dilution assay, and given to a trained sensory panel. This sensory panel determines how close the reconstituted food aroma is to the real food. Aroma-recombination studies are, therefore, a very important last step in verifying the analytical data on key odorants of foods. Aroma-recombination studies will verify and correct for the limitations of the GCO methods and threshold determinations (limitations discussed in previous sections).

So far, information on aroma-recombination studies has been published for tomato (10,11), dill herb (12), butter flavors (13), and Emmentaler cheese (14). Buttery et al. (10,11) determined the odor thresholds and log odor units (i.e., log [concentration in the food vs. odor threshold]) of major volatile compounds in fresh tomatoes and in tomato pastes. In fresh tomatoes, log odor units of 15 volatile compounds were determined. Out of these 15 compounds, a water solution of only the first 8 compounds with the highest log odor units (4.3 to 0.9) was required to simulate the flavor of fresh tomatoes. Also, in a similar study on tomato pastes, Buttery et al. (11) determined that a water solution containing a mixture of 7 volatile compounds (out of 40 volatile compounds they identified) with the highest log odor unit values (3.8 to 0.9) was found to closely duplicate the odor of tomato paste.

In studies on dill herb (12), four odor active compounds, (3R, 4S, 8S)-3,9-epoxy-1-p-methene, (S)-α-phellandrene, methyl-2-methylbutanoate and myristicin, had the highest FD factors by AEDA. When these four compounds were dissolved in water at the same concentrations found in dill herb, the overall odor of this mixture resembled that of the dill herb. Schieberle et al. (13) in a study on butter flavor observed that diacetyl, δ-decalactone, and butanoic acid showed the highest OAVs in an Irish sour cream butter. They combined diacetyl, δ-decalactone, and butanoic acid in sunflower oil and found that the odor of this synthetic mixture very closely resembled that of the cultured butter. In similar work on two samples of Emmentaler cheese, odor active compounds with high OAVs were selected for aroma-recombination studies (14). These compounds, methional (OAV 660, 306), 4-hydroxy-2,5-dimethyl-3(2H)-furanone (OAV 509, 206), and 5-ethyl-4-hydroxy-2-methyl-3(2H)-furanone (OAV 94, 148), along with acetic, propionic, and lactic acids, were added to unripened cheese (similar to mozzarella) in concentrations found in Emmentaler cheese. Sensory studies showed that the model mixture simulated the odor of Emmentaler cheese. Grosch (14) also indicated that odor active compounds with OAVs between 3 and 14 did not have any effect on the overall odor of the cheese.

IX. CONCLUSIONS

Great strides have been made in the last decade on modifications of GCO techniques to determine the overall contributions of key odorants in foods. Three ingenious methods—AEDA/OAV values, CharmAnalysis, and Osme—have gained popularity in the field of flavor research. When using these tools to obtain information on intensities or contributions of key odorants in foods, one should be aware of the strengths and limitations of each of these methods. We are hopeful that more aroma-recombination studies will be forthcoming since these studies provide an invaluable tool in determining the roles of individual odor active compounds and various combinations of these compounds in foods.

REFERENCES

1. H. Maarse, in *Volatile Compuonds in Foods and Beverages* (H. Maarse, ed.), Marcel Dekker, New York, 1991, p. 1.
2. F. Tiemann and W. Haarmann, *Ber. Dtsch. Chem. Ges. 7:*608 (1874) (original not seen).
3. K. Reimer, *Ber. Dtsch. Chem. Ges. 9:*423 (1876) (original not seen).
4. *Volatile Compounds in Food, Qualitative and Quantitative Data*, 6th ed., TNO Nutrition and Food Research in Zeist, the Netherlands, 1989–1994 and supplements.
5. S. Patton and D. Josephson, *Food Res. 22:*316 (1957).
6. D. Guadagni, S. Okano, R. Buttery, and H. Burr, *Food Technol. 20:*166 (1966).
7. E. Mulders, *Z. Lebensm. Unters. Forsch. 151:*310 (1973).
8. M. Rothe and B. Thomas, *Z. Lebensm. Unters. Forsch. 219:*302 (1963).
9. E. Keith and J. Powers, *J. Food Sci. 33:*213 (1968).
10. R. Buttery, R. Teranishi, and L. Ling, *J. Agric. Food Chem. 35:*540 (1987).
11. R. Buttery, R. Teranishi, L. Ling, and J. Turnbaugh, *J. Agric. Food Chem 38:*336 (1990).
12. I. Blank and W. Grosch, *J. Food Sci. 56:*63 (1991).
13. P. Schieberle, K. Gassenmeier, H. Guth, A. Sen, and W. Grosch, *Lebensm. Wiss. Technol., 26:*347 (1993).

14. W. Grosch, *Flavor Fragrance J. 9:*1 (1994).
15. F. Ullrich and W. Grosch, *Z. Lebensm. Unters. Forsch. 184:*277 (1987).
16. T. Acree, J. Barnard, and D. Cunningham, *Food Chem. 14:*273 (1984).
17. M. McDaniel, R. Miranda-Lopez, B. Watson, N. Micheals, and L. Libbey, in *Flavors and Off-Flavors—Proceedings of the 6th International Flavor Conference* (G. Charalambous, ed.), Elsevier Science Publishers B.V., Amsterdam, 1990, p. 23.
18. G. Reineccius, in *Flavor Measurement* (C.-T. Ho and C. Manley, eds.), Marcel Dekker, New York, 1993, p. 61.
19. H. Guth and W. Grosch, *Lebensm. Wiss. Technol. 23:*513 (1990).
20. M. Leahy and G. Reineccius, in *Analysis of Volatiles: Methods and Application* (P. Schreier, ed.), Walter de Gruyter, Berlin, 1984, p. 19.
21. R. Nelson, T. Acree, C. Lee, and R. Butts, *J. Food Sci. 42*(1):57 (1977).
22. G. Reineccius, in *Source Book of Flavors* (G. Reineccius, ed.), Chapman & Hall, New York, 1994, p. 24.
23. T. Acree, in *Flavor Measurement* (C.-T. Ho and C. Manley, eds.), Marcel Dekker, New York, 1993, p. 77.
24. S. Nitz and F. Drawert, *Chem. Mikrobiol. Technol. Lebensm., 7:*148 (1982).
25. M. Gillette, in *Source Book of Flavors* (G. Reineccius, ed.), Chapman & Hall, New York, 1994, p. 824.
26. M. Amerine, R. Pangborn, and E. Roessler, in *Principles of Sensory Evauation of Food* (M. Amerine, ed.), Academic Press, New York, 1965.
27. M. Meilgaard, G. Civille, and B. Carr, in *Sensory Evaluation Techniques* (M. Meilgaard, ed.), CRC Press, New York, 1987.
28. P. Schieberle and W. Grosch, *Z. Lebensm. Unters. Forsch, 185:*111 (1987).
29. I. Blank, A. Sen, and W. Grosch, *Z. Lebensm. Unters. Forsch., 195:*239 (1992).
30. P. Schieberle, in *Characterization of Food: Emerging Methods* (A. Gaonkar, ed.), Elsevier Science, 1995.
31. N. Abbott, P. Etievant, S. Issanchou, and D. Langlois, *J. Agric. Food Chem., 41:*1698 (1993).
32. P. Darriet, V. Lavigne, J. Boidron, and D. Dubourdieu, *J. Int. Sci. Vigne Vin 25:*167 (1991) (original not seen).
33. C. Cerny and W. Grosch, *Z. Lebensm. Unters. Forsch., 194:*322 (1992).
34. U. Gasser and W. Grosch, *Z. Lebensm. Unters. Forsch. 186:*489 (1988).
35. H. Guth and W. Grosch, *Lebensm. Wiss. Technol. 26:*171 (1993).
36. P. Schieberle, *Z. Lebensm. Unters. Forsch. 193:*558 (1991).
37. S. Widder, A. Sen, and W. Grosch, *Z. Lebensm. Unters. Forsch. 193:*32 (1991).
38. M. Preininger and W. Grosch, *Lebensm. Wiss. Technol. 27*(3):237 (1994).
39. I. Blank, A. Sen, and W. Grosch, *Z. Lebensm. Unters. Forsch. 195:*239 (1992).
40. P. Schieberle, S. Ofner, and W. Grosch, *J. Food Sci. 55:*193 (1990).
41. I. Blank, K. Fischer, and W. Grosch, *Z. Lebensm. Unters. Forsch. 189:*426 (1989).
42. P. Schieberle and W. Grosch, *J. Agric. Food Chem. 36:*797 (1988).

43. I. Blank and P. Schieberle, *Flavor Fragrance J. 8:*191 (1993).
44. K. Fischer and W. Grosch, *Lebensm. Wiss. Technol. 20:*233 (1987).
45. H. Guth and W. Grosch, *Z. Lebensm. Unters. Forsch. 196:*22 (1993).
46. H. Guth and W. Grosch, *Fat Sci. Technol. 93:*335 (1991) (original not seen).
47. H. Jung, A. Sen, and W. Grosch, *Lebensm. Wiss. Technol. 25:*55 (1992).
48. P. Schieberle, *J. Agric. Food Chem., 39:*1141 (1991).
49. K. Gassenmeier and P. Schieberle, *Lebensm. Wiss. Technol., 27*(3):282 (1994).
50. P. Schieberle and W. Grosch, *Z. Lebensm. Unters. Forsch., 198:*292 (1994).
51. P. Schieberle, in *Progress in Flavor Precursor Studies* (P. Schreier and P. Winterhalter, eds.), Allured Publishing Corp., IL, 1993, p. 343.
52. P. Schieberle, in *Trends in Flavor Research* (H. Maarse and D. Van der Heij, eds.), Elsevier Press, Amsterdam, 1994, p. 345.
53. H. Guth and W. Grosch, *Flavor Fragrance J. 8:*173 (1993).
54. W. Grosch, C. Milo, and S. Widder, in *Trends in Flavor Research* (H. Maarse and D. Van der Heij, eds.), Elsevier Press, Amsterdam, 1994, p. 409.
55. P. Schieberle and W. Grosch, *Z. Lebensm. Unters. Forsch. 185:*111 (1987).
56. P. Schieberle and W. Grosch, *Z. Lebensm. Unters. Forsch. 192:*130 (1991).
57. H. Guth and W. Grosch, *Lebensm. Wiss. Technol. 23:*59 (1990).
58. P. Schieberle and W. Grosch, *Flavor Fragrance J. 7:*213 (1992).
59. W. Grosch, *Lebensmittelchemie 47:*129 (1993).
60. H. Guth and W. Grosch, in *Trends in Flavor Research* (H. Maarse and D. Van der Heij, eds.), Elsevier Press, Amsterdam, 1994, p. 395.
61. C. Milo and W. Grosch, *J. Agric. Food Chem. 43:*459 (1995).
62. T. Acree, in *Flavor Science: Sensible Principles and Techniques* (T. Acree and R. Teranishi, eds.), American Chemical Society, Washington, DC, 1993, p. 1.
63. A. Marin, T. Acree, J. Hotchkiss, and S. Nagy, *J. Agric. Food Chem. 40:*650 (1992).
64. R. Miranda-Lopez, Master's Thesis, Oregon State University, Corvalis, OR, 1990.
65. N. Sanchez, Master's Thesis, Oregon State University, Corvalis, OR, 1990.
66. R. Miranda-Lopez, L. Libbey, B. Watson, and M. McDaniel, *J. Food Sci. 57*(4):985 (1992).
67. H. Guichard, E. Guichard, D. Langlois, S. Tssanchou, and N. Abbott, *Z. Lebensm. Unters. Forsch. 210:*344 (1995).
68. W. Grosch, *Trends Food Sci. Technol. 4*(3):68 (1993).
69. A. Sen, P. Schieberle, and W. Grosch, *Lebensm. Wiss. Technol. 24:*364 (1991).
70. I. Blank, P. Schieberle, and W. Grosch, in *Progress in Flavor Precursor Studies* (P. Schreier and P. Winterhalter, eds.), Allured Publishing Co., IL, 1993, p. 103.
71. J. Bakker, in *Ingredient Interactions: Effects on Food Quality* (A. Gaonkar, ed.), Marcel Dekker, Inc., New York, 1995, p. 411.
72. R. Buttery, J. Bomben, D. Guadagni, and L. Ling, *J. Agric. Food Chem. 19:*1045 (1971).

73. J. Kinsella, in *Flavor Chemistry of Lipid Foods* (D. Min and T. Smouse, eds.), American Oil Chemists' Society, Champaign, IL, 1989, p. 376.
74. J. Solms, in *Interactions of Food Components* (G. Birch and M. Lindley, eds.), Elsevier Applied Science Publishers, London, 1986, p. 189.
75. R. Pangborn and A. Szczesniak, *J. Texture Stud. 4:*467 (1974).
76. M. Boelens and L. J. van Gemert, in *Developments in Food Flavors* (G. Birch and M. Lindley, eds.), Elsevier Applied Science, London, 1986, p. 23.
77. R. Teranishi, R. Buttery, D. Stern, and G. Takeoka, *Lebensm. Wiss. Technol. 24:*1 (1991).
78. M. Devos, F. Patte, J. Rouault, P. Laffort, and L. van Gemert, eds. *Standardized Human Olfactory Thresholds* Oxford University Press, New York, 1990.
79. C. Milo, Ph.D. dissertation, Technical University, Munich, Germany, 1995.
80. L. Van Gemert and A. Nettenbreijer *Compilation of Odour Threshold Values in Air and Water*, National Inst. for Water Supply, Voorburg, The Netherlands and Central Institute for Nutrition and Food Research TNO, Zeist, The Netherlands, 1977.
81. E. Koster and O. Wouters, *Ernahrungs-Umschau 17:*349 (1970) (original not seen).
82. J. Frijters, in *Progress in Flavor Research* (D. Land and H. Nursten, eds.), Applied Science Publishers Ltd., London, 1978, p. 47.
83. F. Sauvageot, *Evaluation sensorielle. Manuel Methodologiques* TEC and APRIA, Paris, 1990, p. 15 (original not seen).
84. W. Wagenaar, *Acta Psychol. 39:*225 (1975) (original not seen).

10

Gas Chromatography–Olfactometry in Food Aroma Analysis

Imre Blank
Nestec Ltd., Lausanne, Switzerland

I. INTRODUCTION

Progress in instrumental analysis has led to long lists of volatiles (1). Unfortunately, the sensory relevance of these volatile compounds has not been as extensively evaluated, although the use of the human nose as a sensitive detector in gas chromatography (GC) was proposed by Fuller and coworkers as early as 1964 (2). In the meantime, much has been published on food aroma, often without identifying the impact compounds. Therefore, one of the major problems in aroma research is to select those compounds that significantly contribute to the aroma of a food.

Flavor is usually divided into the subsets of taste and smell, which are perceived in the month and the nose, respectively. However, "flavor" is frequently used in publications exclusively dealing with volatiles. The terms "aroma" and "odor" are not well defined and are often used as synonyms.

Odor is best reserved for the smell of food before it is put into the mouth (nasal perception) and aroma for the retronasal smell of food in the mouth.

In general, the aroma of a food consists of many volatile compounds, only a few of which are sensorially relevant. A first essential step in aroma analysis is the distinction of the more potent odorants from volatiles having low or no aroma activity. In 1963, Rothe and Thomas calculated the ratio of the concentration of an odorant to its odor threshold and denoted it "aroma value" (3). This approach was the first attempt to estimate the sensory contribution of single odorants to the overall aroma of a food. Since that time, similar methods have been developed: odor unit (4) based on nasal odor thresholds, flavor unit (5) using retronasal odor thresholds, and odor activity value (OAV) (6). However, this concept requires identification and quantification of a great number of volatile compounds and determination of their threshold values, which is time-consuming. Furthermore, there is no guarantee that all of the important odorants were considered, unless a screening step for the most important aroma compounds was used.

GC in combination with olfactometric techniques (GC-O) is a valuable method for the selection of aroma-active components from a complex mixture (7). Experiments based on human subjects sniffing GC effluents are described as GC-O. This technique helps to detect potent odorants, without knowing their chemical structures, which might be overlooked by the OAV concept (ratio of concentration to threshold) if the sensory aspect is not considered from the very beginning of the analysis. Experience shows that many key aroma compounds occur at very low concentrations; their sensory relevance is due to low odor thresholds. Thus, the peak profile obtained by GC does not necessarily reflect the aroma profile of the food.

The purpose of this contribution is to discuss recent developments in food aroma analysis from the chemist's point of view. It will particularly focus on qualitative aroma composition obtained by GC-O. Potential and limitations of the GC-O approach will be discussed and comments made to allow a more realistic interpretation of data. This overview is addressed to flavor scientists from both industry and academia.

II. GAS CHROMATOGRAPHY–OLFACTOMETRY TECHNIQUES

In general, it is very difficult to judge the sensory relevance of volatiles from a single GC-O run. Several techniques have been developed to objectify GC-O data and to estimate the sensory contribution of single aroma components. This issue seems to be of great concern, as a considerable part of the 7th

Weurman Symposium was dedicated to this topic (8). Dilution techniques and time-intensity measurements are the two main GC-O methods.

A. Time-Intensity Measurements

McDaniel et al. (9) have developed the technique Osme, measuring the perceived odor intensity of a compound in the GC effluent. The subject rates the aroma intensity by using a computerized 16-point scale time-intensity device and indicates the corresponding aroma characteristics. This technique provides an FID-style aromagram called an osmegram (Fig. 1). Ideally, it requires only one injection when working with well-trained assessors. Human subjects were found to be reliable "instruments" for reporting odor intensity changes in response to changes in odorant concentration (10). Similar methods based on olfactive intensity measurements have recently been reported (11).

B. Dilution Techniques

Two techniques based on dilution have been developed: CharmAnalysis by Acree and coworkers (6,12,13) and aroma extract dilution analysis (AEDA) by Grosch and his group (7,14,15). Both evaluate the odor activity of individual compounds by sniffing the GC effluent of a series of dilutions of the origi-

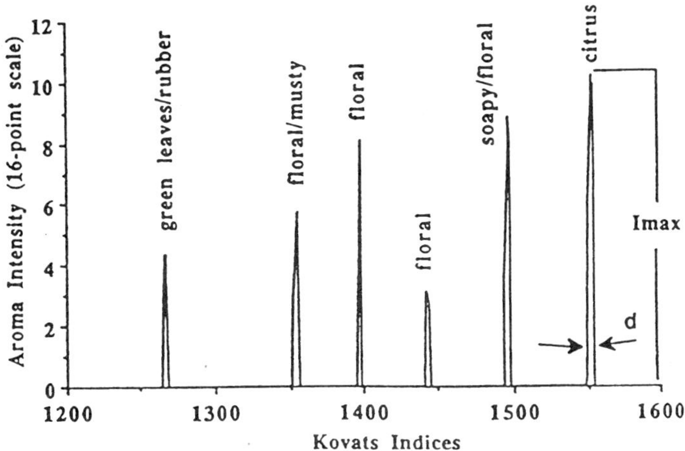

FIGURE 1 Osmegram with odor duration time (d) and maximum odor intensity (I_{max}). (From Ref. 10.)

nal aroma extract. Both methods are based on the odor-detection threshold. The dilution value obtained for each compound is proportional to its OAV in air, i.e., its concentration. Several injections are required to reach a dilution of the aroma extract in which odorous regions are no longer detected.

In CharmAnalysis, the dilutions are presented in randomized order to avoid bias introduced by knowledge of the samples. The assessor detects the beginning and the end of each aroma perception (duration of the smell) and notes the sensory attributes (Fig. 2). The dilution value is measured over the entire time of the eluting peak. From these data, the computerized system constructs chromatographic peaks where the peak areas are proportional to the amount of the odorant in the extract. The Charm value is calculated according to the formula $c = d^{n-1}$, where n is the number of coincident responses and d the dilution value. The result of the CharmAnalysis is displayed in a Charm chromatogram. As shown in Figure 3, the sensory relevant volatile glucose-proline reaction products were detected by Charm analysis and then, based on these results, identified as detailed in Figure 4. The major peak found in the sample, 5-acetyl-2,3-1H-pyrrolizine, was almost odorless (16).

In AEDA, the assessor indicates whether or not an aroma can be perceived and notes the sensory descriptor. The result is expressed as the flavor dilution (FD) factor that corresponds to the maximum dilution value detected, i.e., the peak height obtained in CharmAnalysis. The FD factor is a relative measure and represents the odor threshold of the compound at a given concentration. The data are presented in an FD chromatogram (Fig. 5) indicating the retention indices (x-axis) and FD factors in a logarithmic scale (y-axis).

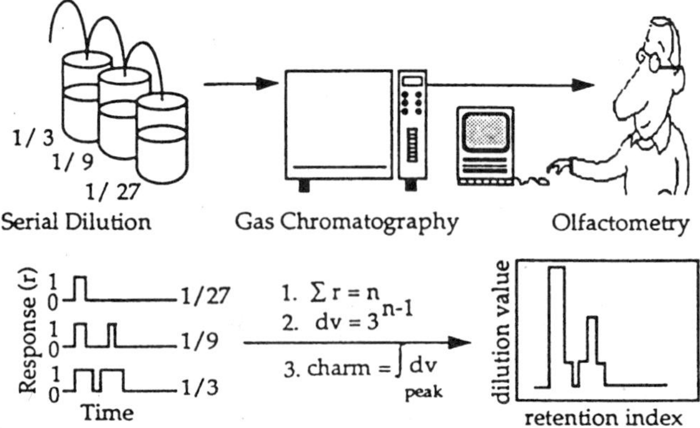

FIGURE 2 Schematic procedure for gas chromatography–olfactometry using CharmAnalysis. (From Ref. 12.)

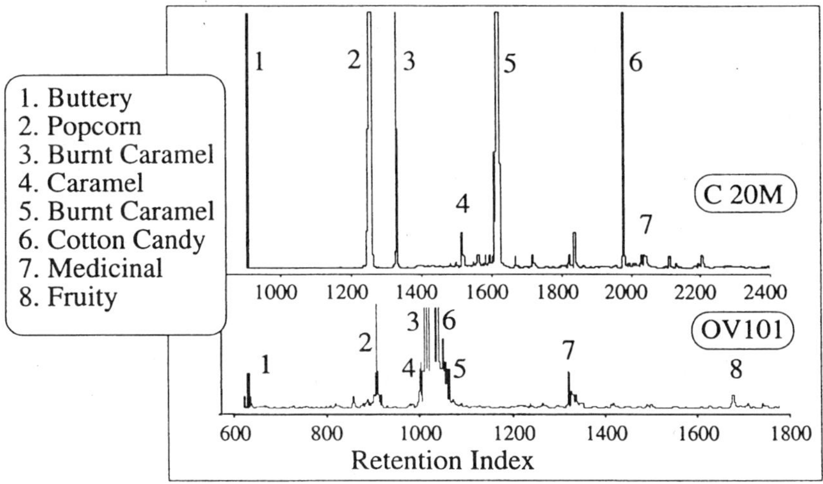

FIGURE 3 Charm chromatograms of the volatile 200°C glucose-proline reaction products on OV 101 and Carbowax 20M columns. (From Ref. 16.)

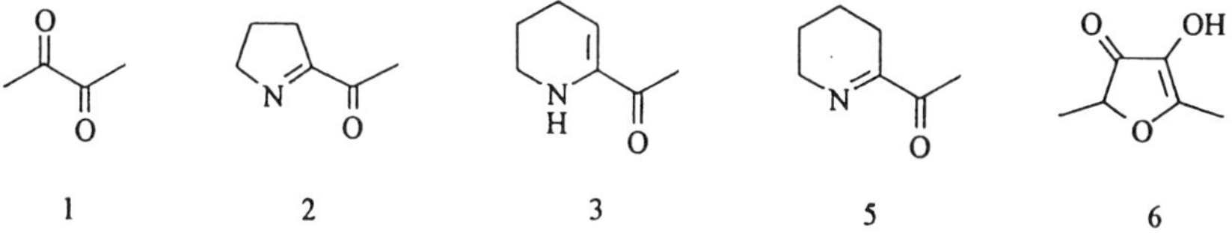

FIGURE 4 Major odor-potent compounds in the glucose-proline reaction detected by CharmAnalysis: diacetyl (no. 1), 2-acetyl-1-pyrroline (no. 2), 2-acetyl-1,4,5,6-tetrahydropyridine (no. 3), 2-acetyl-3,4,5,6-tetrahydropyridine (no. 5), and furaneol (no. 6). Compound numbers refer to Figure 3.

AEDA has been proposed as a screening method for potent odorants as the results are not corrected for losses during isolation (7).

The results obtained for freshly roasted *Arabica* coffee are illustrated in Figure 5 (17). From more than 1000 volatiles detected in the original aroma extract by FID, only about 60 odor-active regions were selected by GC-O. AEDA revealed 38 odorants with FD factors of 16 or higher. Odorants 5, 14, 19, 26, 30, and 32 have been newly identified in coffee aroma. Their identification stemmed from the high FD factors. They would most likely have been overlooked without using GC-O as a screening method for odor-active compounds. Odorants with FD factors of 128 or higher are shown in Figure 6.

C. Static Headspace GC-O

The GC-O techniques described above mainly deal with aroma extracts (liquids) isolated from the food. Recently, Guth and Grosch reported a new concept in aroma research using static headspace in combination with GC-O (18). The equipment is composed of a purge-and-trap system for introducing various volumes of gaseous samples without artefact formation, a suitable capillary column, and an effluent splitter to simultaneously perform GC-O and detection by

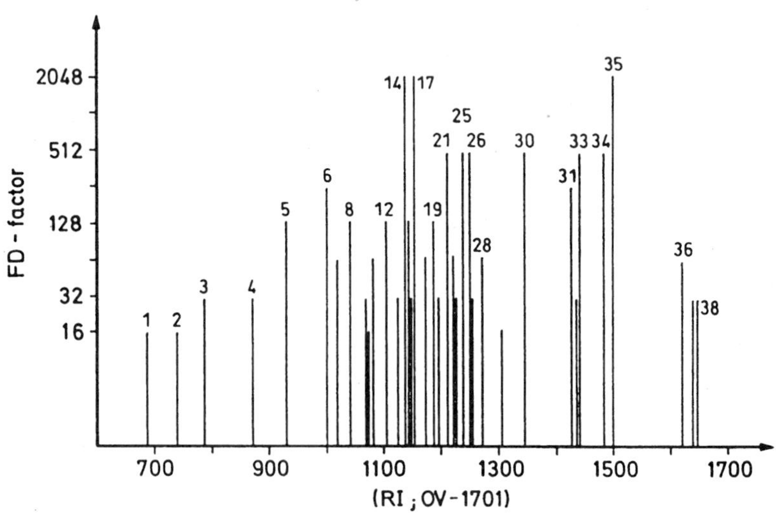

Figure 5 FD chromatogram of an aroma extract obtained from roast and ground *Arabica* coffee. (From Ref. 17.)

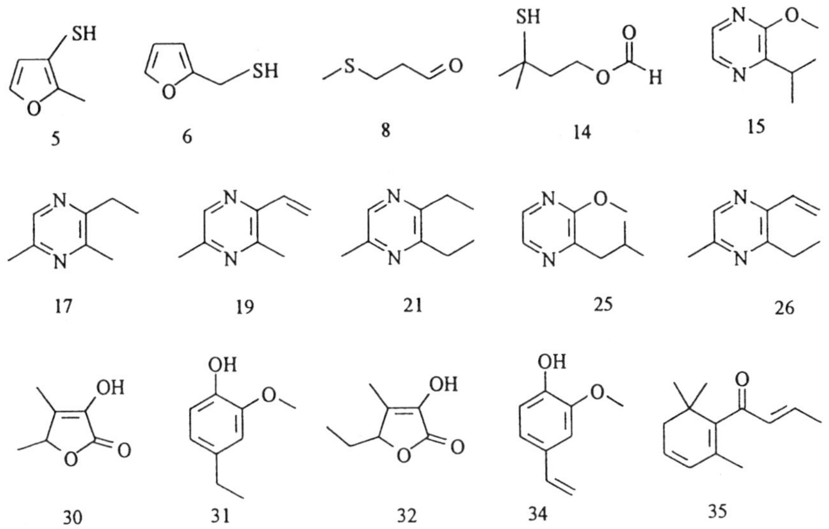

FIGURE 6 Chemical structures of some aroma impact compounds (FD ≥ 128) found in an aroma extract of roast and ground *Arabica* coffee: 2-methyl-3-furanthiol (no. 5), 2-furfurylthiol (no. 6), methional (no. 8), 3-mercapto-3-methylbutyl formate (no. 14), 3-isopropyl-2-methoxypyrazine (no. 15), 2-ethyl-3,5-dimethylpyrazine (no. 17), 2-ethenyl-3,5-dimethyl-pyrazine (no. 19, W. Grosch, personal communication), 2,3-diethyl-5-methylpyrazine (no. 21), 3-isobutyl-2-methoxypyrazine (no. 25), 2-ethenyl-3-ethyl-5-metylpyrazine (no. 26, W. Grosch, personal communication), sotolon (no. 30), 4-ethylguaiacol (no. 31), abhexon (no. 32), 4-vinylguaiacol (no. 34), and (*E*)-β-damascenone (no. 35). The numbering corresponds to that in Figure 5.

FID or MS (Fig. 7). A defined volume of the headspace is injected into a pre-cooled trap to focus the volatiles. After flushing the air present in the gas volume, GC separation is started by raising the oven temperature. Dilution steps are made by injecting decreasing headspace volumes to evaluate the relative odor potencies. The problem of identification is solved by using the same analytical conditions (capillary, temperature program) as for AEDA, so that identification can be performed on the basis of odor qualities and RI values (18).

The sensory relevance of individual odorants can be estimated by injecting various headspace volumes. This is equivalent to AEDA of liquid samples. In contrast to AEDA where aroma compounds are separated from the food matrix,

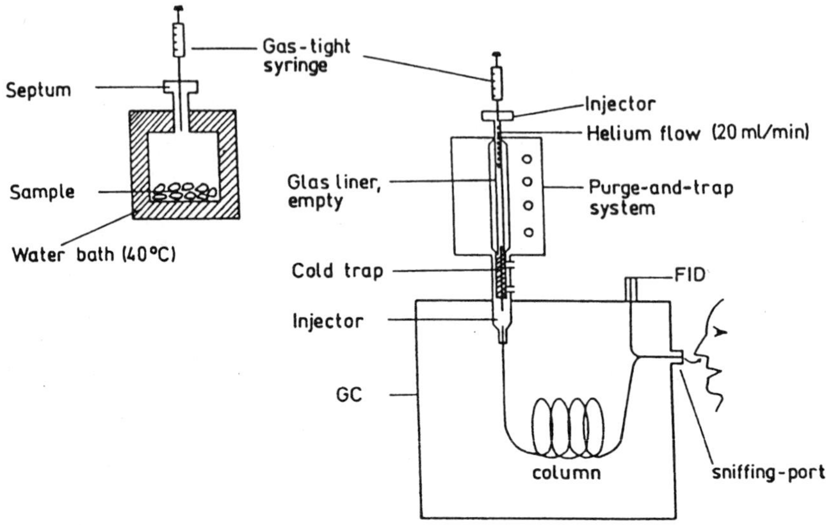

FIGURE 7 Schematic presentation of the static headspace GC-O technique. (Adapted from Guth and Grosch, Annual Report of the Deutsche Forschungsanstalt für Lebensmittelchemie, 1993, p. 27.)

static headspace GC-O provides data about the aroma above the food. This technique is suitable for studying the effect of the food matrix on the aroma profile. Therefore, AEDA and static headspace GC-O result in complementary data.

The analysis of coffee aroma is an excellent example of the potential of static headspace GC-O (19). Compared to AEDA (17), compounds 1–4 and 7 were additionally detected (Table 1). The sensory contribution of odorants was different from that obtained by AEDA. In general, very volatile compounds were underestimated by AEDA, most likely due to losses during sample preparation. 2,3-Pentanedione (no. 8), diacetyl (no. 5), 3-methyl-2-butene-1-thiol (no. 9), acetaldehyde (no. 1), and 3-methylbutanal (no. 6) are key odorants of *Arabica* coffee (Fig. 8). Methanethiol (no. 2) and 2-methylbutanal (no. 7) contribute more significantly to the aroma of *Robusta* coffee.

III. POTENTIAL OF THE GC-O APPROACH

A. Screening and Identification of Potent Odorants

Detection of odorous regions in a gas chromatogram is the first useful information that can be obtained from a single GC-O run. In the first GC-O run, all

TABLE 1 Aroma Impact Odorants of Roast and Ground *Arabica* and *Robusta* Coffee Detected by Static Headspace GC-O[a] and Expressed as FD Factors[b]

No.	Compound	Aroma quality (on GC-O)	FD factor	
			Arabica	*Robusta*
1.	Acetaldehyde	Fruity, pungent	25	25
2.	Methanethiol	Cabbagelike, sulfury	5	12.5
3.	Propanal	Fruity	5	5
4.	Methylpropanal	Fruity, malty	5	5
5.	Diacetyl	Buttery	62.5	125
6.	3-Methylbutanal	Malty	12.5	25
7.	2-Methylbutanal	Malty	5	12.5
8.	2,3-Pentanedione	Buttery	125	125
9.	3-Methyl-2-butene-1-thiol	Sulfury, *Allium*-like, foxy[c]	62.5	62.5

[a]Modified from Ref. 19.
[b]The headspace volumes of 25, 5, 2, 1, 0.4, and 0.2 ml correspond to the FD factors of 1, 5, 12.5, 25, 62.5, and 125, respectively.
[c]Aroma qualities depend on concentration.

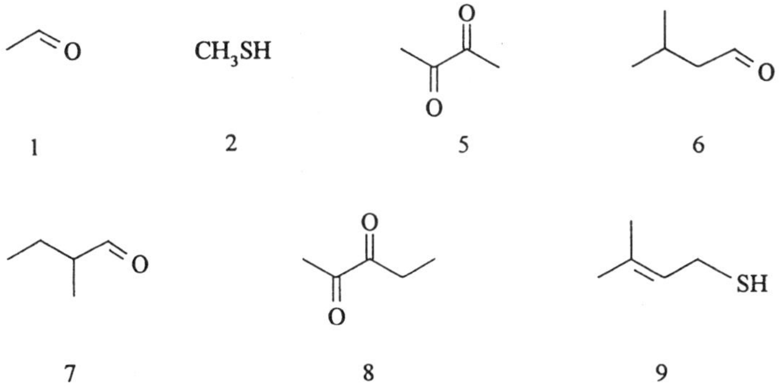

O

CH_3SH

1 2 5 6

7 8 9

FIGURE 8 Chemical structures of some aroma impact compounds (FD ≥ 12.5) found in the headspace of roast and ground *Arabica* and *Robusta* coffee: acetaldehyde (no. 1), methanethiol (no. 2), diacetyl (no. 5), 3-methylbutanal (no. 6), 2-methylbutanal (no. 7), 2,3-pentanedione (no. 8), and 3-methyl-2-butene-1-thiol (no. 9). The numbers correspond to those in Table 1.

volatiles are detected whose concentrations in the GC effluent are higher than their odor thresholds. The corresponding volatiles are then characterized by their aroma quality and intensity as well as by their chromatographic properties, i.e., retention index (RI). The RI increments, obtained on stationary phases with different polarities, provide additional information about the nature of the aroma-active component, such as functional groups. Aroma qualities and intensities are very useful data for flavorists, who can then use these to create characteristic and complex aroma notes.

As mentioned in Section II, chromatograms obtained by FID detection and olfactory response are different. Aroma-active compounds usually do not correspond to the major volatile components in the food. As shown in Figure 9, many important odorants of white bread crust were not visible in the gas chromatogram, for example, 2-acetyl-1-pyrroline (no. 11) (20). This can be explained by the low odor threshold of these compounds. Identification of such minor components (Fig. 10) is a challenging task.

Once the aroma-active regions have been selected by a dilution analysis, the often time-consuming identification experiments can be focused on the most potent odorants. If further fractionation and clean-up steps are required, GC-O may again serve as a screening method and guide sample-purification work. This approach, called sensory directed chemical analysis, is particularly useful when identifying unknown compounds with very low threshold values. An impressive example is the identification of 1-*p*-menthene-8-thiol as the aroma principle of grapefruit juice (21). Its threshold is the lowest ever reported for a naturally occurring compound: 2×10^{-8} mg/liter water. More examples are listed in Table 2. Most of these compounds occur at very low concentrations and are difficult to identify using conventional analytical techniques.

In general, the aroma quality of a volatile component combined with more than one RI value is considered as equivalent to identification by GC-MS. However, the reference compound should be available because of shifts of RI values, especially on polar capillaries. The presence of an odorant can be verified by coelution with the reference compound on capillaries of differing polarity. This approach is helpful for the identification of odorants with very low threshold values and unique aroma qualities (Table 3). RI values may also provide crucial data for the identification of unknown odorants, even if the reference compound is not available. In some cases, verification by GC-MS is possible by tuning the detection technique, e.g., looking at typical fragments of the target molecule in a well-defined region of the gas chromatogram, recording in the SIM mode, and applying GC-MS/MS. It should be mentioned that, with certain experience, time-consuming identification work can be limited to a few, still unknown, compounds.

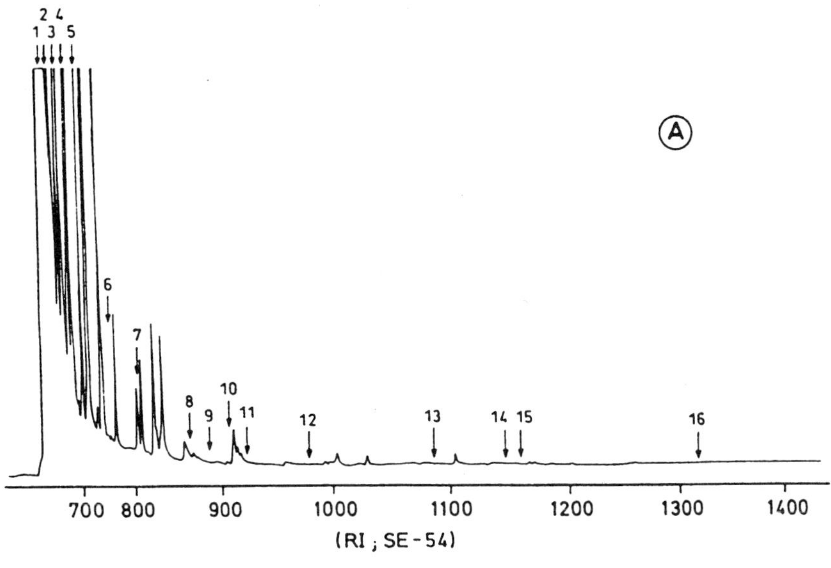

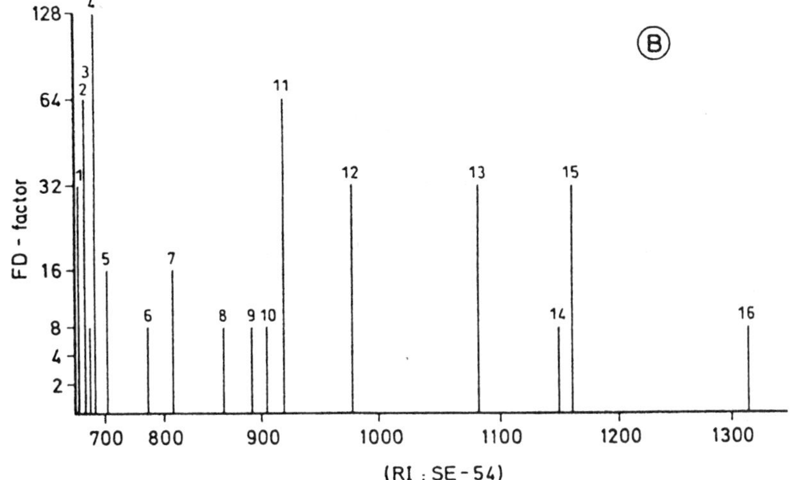

FIGURE 9 Gas chromatogram (A) and FD chromatogram (B) of the headspace volatiles of fresh white bread crust. (From Ref. 20.)

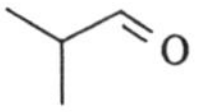

FIGURE 10 Chemical structures of the odor-active components identified in the headspace of fresh white bread crust: 2-methylpropanal (no. 1), diacetyl (no. 2), 3-methylbutanal (no. 4), 2-acetyl-1-pyrroline (no. 11), 1-octene-3-one (no. 12), 2-ethyl-3,5-dimethylpyrazine (no. 13), and (*E*)-2-nonenal (no. 15). The numbering corresponds to that in Figure 9.

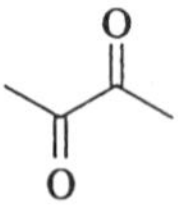

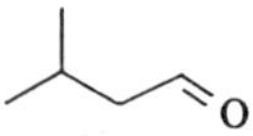

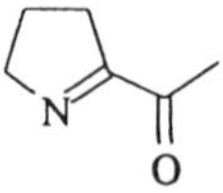

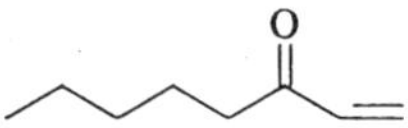

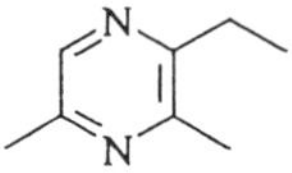

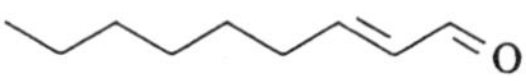

TABLE 2 Aroma Impact Components Newly Identified in Foods on the Basis of GC-O

Food	Compound	Ref.
Bread crust, wheat	2-Acetyl-1-pyrroline	22
Beef meat, boiled	2-Methyl-3-furanthiol[a]	23
Beef meat, roasted	2-Acetyl-2-thiazoline	24
Beef meat, stewed	12-Methyltridecanal[a]	25
Coffee, roasted	3-Mercapto-3-methylbutyl formate[a]	26
Cheese (Emmentaler)	Furaneol, homofuraneol	27
Grapefruit	1-*p*-Menthene-8-thiol[a]	21
Wine (Sauvignon)	4-Mercapto-4-methyl-2-pentanone	28
Tea, green	3-Methyl-2,4-nonanedione	18
Lovage	Sotolon	29

[a]Odorant was reported for the first time as food constituent.

TABLE 3 Selected Examples for Compounds that Can Be Identified by GC-O on the Basis of Aroma Quality and Retention Indices

Compound	Aroma quality (at sniffing port)	Linear retention indices		
		SE-54	OV-1701	FFAP
1-Octene-3-one[a]	Mushroomlike	982	1065	1315
(*Z*)-1,5-Octadiene-3-one[a]	Metallic, geranium-like	985	1085	1395
trans-4,5-Epoxy-(*E*)-2-decenal[a]	Fatty, metallic	1385	1550	1990
3-Methyl-2,4-nonanedione[a]	Strawy, haylike	1316	1400	1700
δ-Decalactone	Coconutlike	1685	1733	2185
(*E*)-β-Damascenone[a]	Honeylike, cooked apples	1395	1500	1825
Sotolon	Seasoninglike	1107	1350	2215
Furaneol	Caramellike	1065	1240	2045
2-Isopropyl-3-methoxypyrazine	Earthy, potatolike	1097	1146	1430
2-Isobutyl-3-methoxypyrazine	Earthy, paprikalike	1186	1237	1520
2-Ethyl-3,5-dimethylpyrazine	Earthy, roasty	1083	1150	1455
2,3-Diethyl-5-methylpyrazine	Earthy, roasty	1155	1219	1485
2-Acetyl-1-pyrroline[a]	Roasty	923	1013	1345
2-Acetyl-2-thiazoline	Roasty, popcornlike	1110	1245	1720
Methional	Cooked potato–like	909	1042	1465
3-Mercapto-2-pentanone[a]	Catty, sulfury	907	1018	1365
2-Furfurylthiol	Roasty, sulfury	913	1000	1445
2-Methyl-3-furanthiol	Meaty, roasty, sweet	870	932	1325
3-Methyl-2-butene-1-thiol[a]	Sulfury, *Allium*-like, foxy	821	874	1105
3-Mercapto-3-methylbutyl formate[a]	Catty, sulfury	1023	1138	1515

[a]Compound is not commercially available.

B. Formation of Potent Odorants

The identity of a key aroma compound is a flavor chemist's first information. However, it will not automatically lead to product quality improvement. Additional work on precursors and formation mechanisms is required (Table 4). This may result in conditions favoring the generation of positive aromas by processing. It may also support selection of raw materials and give some indications for a more efficient enzymatic and/or thermal treatment to liberate precursors of key aroma components.

TABLE 4 Precursors of Some Aroma Impact Compounds Found in Food

Compounds	Food	Precursor systems	Ref.[a]
12-Methyltridecanal	Stewed beef	Plasmaologens	25
2-Methyl-3-furanthiol	Boiled beef	Thiamine/Cysteine (H_2S)	31
2-Ethyl-3,5-dimethylpyrazine	Roasted beef, coffee	Alanine/Methylglyoxal	32
2-Acetyl-2-thiazoline	Meatlike model system	Cysteamine/Methylglyoxal[b]	33
3-Methyl-2-butene-1-thiol	Roasted coffee	Prenyl alcohol/H_2S	34
2-Acetyl-1-pyrroline	Wheat bread crust	Ornithine/Methylglyoxal[c]	35
Furaneol	Wheat bread crust	Fructose-1,6-bisphosphate	36
Homofuraneol	Soy sauce	Sedoheptulose-7-phosphate	37
Sotolon	Fenugreek	4-Hydroxy-L-isoleucine	38
3-Methyl-2,4-nonanedione	Soy beans, green tea	Furanoid fatty acids	39

[a]Recently published references are preferably cited.
[b]2-(1-Hydroxyethyl)-4,5-dihydrothiazole is the key intermediate.
[c]1-Pyrroline is an important intermediate.

Recently, furaneol and homofuraneol were detected by GC-O in Maillard model reactions based on pentoses and different amino acids. This initiated a systematic study to explain these surprising findings (30). As shown in Figure 11, the Strecker aldehydes of glycine and alanine were actively involved in the formation of furaneol and homofuraneol, respectively. The results were obtained using the ^{13}C-labeled precursors and GC-MS/MS as a selective and sensitive detection technique.

C. Off-Flavor Analysis

GC-O is the method of choice for selecting those components that are responsible for aroma deviation in food, i.e., an off-flavor. In general, it can be applied to both foodborne off-flavor formation and off-flavor problems related to contamination. The latter is caused by odorants that normally do not belong to the overall aroma of the product, i.e., external contaminants (e.g., packaging) or compounds formed upon processing and storage (e.g., microbial spoilage). In both cases, the comparison of the off-flavor of the contaminated food with the reference product usually results in a limited number of sensory relevant compounds, which reflect the difference in aroma profiles. Identification work can then be focused on these odorants.

Recent work by Spadone et al. (40) on the Rio defect in green coffee from Brazil and by Marsili et al. (41) on the off-flavor of sugar beet impres-

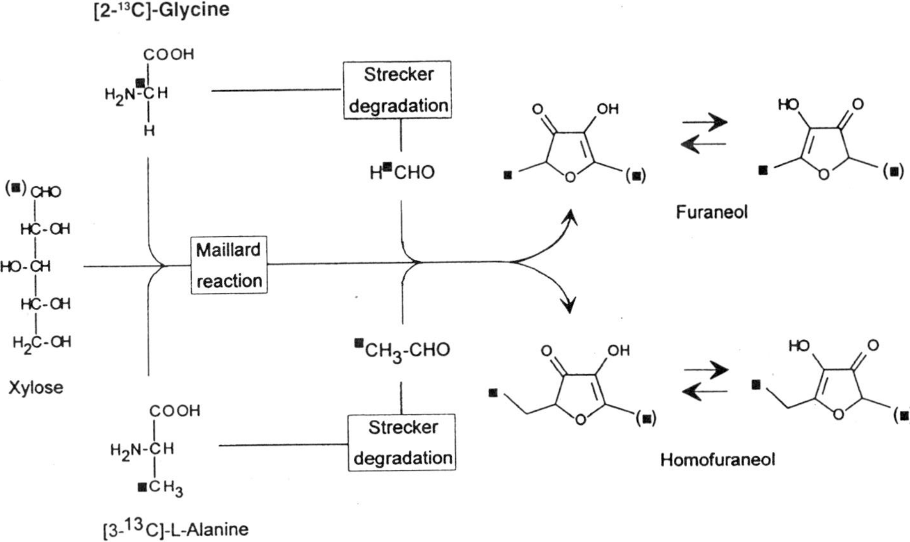

FIGURE 11 Schematic formation of furaneol and homofuraneol from pentoses (e.g., xylose) in the presence of glycine and alanine elucidated by labeling experiments. The marked positions (■) represent ^{13}C-atoms. (Adapted from Ref. 30.)

sively illustrates the potential of this approach: 2,4,6-trichloroanisole and geosmin were identified as off-flavor compounds, respectively. Both odorants have very low odor thresholds in water: 5×10^{-8} and 5×10^{-7} mg/liter, respectively. Identification work was completed by quantitative data, and the off-flavor activity was confirmed by sensory evaluation. The approach, based on sensory techniques and a strong analytical support, provides a good basis for solving off-flavor problems in a reasonable time (Table 5).

Foodborne off-flavor is mainly caused by concentration shifts in aroma-active food constituents. This is much more difficult to handle due to the subtle changes that finally result in an unbalanced aroma. The warmed-over flavor (WOF) of cooked meat is a well-known example in the food industry. Quantitative results of odorants contributing to the off-flavor are indispensable for obtaining reliable data about changes in the aroma profile. Using this approach, hexanal and *trans*-4,5-epoxy-(*E*)-2-decenal have recently been found to be the main contributors of WOF (48).

TABLE 5 Examples of GC-O Recently Applied to Off-Flavors Caused by Direct or Storage-Related Contamination

Product	Off-flavor compound	Ref.[a]
Coffee, green	2,4,6-Trichloroanisole	40
Beet sugar	Geosmin, butyric, and isovaleric acids	41
Water, river	2-Methylisoborneol, geosmin	42
Water, mineral	C_3-Alkyl benzenes	43
Cognac, cork taint	2,4,6-Trichloroanisole, 2,3,4,6-tetrachlorophenol	44
Wine	2-Acetyletetrhydropyridines, furaneol	45,46
Pearl millet, ground, wetted	2-Acetyl-1-pyrroline	47

[a]Recently published references are given preference.

IV. ANALYTICAL CONSIDERATIONS RELATED TO GC-O

A. Representativeness of the Aroma Extract

An excellent review of sample preparation has recently been published by Teranishi and Kint (49). In general, heat treatment should be limited to avoid formation of artefacts and decomposition of aroma impact components. Enzymatic activity in natural products is another critical parameter that should be controlled during sample preparation. In general, there is no ideal extraction method in food aroma analysis. The choice of an extraction procedure depends on the food and is always a compromise.

The issue of representativeness of the aroma extract has recently been discussed in detail by Etiévant and coworkers (50,51). Apparently, little attention is paid in the literature to the quality of the aroma extract, although it is well known that aroma composition depends on the extraction method used. Indeed, the first objective in aroma analysis is to ensure that the extract is representative of the original product. The conditions of extraction and concentration should be designed in such a way as to obtain a sample with an authentic aroma. To make sure that an aroma extract merits further analytical and sensory characterization, it is highly recommended to check its representativeness, e.g., using triangle, similarity scaling, descriptive, or matching tests. This is the basis for obtaining reliable results.

As illustrated in Table 6, the isolation method used to prepare sample B changed the unique meaty/savory note of the original product (sample A) to "boiled vegetables, grilled, burnt." In contrast, the isolation method used to obtain sample C resulted in an extract that revealed the authentic aroma of the

TABLE 6 Sensory Evaluation to Check the Representativeness of the Aroma Extract Obtained from a Commercially Available Food Flavoring with Savory Character

Sample	Isolation method	Sensory attributes
A (original product)		Meaty, roasty, savory, onionlike
B (extract of A)	SDE (boiling conditions)	Cooked vegetables, burnt, meaty
C (extract of A)	SDE (static vacuum at 35°C)	Meaty, roasty, savory, onionlike
D (extract of SDE residue)[a]	Direct solvent extraction	Caramel-like, savory, acidic

[a]Sample D was obtained from the SDE residue of sample C by extraction with diethyl ether.
SDE = simultaneous distillation-extraction.
Source: Modified from Ref. 52.

original product. Consequently, this extract was further characterized by GC-O and other instrumental and analytical techniques. The results and the isolation techniques used will be discussed in the following section.

B. Comparison of Different Isolation Techniques

1. SDE Under Reduced Pressure

The simultaneous distillation-extraction (SDE) under atmospheric pressure (53) is not always the most appropriate technique, and its use should be carefully considered. This technique is an elegant and rapid extraction method resulting in an aroma extract that is ready to be injected into a GC system after concentration. However, heat-induced artefact formation, decomposition of labile compounds, and loss of very volatile compounds are serious drawbacks. Furthermore, only steam-distillable volatiles are extracted. Polar compounds, such as hydroxyfuranones and phenols, are particularly poorly recovered.

Considerable effort has been made to overcome at least one of the limitations of the SDE technique, i.e., heat-induced changes of the aroma extract. A modified SDE apparatus was designed to work under static vacuum (SDE-SV), thus allowing extraction at 30–35°C (54). Several solvents were tested, of which butylethyl ether showed good results for various classes of substances (52). The extract (SDE fraction) can be directly analyzed by GC without any concentration step. SDE-SV is more time-consuming than conventional SDE and also more delicate in handling: exact control of three temperatures (aqueous sample, organic solvent, cooling by cryostat) is necessary, but results in a ready-to-inject aroma extract free of artefacts.

GC-O of the SDE-SV extract of a commercial meaty/savory flavoring (sample C, Table 6) revealed 15 odor-active components out of about 100 volatiles. However, only 6 odorants showed FD factors of 2^8 and higher (Table 7). The meaty/savory note was mainly imparted by odorants containing sulfur. The *cis*-isomer of 2-methyl-3-tetrahydrofuranthiol was also found, but did not contribute to the overall aroma. Identification was mainly based on GC-MS and NMR and was verified by commercially available or synthesized reference compounds. These are essential for unequivocal identification. The chemical structures of the aroma impact compounds identified in the flavoring are shown in Figure 12.

2. SDE Combined with Direct Solvent Extraction

As shown in Table 8, the acidic fraction (sample D in Table 6) obtained from the residue after extraction by SDE-SV was a good source of additional information, particularly about polar aroma compounds. They were isolated from the SDE residue by direct solvent extraction with diethyl ether, purified by extraction with sodium carbonate (0.5 mol/liter) and after acidification reextracted with the solvent. Furaneol (no. 8) was the dominating odorant in this extract; accordingly sample D was mainly described as caramel-like.

3. SDE Versus Static Headspace

As mentioned earlier (Sec. II.C.), headspace GC analysis yields additional data about very volatile compounds, which are usually lost during conventional sample preparation. The sensory relevance of odorants present in the

TABLE 7 Odorants Identified on the Basis of AEDA in the SDE-SV Extract (sample C) of a Commercially Available Food Flavoring with Savory Character

No.	Compound[a]	Retention index OV-1701	Retention index FFAP	Odor quality (GC-O)	FD factor (2^n)
1	2-Methyl-3-furanthiol (MFT)	931	1325	Meaty, roasty, sweet	10–11
2	*trans*-2-Methyl-3-tetrahydrofuranthiol	992	1315	Meaty, savory, onion	10–11
3	2-Furfurylthiol	1000	1450	Sulfury, roasty	14–15
4	Methional	1044	1465	Cooked potato, boiled	10–11
5	S-(2-methyl-3-furyl)-ethanethioate	1238	1700	Meaty, roasty	10–11
6	4-Acetyloxy-2,5-dimethyl-3(2H)-furanone	1430	2005	Caramel-like, savory	8–9

[a]Compounds nos. 1–6 were detected in the SDE fraction obtained under static vacuum.
Source: Modified from Ref. 52.

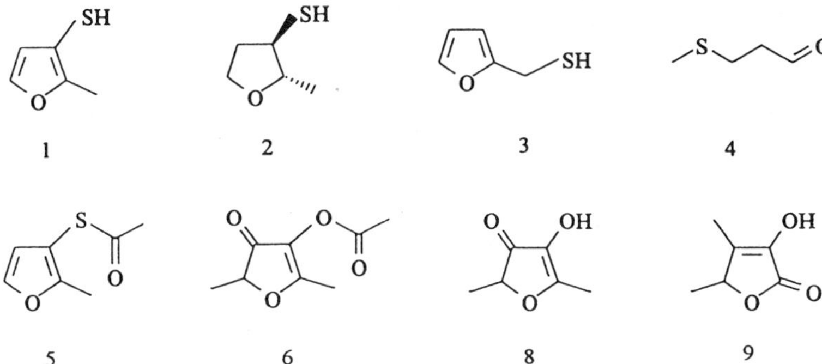

FIGURE 12 Aroma impact compounds identified in a meaty/savory food flavoring: 3-methyl-2-furanthiol (no. 1), *trans*-2-methyl-3-tetrahydrofuranthiol (no. 2), 2-furfurylthiol (no. 3), methional (no. 4), S-(2-methyl-3-furyl)-ethanethioate (no. 5), 4-acetyloxy-2,5-dimethyl-3(2H)-furanone (no. 6), furaneol (no. 8), and sotolon (no. 9). Acetic acid (no. 7) is not shown. The numbering corresponds to that in Tables 7–9.

TABLE 8 Odorants Identified on the Basis of AEDA in the Acidic Fraction (sample D) of a Commercially Available Food Flavoring with Savory Character

No.	Compound[a]	Retention index OV-1701	Retention index FFAP	Odor quality (GC-O)	FD factor (2^n)
7	Acetic acid	785	1460	Acetic, pungent	10–11
8	Furaneol	1240	2045	Caramel-like, sweet	16–17
9	Sotolon	1350	2220	Seasoninglike	11–12

[a]Compounds nos. 7–9 were detected in the acidic fraction (SDE residue of sample C).
Source: Modified from Ref. 52.

headspace above a food can be evaluated by combining AEDA with the static headspace technique (18). This new approach, called static headspace GC-O, was applied to the food flavoring discussed above.

The odorants listed in Table 9 were identified on the basis of their chromatographic and sensory properties using the same analytical conditions as applied to AEDA. A stepwise reduction of the headspace volume revealed the most potent odorants. The medium, dry or aqueous, significantly influenced the results. For example, thiols nos. 1 and 2 were completely lacking in the headspace of the solid product, while in the aqueous medium they showed high odor potencies. These compounds could have been either efficiently encapsulated or liberated from nonvolatile percursors by hydrolysis.

Compounds 1–4 and 10–13 were more abundant in the headspace of the aqueous sample. Others dominated in the headspace of the dry product, such

TABLE 9 Static Headspace GC-O of a Commercially Available Food Flavoring with Savory Aroma Character

No.	Compound[a]	Aroma quality (on GC-O)	FD factor (2^n)[b]	
			Solid sample	Aqueous sample
1+2	MFT + *trans*-2-methyl-3-tetrahydrofuranthiol	Meaty, savory	—	8
3	2-Furfurylthiol	Sulfury, roasty	4	8
4	Methional	Cooked potato	4	8
5	S-(2-Methyl-3-furyl)-ethanethioate	Meaty, roasty	2	2
6	4-Acetyloxy-2,5-dimethyl-3(2H)-furanone	Carmel-like	5	2
7	Acetic acid	Acidic, pungent	2	—
8	Furaneol	Carmel-like	2	—
9	Sotolon	Seasoninglike	—	—
10	Diacetyl	Buttery, sweet	<2	4
11	Hexanal	Green, fatty	<2	4
12	1-Octene-3-one	Mushroomlike	3	7
13	(E)-2-Nonenal	Fatty	2	7

[a]Numbering corresponds to that in Tables 7 and 8.
[b]The initial headspace volume of 20 ml was set as FD = 1. The headspace volume was stepwise reduced and the GC-O procedure repeated to 0.1 ml, which corresponds to FD = 2^8.
Source: Modified from Ref. 52.

as the polar and well water-soluble compounds 6–8. Diacetyl and the lipid degradation products 11–13 contributed more significantly to the aroma of the headspace than the liquid aroma extract obtained by SDE-SV.

4. Vacuum Distillation Versus Direct Solvent Extraction

The analysis of furaneol is an excellent example to illustrate that, unless appropriate isolation techniques are used, an important odorant may be missed. Contradictory results have been published concerning the occurrence and concentration of furaneol and its methylether (MDMF) in strawberries. Therefore, no clear conclusion can be drawn about their sensory relevance. As shown in Table 10, it was rather difficult to detect furaneol in vacuum distillats (Refs. A and B). It is highly oxygenated and, therefore, does not steam-distil due to its low vapor pressure in aqueous samples (58). Consequently, furaneol must be extracted with solvent (Refs. C and D). Cold on-column injection should ideally be used to avoid thermally induced decomposition of furaneol (59) (see Sec. IV.C).

C. Optimized Chromatographic Conditions

1. Aroma Alteration Prior to Chromatography

As many odorants are rather labile and occur at low concentrations, a long storage period between sample preparation and GC-O should be avoided. The choice of solvent is another critical parameter. Certain thiols rapidly dimerize

TABLE 10 Results Reported in the Literature on the Presence of Furaneol and Its Methylether in Strawberries—Effect of Analytical Conditions

Analytical parameter	Ref. A (56)	Ref. B (57)	Ref. C (58)	Ref. D (59)
Extraction				
Vacuum distillation	x	x		
Direct solvent extraction			x	x
Injection mode				
Split/Splitless	x	x	x	
Cold on-column				x
Concentration (mg/kg)				
Furaneol	<0.01	—	2.2–6.3	2.7–16.2
MDMF	0.2	0.1–2.6	0.5–10.9	Not determined

in diethyl ether upon refrigerated storage (60), for example, 2-methyl-3-furanthiol, which is an aroma impact compound of boiled beef (23). In such cases, the aroma concentrate should preferably be stored in pentane at –30°C, if possible under an inert gas, to avoid alteration of the aroma profile.

Furthermore, the aroma extract should be injected using the cold on-column technique. Unstable volatiles readily decompose in a heated injector block and form artefacts, e.g., hydroxyfuranones and thiols. Sulfur-containing compounds are particularly susceptible to heat-induced decomposition that can take place during split/splitless injection, GC separation, or in the GC-MS interface (61). Indeed, many newly reported constituents in *Allium* chemistry are artefacts (Fig. 13). HPLC and low-temperature GC and GC-MS conditions have been proposed for their analysis (62,63).

2. Effect of Chromatography on GC-O Data

The problems involved in analyzing very low amounts of often labile components should not be neglected in GC-O (64). Testing column quality on a regular basis is indispensable. Several mixtures are commercially available for testing polar and apolar capillaries. The so-called Grob test is highly recom-

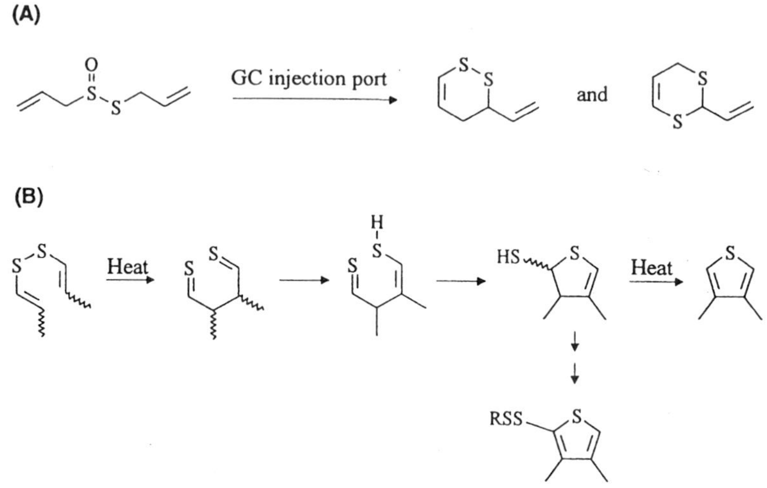

(A)

GC injection port

and

(B)

Heat

Heat

HS

RSS

FIGURE 13 Formatin of artefacts in *Allium* chemistry. (A) Allicin readily decomposes in a heated injector block forming two thioacrolein isomers before GC separation (62). (B) Bis-(1-propenyl)-disulfide rearranges at 85°C to thienyl compounds commonly found in *Allium* distillates (63).

mended, as it rapidly indicates the quality of the analytical capillary (65). For example, adsorption effects due to active surfaces are indicated by tailing of the 1-octanol peak. The quality of an FFAP column can be tested by injecting mixtures of alkanes and free fatty acids.

Many products, especially heat-processed and fermented foods, contain a large variety of substance classes. Therefore, an aroma extract should be analyzed on at least two capillaries of different polarity: an apolar phase (e.g., OV-1, SE-54) and a polar phase (e.g., Carbowax, FFAP). This may help to achieve a better separation of odor-active compounds, as shown in Figure 3. The medium polar capillary OV-1701 is a good compromise for analyzing both apolar and rather polar compounds. In general, chromatography may affect the FD factor and Charm value, particularly at high dilution levels when picogram amounts are analyzed.

As shown in Table 11, odor thresholds determined by GC-O may vary by several orders of magnitude depending on the stationary phase used. Consequently, such effects will also influence the FD factor and Charm value since they represent the odor threshold of the compound at a given concentration. Indeed, different FD factors were determined for MFT on SE-54 and FFAP: 2^{14} and 2^{6}, respectively. On the contrary, abhexon showed higher FD factors on FFAP than SE-54: 2^{16} and 2^{5}, respectively. Consequently, FD factors should be determined on suitable capillaries (64). Compounds with low threshold values are much more affected by this phenomenon, i.e., sotolon compared to furaneol. This can be explained by a chromatographic discrimination at low concentration as discussed below.

TABLE 11 Odor Thresholds[a] (ng/liter air) of Some Selected Odorants as Affected by the Stationary Phase[b]

Compound	SE-54	OV-1701	FFAP
2-Methyl-3-furanthiol (MFT)	0.001–0.002	n.d.	5–10
Abhexon	2–4	n.d.	0.002–0.004
Sotolon	n.d.	0.6–1.2	0.01–0.02
Furaneol	n.d.	1–2	0.5–1.5
3,4-Dimethylcyclopentenolone	n.d.	1–2	0.05–0.1
Cyclotene	n.d.	10–20	10–20

[a]Odor thresholds were determined by GC-O (14) using (*E*)-2-decenal as internal standard.

[b]Capillaries were selected using the Grob test.

3. Discrimination of Odorants on Stationary Phases

The phenomenon of adsorption/instability of enoloxo compounds during GC analysis is illustrated in Figure 14. Furaneol and its methylether were analyzed at different concentrations by diluting the samples 1:1, i.e. FD-1, FD-2, FD-4, and FD-8. The chromatography of 4-methoxy-2,5-dimethyl-3(2H)-furanone (no. 1) was not affected by the stationary phase. On the contrary, furaneol (no. 2) was partially 'lost' on SE-54. Chromatographic behavior on FFAP was acceptable.

Discrimination of several compounds at low concentrations on different stationary phases was studied using furaneol, cyclotene, and their methylethers (Fig. 15). Decreasing amounts were injected via cold on-column, and the yields were determined by projecting the peak areas onto that of the undiluted sample, which was set at 100%. These experiments were continued until the detection limit of the FID was reached. FFAP was found to be the most suitable stationary phase for the analysis of polar compounds followed by Carbowax. On the contrary, yields on SE-54 and OV-1701 decreased strongly with increasing dilution. The corresponding methylethers showed much better chromatographic properties, most likely due to the blocked hydroxyl group, which reduces interaction with the stationary phase.

About 1 ng of furaneol injected on-column onto a FFAP still revealed a symmetrical peak by FID detection which can be integrated for quantification. It has been reported that, using a heated injector block, 10 ng of furaneol still gives a well-defined, sharp peak on a Carbowax fused silica capillary (66). However, we found that about 20–30 ng of furaneol on a OV-1701 resulted in an almost undetectable broad peak. Therefore, the FD factors of furaneol determined on FFAP are usually higher than those on OV-1701. The same phenomenon was observed for homofuraneol, sotolon, and abhexon, which are potent odorants and contribute to the flavor of several heat-processed and fermented foods.

V. SENSORY ASPECT OF GC-O

A. Role of Odor Thresholds in GC-O

It is very useful to have an approximate idea about the threshold value of odorants. The odor threshold of a compound (O_x), measured as ng/liter of air, can be determined by GC-O using (*E*)-2-decenal as "sensory" internal standard according to the following equation (14):

$$O_x = \frac{O_I \cdot D_I}{C_I} \cdot \frac{C_x}{D_x} \tag{1}$$

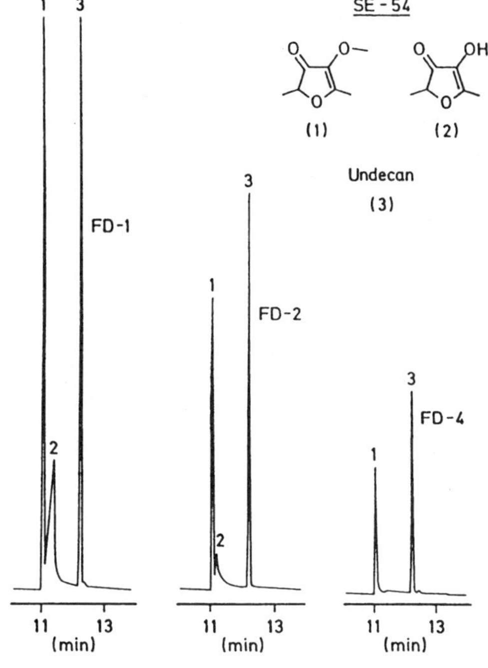

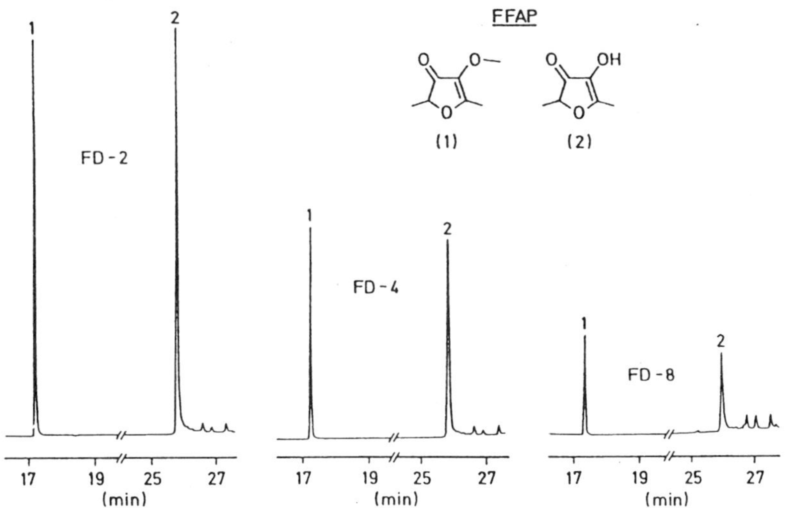

FIGURE 14 Gas chromatography of 4-methoxy-2,5-dimethyl-3(2H)-furanone (no. 1) and furaneol (2) on SE-54 and FFAP fused silica capillaries (I. Blank and W. Grosch, unpublished results). The original sample (FD-1) was stepwise diluted (FD-2, FD-4, FD-8) and analyzed using the same conditions (injection: cold on-column).

where C_I and C_x represent the concentrations and D_I and D_x the dilution values of the internal standard and the odorant, respectively. The term O_I is the odor threshold of the internal standard, (*E*)-2-decenal, which has previously been determined: 2.7 ng/liter air (67). This compound must be present in the solution containing the odorant(s). Therefore, all thresholds listed in Table 12 are related to the "sensory" internal standard, which allows an objective comparison of the values.

The information about odor thresholds determined by GC-O can be of great help in identifying sensory relevant compounds of both positive and off-flavors, particularly in case of separation problems (peak overlapping) or similar mass spectra. 2-Ethyl-3,5-dimethylpyrazine and 2-ethyl-3,6-dimethylpyrazine have similar mass spectra but can easily be distinguished based on

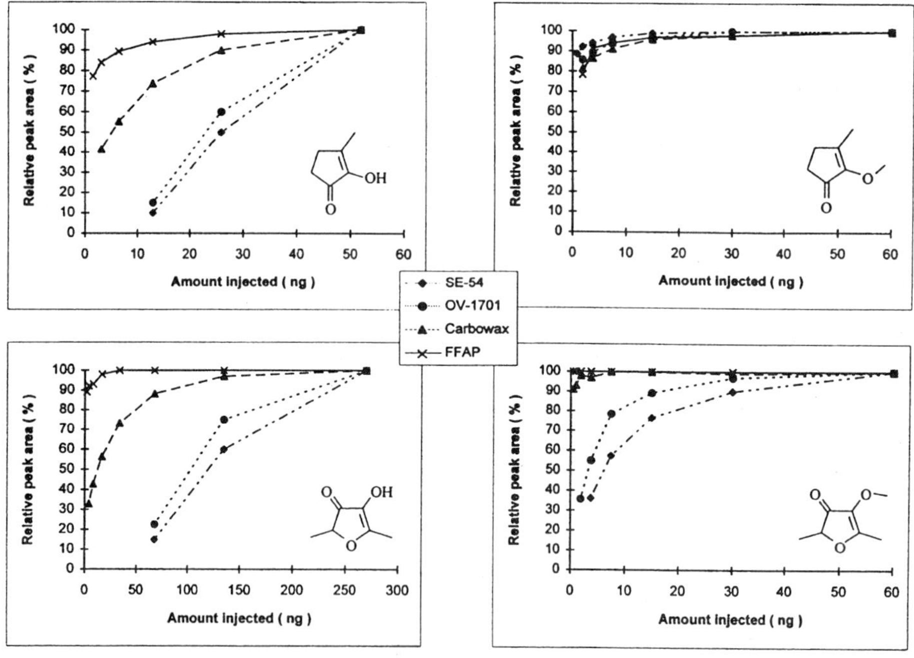

FIGURE 15 Yields of cyclotene, 2-methoxy-3-methyl-2-cyclopentene-1-one, furaneol, and 4-methoxy-2,5-dimethyl-3(2H)-furanone as a function of different polar stationary phases on GC with fused silica capillaries (injection: cold on-column). (Adapted from Ref. 64.)

TABLE 12 Odor Thresholds Determined by GC-O[a] of Some Aroma Impact Components[b] Found in Thermally Processed Foods[c]

Compound	Odor threshold (ng/liter air)
trans-4,5-Epoxy-(*E*)-2-decenal	0.0005–0.005
(*Z*)-2-Nonenal	0.002–0.008
(*E*)-2-Nonenal	0.04–0.16
(*E*,*E*)-2,4-Decadienal	0.05–0.2
(*E*,*Z*)-2,6-Nonadienal	0.1–0.4
Hexanal	15–45
(*E*)-β-Damascenone	0.002–0.004
(*Z*)-1,5-Octadiene-3-one	0.003–0.006
3-Methyl-2,4-nonanedione[d]	0.007–0.014
1-Octene-3-one	0.05–0.1
4-Methylacetophenone	2–4
Diacetyl	10–20
4-Ethylguaiacol	0.01–0.03
4-Vinylguaiacol	0.4–0.8
Eugenol	0.2–0.4
Vanillin	0.6–1.2
4-Methylphenol	0.3–1
Myristicin	1–2
2-Isopropyl-3-methoxypyrazine	0.0005–0.001
2,3-Diethyl-5-methylpyrazine	0.009–0.018
2-Ethyl-3,5-dimethylpyrazine	0.007–0.014
2-Isobutyl-3-methoxypyrazine	0.002–0.004
2-Acetyl-1-pyrroline	0.02–0.04
2-Acetyltetrahydropyridine	0.1–0.2
3-Mercapto-3-methylbutyl formate	0.0002–0.0004
2-Methyl-3-furanthiol[e]	0.001–0.002
2-Furfurylthiol	0.01–0.02
Dimethyltrisulfide	0.06–0.12
Methional	0.1–0.2
2-Acetylthiazol	2–5

[a]Odor thresholds were determined by GC-O (14) on an OV-1701 using (*E*)-2-decenal as 'sensory' internal standard.
[b]From Refs. 32, 64, 68–70.
[c]The threshold values of enoloxo compounds determined on FFAP are listed in Table 11, i.e., abhexon, sotolon, furaneol, cyclotene, and 3,4-dimethylcyclopentenolone.
[d]Odor threshold was determined on a Carbowax.
[e]Odor threshold was determined on a SE-54.

their odor thresholds: 0.007–0.014 and 2.5–5 ng/liter air, respectively (32). Although 1-octene-3-ol and 1-octene-3-one coelute on apolar capillaries, the presence of the latter can be verified by dilution of the sample due to its 100-fold lower threshold. Thus, dilution techniques provide additional data for positive identification. Compounds with odor thresholds lower than 1 ng/liter air are usually below the detection limit of an FID.

B. Limitations of the GC-O Approach

The importance of the representativeness of the aroma extract and the possible effects of the GC analysis on GC-O data have already been discussed in detail (see Sec. IV). Several recently published articles are recommended regarding practical aspects of the GC-O procedure (12,13,71–73). Therefore, only a few additional remarks will be made here.

All GC-O runs of a dilution analysis should be performed within one week to reduce variability in GC analysis and sensorial perception. If analysis takes longer to complete, assessors can have "gaps" during sniffing, i.e., they do not detect a substance at a certain dilution, but detect it again at a higher dilution (73). The first step is to establish a profile of the original aroma extract by detecting the odor-active regions and describing their aroma characteristics. This should be done on two capillaries of different polarity. A medium polar capillary is proposed for the dilution analysis. All odor-active regions detected in the original aroma extract should be sniffed throughout the entire dilution series, consisting of not more than 10 samples. The last 5 dilutions should be repeated on the second capillary, preferably an FFAP. Some of the dilutions should be evaluated by additional assessors. The use of humidified air is recommended to reduce olfactory fatigue by nasal dehydration. Consider that the number of odorants detectable by GC-O depends on the extraction method and the threshold of the volatiles, but also on parameters that are arbitrarily selected, i.e., amount of food sample, concentration factor, sample volume injected.

Problems such as representativeness, GC analysis, and "gaps" during sniffing can be solved by taking the necessary precautions. More serious limitations of the GC-O approach originate from the sensory area. Methods based on odor threshold detection, i.e., GC-O using dilution techniques (Charm, AEDA) and the OAV concept (ratio of concentration to threshold), are not consistent with psychophysical views (74). The major problems are that thresholds vary depending on the experimental conditions, differing intensity functions for volatiles above the threshold are not accommodated, and no prediction about the activity of volatiles in a mixture is possible, especially if they occur at concentrations below threshold.

Differing intensity functions for volatiles account for a well-known phenomenon in GC-O: some intensely smelling compounds disappear after a few dilution steps (e.g., vanillin), while others with a lower aroma intensity in the original extract have the highest FD factors. The sensory relevance of the latter is overestimated. (*E*)-β-Damascenone is a typical representative for such compounds, which are characterized by a relatively flat dose/intensity function. This is most likely why (*E*)-β-damascenone does not play a major role in the aroma of coffee, despite low threshold values (Table 12), i.e., high FD factors and OAVs. In other words, threshold concentration does not necessarily correlate with aroma potency.

A more satisfactory but more difficult approach is to provide intensity measures, which can only be carried out with a well-trained panel (75). A fundamental weakness of all of these techniques is that they do not account for interactions arising in the olfactory system or between taste and smell. The chemical bases of these senses are still not sufficiently understood.

C. Interpretation of GC-O Data

Properly performed GC-O and adequate knowledge about the possible limitations of the technique are the basis for a realistic interpretation of the results. The flavor scientist's major questions are: "What can be concluded from GC-O data?" and "Where is the limit of a realistic interpretation?"

Certainly, GC-O is a first essential step for distinguishing odor-active compounds from volatiles without odor impact. This screening procedure is the basis for identification experiments. GC-O also provides a first indication about the odor potency of volatile compounds, i.e., to what extent they individually contribute to the overall aroma. However, in most cases final conclusions about their sensory relevance cannot be drawn and further work is necessary (see Sec. VI.).

Analytical and sensorial data cannot be presented with the same precision. While RI values and mass spectra can be precisely determined, GC-O data lack comparable accuracy and reproducibility. FD factors and Charm values are approximations of the sensory relevance of an odorant. In fact, a 256-fold dilution is a rough estimation, depending on extraction yields and the assessor, and could also be 128 or 512. Such exact values are rather misleading: GC-O techniques are not this accurate. The use of 2^n, where n is the number of dilution steps, may help to avoid overinterpretation of GC-O data (76). Though 256 and 2^8 represent the same value, the latter gives a more realistic idea of the odor potency of a compound. It should be mentioned, however, that FD factors do not normally differ by more than two dilution steps.

Furthermore, Charm or FD chromatograms can be divided into three regions, represented by compounds with high, medium, or low dilution values. This classification of odorants could be used as selection criteria for identification, which would be focused on the first two categories, i.e., odorants of high and medium potencies. Less effort would be attributed to those odorants contributing to the "background" aroma. However, the role of the aroma quality should not be neglected in this context: several background odorants with a typical note may also contribute to the overall aroma.

The approach presented above could be standardized by setting the highest dilution value at 2^{10} (= 1024) and relating the remaining values accordingly. Odorants of high and medium potencies would be grouped depending on their dilution values, i.e., 2^{8-10} and 2^{5-7}, respectively. In this way, the role of an odorant in different foods could easily be estimated. Moreover, it would allow a better comparison of GC-O data from different laboratories.

In summary, GC-O techniques should be seen as screening methods to gain an insight into important contributors to a characteristic aroma (7,71). GC-O performed as Charm analysis and Osme have also been claimed as quantitative bioassays (10,77). However, more time is needed for training of assessors and verification using statistical means.

VI. OUTLOOK

The aim of GC-O techniques in food aroma research is to determine the relative odor potency of compounds present in the aroma extract. This method gives the order of priority for identification and thus indicates the chemical origin of olfactory differences (7). The value of the results obtained by GC-O depends directly on the effort invested in sample preparation and analytical conditions. Analysis of an aroma extract by dilution techniques (AEDA, Charm) combined with static headspace GC-O provides a complete characterization of the qualitative aroma composition of a food. However, this is only the first step in understanding the complex aroma of a food.

State of the art in food aroma research today is based on a combined sensory and analytical approach. It is basically composed of the following three steps, which can be applied to the characterization of both positive aroma and off-flavors:

1. Qualitative aroma composition (based on GC-Olfactometry)
2. Quantitative aroma composition (odor activity value concept)
3. Aroma recombination studies (aroma simulation based on quantitative data)

Work starts with the analysis of the aroma composition and is completed when the aroma of the food can be simulated in an appropriate matrix on the basis of the quantitative data obtained. The last step is essential and validates the analytical results. Recently published data on stewed beef (78) and coffee brew (79) impressively demonstrate the potential of this approach. However, a crucial step is accurate quantification of the aroma impact compounds. Special techniques are necessary to quantify labile odorants at low concentrations, i.e., isotope dilution assay using the labeled odorant as internal standard. A major concern is the availability of these labeled compounds. The recently published review articles of Grosch (80) and Schieberle (72) are recommended for more details.

In conclusion, there is a clear need to improve the quality and stability of food aromas and flavors. The techniques presented above represent an attractive approach for analyzing aromas more purposefully. Depending on the case, it is possible to simplify the approach and find compromises in all three phases so that essential work can be done in a reasonable time. The food and flavor industry is well advised to profit from this development and to adapt the different techniques to their specific needs.

ACKNOWLEDGMENTS

The author is grateful to Drs. E. Prior, D. Roberts, L. Fay, and J. Löliger for their helpful suggestions in preparing this manuscript.

APPENDIX: ABBREVIATIONS AND TRIVIAL AND TRADE NAMES

Chemicals

Abhexon	5-Ethyl-3-hydroxy-4-methyl-2(5H)-furanone
Cyclotene	2-Hydroxy-3-methyl-2-cyclopentene-1-one
(*E*)-β-Damascenone	1-(2,6,6-Trimethyl-1,3-cyclohexadienyl)-(*E*)-2-butene-1-one
3,4-Dimethylcyclopentenolone	2-Hydroxy-3,4-dimethyl-2-cyclopentene-1-one
4-Ethylguaiacol	4-Ethyl-2-methoxyphenol
Eugenol	4-(1-Propenyl)-2-methoxyphenol
Furaneol®	4-Hydroxy-2,5-dimethyl-3(2H)-furanone Furaneol is a trade name of Firmenich, Geneva, Switzerland

Homofuraneol	2(5)-Ethyl-4-hydroxy-5(2)-methyl-3(2H)-furanone
Isovaleric acid	3-Methylbutanoic acid
MDMF	4-Methoxy-2,5-dimethyl-3(2H)-furanone
Methional	3-Methylthio-1-propanal
Methylglyoxal	2-Oxopropanal
MFT	2-Methyl-3-furanthiol
Sotolon	3-Hydroxy-4,5-dimethyl-2(5H)-furanone
4-Vinylguaiacol	4-Vinyl-2-methoxyphenol

Analytical Techniques

AEDA	Aroma Extract Dilution Analysis
Charm	Combined Hedonic and Response Measurement
FID	Flame Ionization Detector
FFAP	Free Fatty Acid Phase (polar stationary phase for GC)
GC	Gas Chromatography (using capillary columns)
GC-O	GC-Olfactometry
GC-MS	GC–Mass Spectrometry
GC-MS/MS	GC–Tandem-MS
HPLC	High-Performance Liquid Chromatography
MS	Mass Spectrometry
OAV	Odor Activity Value (ratio of concentration to odor threshold)
Osme	from the Greek word δμη, meaning 'smell'
OV-101	Ohio Valley apolar stationary phase for GC
OV-1701	Ohio Valley medium polar stationary phase for GC
RI	Retention Index
SDE	Simultaneous Distillation Extraction
SDE-SV	SDE under Static Vacuum
SE-54	Apolar stationary phase for GC
SIM	Selective Ion Monitoring (GC-MS technique)

REFERENCES

1. H. Maarse and C. A. Visscher (eds.), Volatile compounds in food. Qualitative and quantitative data, *TNO-CIVO*, Food Analysis Institute, Vol. I-III, 6th ed., Zeist, 1989.
2. G. H. Fuller, R. Steltenkamp, and G. A. Tisserand, The gas chromatograph with human sensor: perfumer model, *Ann. NY Acad. Sci. 116:*711 (1964).
3. M. Rothe and B. Thomas, Aromastoffe des Brotes, *Z. Lebensm. Unters. Forsch. 119:*302 (1963) (in German).
4. D. G. Guadagni, R. G. Buttery, and J. Harris, Odour intensities of hop oil compo-

nents, *J. Sci. Food Agric. 17:*142 (1966).
5. M. C. Meilgaard, Aroma volatiles in beer: purification, flavor threshold and interaction, *Geruch- und Geschmacksstoffe* (F. Drawert, ed.), Verlag Hans Carl, Nürnberg, 1975, p. 210.
6. T. E. Acree, J. Barnard, and D. G. Cunningham, A procedure for the sensory analysis of gas chromatographic effluents, *Food Chem. 14:*273 (1984).
7. W. Grosch, Detection of potent odorants in foods by aroma extract dilution analysis, *Trends Food Sci. Technol. 4:*68 (1993).
8. H. Maarse and D. G. van der Heij (eds.), *Trends in Flavour Research*, Elsevier Science, Amsterdam, 1994, pp. 179–190, 191–209, 211–220, 267–270, 271–276, 305–309, 345–351, 409–415.
9. M. R. McDaniel, R. Miranda-López, B. T. Watson, N. J. Micheals, and L. M. Libbey, Pinot noir aroma: a sensory/gas chromatographic approach, *Flavors and Off-Flavors* (G. Charalambous, ed.), Elsevier, Amsterdam, 1990, p. 23.
10. M. A. A. P. da Silva, D. S. Lundahl, and M. R. McDaniel, The capability and psychophysics of Osme: a new GC-olfactometry technique, *Trends in Flavour Research* (H. Maarse and van der Heij D. G., eds.), Elsevier, Amsterdam, 1994, p. 191.
11. H. Guichard, E. Guichard, D. Langlois, S. Issanchou and N. Abbott, GC sniffing analysis: olfactive intensity measurements by two methods, *Z. Lebensm. Unters. Forsch. 201:*344–350 (1995).
12. T. E. Acree, Bioassays for flavor, *Flavor Science. Sensible Principles and Techniques* (T. E. Acree and R. Teranishi, eds.), ACS Professional Reference Book, American Chemical Society, Washington, DC, 1993, p. 1.
13. T. E. Acree, Gas chromatography-olfactometry, *Flavor Measurement* (C. T. Ho and C. H. Manley, eds.), Marcel Dekker, New York, 1993, p. 77.
14. F. Ullrich and W. Grosch, Identification of the most intense odor compounds formed during autoxidation of linoleic acid, *Z. Lebensm. Unters. Forsch. 184:*277 (1987).
15. W. Grosch and P. Schieberle, Bread flavour: qualitative and quantitative analysis, Characterization, production and application of food flavours., Proceedings of 2nd Wartburg Aroma Symp., Akademie-Verlag, Berlin, 1987, p. 139.
16. D. D. Roberts and T. E. Acree, Gas chromatography-olfactometry of glucose-proline Maillard reaction products, *Thermally Generated Flavors* (T. H. Parliment, M. J. Morello, R. J. McGorrin, eds.), American Chemical Society, Washington, DC, 1994, p. 71.
17. I. Blank, A. Sen, and W. Grosch, Aroma impact compounds of Arabica and Robusta coffee. Qualitative and quantitative investigations, Proc. 14th Int. Conf. Coffee Sci. (ASIC 14), San Francisco, 1992, p. 117.
18. H. Guth and W. Grosch, Identification of potent odourants in static headspace samples of green and black tea powders on the basis of aroma extract dilution analysis (AEDA), *Flav. Fragr. J. 8:*173 (1993).
19. P. Semmelroch and W. Grosch, Analysis of roasted coffee powders and brews by

gas chromatography-olfactometry of headspace samples, *Lebensm. Wiss. Technol. 28:*310 (1995).
20. P. Schieberle and W. Grosch, Changes in the concentration of potent crust odourants during storage of white bread, *Flav. Fragr. J. 7:*213 (1992).
21. E. Demole, P. Enggist, and G. Ohloff, 1-*p*-Menthene-8-thiol: a powerful flavor impact constituent of grapefruit juice (*Citrus paradisi* MacFayden), *Helv. Chim. Acta 65:*1785 (1982).
22. P. Schieberle, and W. Grosch, Identification of the volatile flavour compunds of wheat bread crust—comparison with rye bread crust, *Z. Lebensm. Unters. Forsch. 180:*474 (1985).
23. U. Gasser and W. Grosch, Identification of volatile flavour compounds with high aroma values from cooked beef, *Z. Lebensm. Unters. Forsch. 186:*489 (1988).
24. C. Cerny and W. Grosch, Evaluation of potent odorants in roasted beef by aroma extract dilution analysis, *Z. Lebensm. Unters. Forsch. 194:*322 (1992).
25. H. Guth and W. Grosch, 12-Methyltridecanal, a species-specific odorant of stewed beef, *Lebensm. Wiss. Technol. 26:*171 (1993).
26. W. Holscher, O. G. Vitzthum, and H. Steinhart, Identification and sensorial evaluation of aroma-impact-compounds in roasted Colombian coffee, *Café, Cacao, Thé 34:*205 (1990).
27. M. Preininger and W. Grosch, Evaluation of key odorants of the neutral volatiles of Emmentaler cheese by the calculation of odour activity values, *Lebensm. Wiss. Technol. 27:*237 (1994).
28. P. Darriet, T. Tominaga, V. Lavigne, J. N. Boidron, and D. Dubourdieu, Identification of a powerful aromatic component of *Vitis vinifera* L. var. Sauvignon wines: 4-mercapto-4-methyl-2-pentanone, *Flav. Fragr. J. 10:*385 (1995).
29. I. Blank and P. Schieberle, Analysis of the seasoning-like flavour substances of a commercial lovage extract (*Levisticum officinale* Koch), *Flav. Fragr. J. 8:*191 (1993).
30. I. Blank and L. B. Fay, Formation of 4-hydroxy-2,5-dimethyl-3(2H)-furanone and 4-hydroxy-2(or 5)-ethyl-5(or 2)-methyl-3(2H)-furanone through Maillard reaction based on pentose sugars, *J. Agric. Food Chem. 44:*531 (1996).
31. W. Grosch and G. Zeiler-Hilgart, Formation of meat-like flavor compounds, *Flavor Precursors—Thermal and Enzymatic Conversations* (R. Teranishi, G. R. Takeoka, and M. Güntert, eds.), Washington, DC, 1992, p. 183.
32. C. Cerny and W. Grosch, Precursors of ethyldimethylpyrazine isomers and 2,3-diethyl-5-methylpyrazine formed in roasted beef, *Z. Lebensm. Unters. Forsch. 198:*210 (1994).
33. T. Hofmann and P. Schieberle, Studies on the formation and stability of the roast-flavor compound 2-acetyl-2-thiazoline, *J. Agric. Food Chem. 43:*2946 (1995).
34. W. Holscher, O. G. Vitzthum, and H. Steinhart, Prenyl alcohol—source of odorants in roasted coffee, *Agric. Food Chem. 40:*655 (1992).
35. P. Schieberle, The role of free amino acids present in yeast as precursors of the odorants 2-acetyl-1-pyrroline and 2-acetyltetrahydropyridine in wheat bread crust, *Z. Lebensm. Unters. Forsch. 191:*206 (1990).

36. P. Schieberle, Studies on the formation of furaneol in heat-processed foods, *Flavor Precursors—Thermal and Enzymatic Conversations* (R. Teranishi, G. R. Takeoka, and M. Güntert, eds.), Washington, DC, 1992, p. 164.
37. M. Sasaki, N. Nunomura and T. Matsudo, Biosynthesis of 4-hydroxy-2(or 5)-ethyl-5(or 2)-methyl-3(2H)-furanone by yeasts, *J. Agric. Food Chem. 39:*934 (1991).
38. I. Blank, J. Lin, L. B. Fay, and R. Fumeaux, Formation of 3-hydroxy-4,5-dimethyl-2(5H)-furanone (sotolon) from 4-hydroxy-L-isoleucine, *Bioflavour 95* (P. X. Etiévant and P. Schreier, eds.), INRA Editions (Les Colloques, no. 75), Paris, 1995, p. 385.
39. W. Grosch, U. C. Konopka, and H. Guth, Characterization of off-flavors by aroma extract dilution anaysis, *Lipid Oxidation in Food* (A. J. St. Angelo, ed.), American Chemical Society, Washington, DC, 1992, p. 266.
40. J. C. Spadone, G. Takeoka, and R. Liardon, Analytical investigation of Rio off-flavor in green coffee, *J. Agric. Food Chem. 38:*226 (1990).
41. R. T. Marsili, N. Miller, G. J. Kilmer, and R. E. Simmons, Identification and quantification of the primary chemicals responsible for the characteristic malodor of beet sugar by purge and trap GC-MS-OD techniques. *J. Chromatogr. Sci. 32:*165 (1994).
42. B. Lundgren, H. Borén, A. Grimvall, and R. Sävenhed, Isolation of off-flavour compounds in water by chromatographic sniffing and preparative gas chromatography, *J. Chromatogr. 482:*23 (1989).
43. J. P. H. Linssen, J. L. G. Janssens, J. P. Roozen, and M. A. Posthumus, Combined gas chromatography and sniffing port analysis of volatile compounds of mineral water packed in polyethylene laminated packages, *Food Chem. 46:*367 (1993).
44. R. Cantagrel and J. P. Vidal, Research on compounds responsible for cork taint in cognacs, *Flavors and Off-Flavors* (G. Charalambous, ed.), Elsevier, Amsterdam, 1990, p. 139.
45. C. R. Strauss and T. Heresztyn, 2-Acetyltetrahydropyridines—a cause of the 'mousy' taint in wine, *Chem. Ind.*, 109 (1984).
46. A. Rapp, P. Pretorius, and D. Kugler, Foreign and undesirable flavours in wine, *Off-flavors in Foods and Beverages* (G. Charalambous, ed.), Elsevier, Amsterdam, 1992, p. 485.
47. L. M. Seitz, R. L. Wright, R. D. Waniska, and L. W. Rooney, Contribution of 2-acetyl-1-pyrroline to odors from wetted ground pearl millet, *J. Agric. Food Chem. 41:*955 (1993).
48. U. C. Konopka, H. Guth, and W. Grosch, Potent odorants formed by lipid peroxidation as indicators for the warmed-over-flavor (WOF) of cooked meat, *Z. Lebensm. Unters. Forsch. 201:*339 (1995).
49. R. Teranishi and S. Kint, Sample preparation, *Flavor Science. Sensible Principles and Techniques* (T. E. Acree and R. Teranishi, eds.), American Chemical Society, Washington, DC, 1993, p. 137.
50. N. Abbott, P. X. Etiévant, D. Langlois, I. Lesschaeve, and S. Issanchou, Evalua-

tion of the representativeness of the odor of beer extracts prior to analysis by GC eluate sniffing, *J. Agric. Food Chem. 41:*777 (1993).

51. P. Etiévant, L. Moio, E. Guichard, D. Langlois, I. Lesschaeve, P. Schlich, and E. Chambellant, Aroma extract dilution analysis (AEDA) and the representativeness of the odour of food extracts, *Trends in Flavour Research* (H. Maarse and D. G. van der Heij, eds.), Elsevier, Amsterdam, 1994, p. 179.
52. I. Blank, A. Stämpfli, and W. Eisenreich, Analysis of food flavourings by gas chromatography-olfactometry, *Trends in Flavour Research* (H. Maarse and D. G. van der Heij, eds.), Elsevier, Amsterdam, 1994, p. 271.
53. G. B. Nickerson and S. T. Likens, Gas chromatographic evidence for the occurrence of hop oil components in beer, *J. Chromatogr. 21:*1 (1966).
54. L. Maignial, P. Pibarot, G. Bonetti, A. Chaintreau, and J. P. Marion, Simultaneous distillation-extraction under static vacuum: isolation of volatile compounds at room temperature, *J. Chromatogr. 606:*87 (1992).
55. A. Sen, G. Laskawy, P. Schieberle, and W. Grosch, Quantitative determination of β-damascenone in foods using a stable isotope dilution assay, *J. Agric. Food Chem. 39:*757 (1991).
56. N. Fischer and F. J. Hammerschmidt, A contribution to the analysis of fresh strawberry flavour, *Chem. Mikrobiol. Technol. Lebensm. 14:*141 (1992).
57. P. Schreier, Quantitative composition of volatile constituents in cultivated strawberries, *Fragaria ananassa* cv. Senga Sengana, Senga Litessa and Senga Gourmella, *J. Sci. Food Agric. 31:*487 (1980).
58. W. Pickenhagen, A. Velluz, J. P. Passerat, and G. Ohloff, Estimation of 2,5-dimethyl-4-hydroxy-3(2H)-furanone (FURANEOL) in cultivated and wild strawberries, pineapples and mangoes, *J. Sci. Food Agric. 32:*1132 (1981).
59. P. Schieberle, Heat-induced changes in the most odour-active volatiles of strawberries, *Trends in Flavour Research* (H. Maarse and D. G. van der Heij, eds.), Elsevier, Amsterdam, 1994, p. 345.
60. T. Hofmann, P. Schieberle, and W. Grosch, Oxidative stability of thiols formed by the Maillard reaction, *J. Agric. Food Chem. 44:*251 (1996).
61. E. Block, Flavor artefacts, *J. Agric. Food Chem. 41:*692 (1993).
62. E. Block, S. Naganathan, D. Putman, and S. H. Zhao, *Allium* chemistry: HPLC analysis of thiosulfinates from onion, garlic, wild garlic (Ramsoms), leek, scallion, shallot, elephant (great-headed) garlic, chive, and Chinese chive, *J. Agric. Food Chem. 40:*2418 (1992).
63. E. Block, D. Putman, and S. H. Zhao, *Allium* chemistry: GC-MS analysis of thiosulfinates and related compounds from onion, leek, scallion, shallot, chive, and Chinese chive, *J. Agric. Food Chem. 40:*2431 (1992).
64. I. Blank, A. Sen, and W. Grosch, Potent odorants of the roasted powder and brew of Arabica coffee, *Z. Lebensm. Unters. Forsch. 195:*239 (1992).
65. K. Grob Jr., G. Grob, and K. Grob, Comprehensive, standardized quality test for glass capillary columns, *J. Chromatogr. 156:*1 (1978).

66. A. A. Williams and D. S. Mottram, Gas chromatographic analysis of furaneol, *J. HRC CC 4:*421 (1981).
67. M. H. Boelens and L. J. van Gemert, Physiochemical parameters related to organoleptic properties of flavour components, *Developments in Food Flavours* (G. G. Birch and M. G. Lindley, eds.), Elsevier, London, 1986, p. 23.
68. I. Blank, K. H. Fischer, and W. Grosch, Intensive neutral odorants of linden honey. Differences from honeys of other botanical origin, *Z. Lebensm. Unters. Forsch. 189:*426 (1989).
69. I. Blank and W. Grosch, Evaluation of potent odorants in dill seed and dill herb (*Anethum graveolens* L.) by aroma extract dilution analysis. *J. Food Sci. 56:*63 (1991).
70. H. Guth, Verderb von Sojaöl unter Einwirkung von Licht und Sauerstoff—Identifizierung der Aromastoffe und Vorläufer, Thesis, Technical University of Munich, Munich, 1991, p. 56.
71. L. J. van Gemert, Report of the workshop 'Gas chromatography-olfactometry,' *Trends in Flavour Research* (H. Maarse and D. G. van der Heij, eds.), Elsevier Science, Amsterdam, 1994, p. 305.
72. P. Schieberle, New developments in methods for analysis of volatile flavor compounds and their precursors, *Characterization of Food: Emerging Methods* (A. G. Gaonkar, ed.), Elsevier Science, Amsterdam, 1995, p. 403.
73. N. Abbott, P. X. Etiévant, S. Issanchou, and D. Langlois, Critical evaluation of two commonly used techniques for the treatment of data from extract dilution sniffing analysis, *J. Agric. Food Chem. 41:*1698 (1993).
74. J. E. R. Frijters, A critical analysis of the odor unit number and its use. *Chem. Senses Flav. 3:*227 (1978).
75. J. R. Piggott, Relating sensory and chemical data to understand flavor, *J. Sens. Stud. 4:*261 (1990).
76. M. Güntert, H. J. Bertram, R. Hopp, W. Silberzahn, H. Sommer, and P. Werkhoff, Thermal generation of flavor compounds from thiamin and various amino acids, *Recent Developments in Flavor and Fragrance Chemistry* (R. Hopp and K. Mori, eds.), VCH, Weinheim, 1993, p. 215.
77. T. E. Acree and J. Barnard, Gas chromatography-olfactometry and CharmAnalysis™, *Trends in Flavour Research* (H. Maarse and D. G. van der Heij, eds.), Elsevier, Amsterdam, 1994, p. 211.
78. H. Guth and W. Grosch, Identification of the character impact odorants of stewed beef juice by instrumental analyses and sensory studies, *J. Agric. Food Chem. 42:*2862 (1994).
79. P. Semmelroch and W. Grosch, Studies on character impact odorants of coffee brews, *J. Agric. Food Chem. 44:*537 (1996).
80. W. Grosch, Determination of potent odourants in foods by aroma extract dilution analysis (AEDA) and calculation of odour activity values (OAVs), *Flav. Fragr. J. 9:*147 (1994).

11

The Electronic Nose: Sensor Array-Based Instruments that Emulate the Human Nose

DIANA HODGINS
Wheathampstead, Hertfordshire, England

I. INTRODUCTION

Electronic "noses" are designed to analyze complex vapors as they exist and produce a simple output. It must be recognized, however, that there will be limitations with any analytical tool when compared to the human, and these will be discussed.

The human olfactory system has been investigated by a number of academics worldwide for many years (1–3). Their goal has been to ascertain how the individual sensors in the human nose respond to complex vapors and whether these sensors are interlinked before their signals reach the brain. It is thought that humans may have up to 10,000 individual sensors and that these may be linked to form a significantly smaller number of groups. The brain generates a pattern from the inputs of the sensor or sensor groups. The exact way in which the individual sensors interact with a complex vapor is not well understood, although it is accepted that each sensor does not detect one specific compound. Fortunately it is not necessary to understand exactly how the human responds to complex vapors to be able to develop an electronic instrument that, in the broadest sense of the word, mimics the human olfactory system.

In this chapter the main features for different systems will be described, as well as how they may be used in industry. A more detailed description will then be given of one system designed around the use of conducting polymer materials as sensors, together with results of specific applications. And finally, suggestions will be given as to how this technology may evolve.

II. BASIC REQUIREMENTS FOR AN ELECTRONIC NOSE

Three basic building blocks make up a system, as shown in Figure 1. In humans, the sensor array represents the sensors in the nose. The circuitry represents the conversion of the chemical reactions on the human sensors to electrical signals into the brain. Finally the software analysis represents the brain itself. The electronic nose is therefore analogous to that of the human olfactory sensing system.

A system needs to be able to analyze a complex vapor as it exists without affecting it in any way. The vapor will normally exist as the headspace above a liquid or solid sample, although in some applications, for example, environmental monitoring, the vapor is the sample. In all cases no part of the instrument should interact with either the sample or the headspace above the sample, i.e., all wetted parts need to be inert. Ways in which this can be achieved will be discussed in more detail later in the chapter.

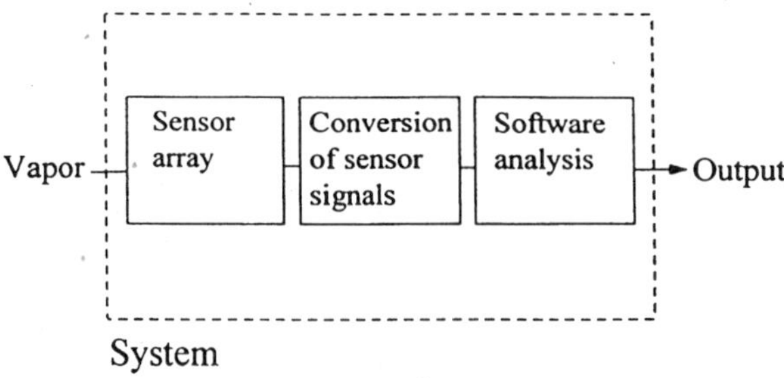

FIGURE 1 System block design.

Analyzing a complex vapor cannot realistically be achieved by using discrete sensors for two primary reasons. First, many thousands of different compounds can and do exist in the headspace above different samples. Some examples where data have been extracted from published papers referring to gas chromatography/mass spectrometry (GC/MS) headspace analysis are given in Table 1. These examples alone indicate how complex some headspace vapors are: to analyze them with discrete sensors, the exact composition would need to be known. A discrete sensor system would therefore be analogous to GC/MS analysis. Second, and perhaps more important, the individual molecules join together to form complex structures. This is difficult to prove since there are no instruments currently available that can specify complex compounds. However, many practical examples support this claim, for example, cocoa. It is known that some compounds present in cocoa have an aroma (4). Using a gas chromatograph with a sniffer port, it can be shown (4) that none of the individual aromatic molecules smell like cocoa to humans (4). However, when all of the aromatic compounds are present, the overall aroma is one of cocoa. Therefore, since the exact form of any complex vapor is neither known nor understood, it would be impossible to design discrete sensors for different applications.

Hence the sensors used in an instrument must be nonselective, i.e., they must respond to many different individual and complex compounds. They must also respond to compounds known to be detected by humans, i.e., aromatic compounds, with a sensitivity similar to that of humans.

The analog circuitry must be designed for the specific sensor technology

TABLE 1 Compounds Found in Vapors

Vapor	Number of compounds
Coffee	670
Scotch whisky	260
Celery seed oil	27 identified 23 unidentified
Carrot oil	79
Potato crisps	42
Potato	>80
Tomato	>250
Basil	37
Tobacco	>600

employed. The outputs will then be digitized before being analyzed using computer software. The front end software must be customized for a particular system. However, as more and more instruments become available, the major component of software analysis may be standardized packages. Currently, however, most software analysis tools are unique to an instrument.

III. HOW THE SYSTEM CAN BE APPLIED TO THE FOOD INDUSTRY

As the commercial environment of the food industry becomes more and more competitive, there is an increasing need for the maintenance and improvement of food and drink quality. When consuming foods, color, texture, and flavor are all important in our appreciation and expectations of a product. However, flavor is generally accepted as the most important sensory characteristic associated with foods. Flavor perception consists of two components: taste and aroma. Taste arises from the presence of nonvolatile compounds, which interact with sensors in the mouth and on the tongue and give rise to the basic tastes of sweet, sour, salt, and bitter. Although important, it is unlikely the flavor of a food can be defined by taste alone. What is far more important are the many hundreds of volatile compounds that are responsible for the aroma of a food. It is these compounds that define the nature of a food and its product identity, as well as contribute to consumer preferences between brands of product. Volatile compounds are also invariably responsible for the occurrence of off-flavor and taints, which arise due to chemical or biochemical changes, microbial action, or contamination.

It is clearly of great importance that the food industry have appropriate techniques for the assessment of the flavor quality from raw material through to final product (see Fig. 2). Currently there are two basic techniques available to assess flavor quality: sensory analysis and GC/MS.

A. Sensory Analysis

Many different types of tests are available for the sensory analysis of foods. However, only some of these are suitable for quality control (QC) analysis.

1. Difference tests

The simplest and perhaps most commonly used sensory analysis tests are difference tests. These tests basically determine whether or not a sensory difference exists between two samples. Determination of sensory threshold values can also be carried out using these procedures. Samples can be presented to

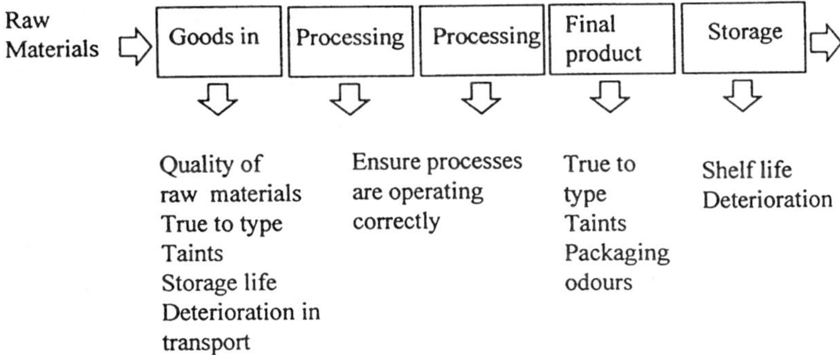

FIGURE 2 Potential application areas for the nose.

panelists in several ways: (a) as a pair of samples that may or may not be different (paired comparison test), (b) as three samples, one of which is different from the other two (triangular test), or (3) where one sample is presented as a standard to which two unknowns are compared (duo-trio test). These types of tests do not require trained panelists and are often used in food QC laboratories.

However, in many instances these tests involve a limited number of panelists (as few as one or two), these people may not be sensitive to some flavors or may have an illness that dulls their sense of smell. Testing is often carried out too infrequently, and some materials (e.g., packaging and many raw materials) are difficult to assess using human panelists.

2. Descriptive Tests

Descriptive tests are normally carried out using a panel of trained experts or selected assessors. There are several methods for carrying out these tests. In sensory profile testing, samples are assessed and ranked using an agreed-upon list of sensory descriptor terms. The data is then analyzed statistically using, for example, principal component analysis. This type of analysis can be used to discriminate between samples and define product type and acceptability with respect to flavor quality. However, it is expensive to train and implement this type of panel system, and the panelists are subject to fatigue.

B. GC-MS

The development of capillary GC has provided the flavor chemist with a technique capable of taking complex mixtures of flavor compounds, quantifying the individual components, and, when linked to a mass spectrometer, identifying them as well. Using this technique, the volatile composition of most foods and drinks have been identified and tabulated. However, this technique remains essentially a research and development technique. Sample extraction and preparation time and GC analysis times can be long. The equipment is expensive and requires a trained technician for both operation and interpretation of the results. Also, it is relatively delicate and not ideally suited to the rigors of a food process hall or QC laboratory. Furthermore, it is difficult to relate the GC/MS trace to the human's perception of the aroma.

C. The Electronic NOSE

The electronic NOSE offers a third technique for analyzing an aroma and is complementary to those discussed, as indicated in Figure 3. The aroma is analyzed as a complex vapor using an array of sensors and the output presented in a simplified form. The system generally gives comparative rather than quantitative or qualitative information and therefore is ideally suited for quick QC/QA checking. Its task is similar to that of the human in that the exact composition of the vapor is not the result. For example, the human smells fresh and stale potato chips and separates them into the two appropriate categories. However, in reality there may be many different compounds present in the two samples at varying concentrations. The main difference between the human and the electronic

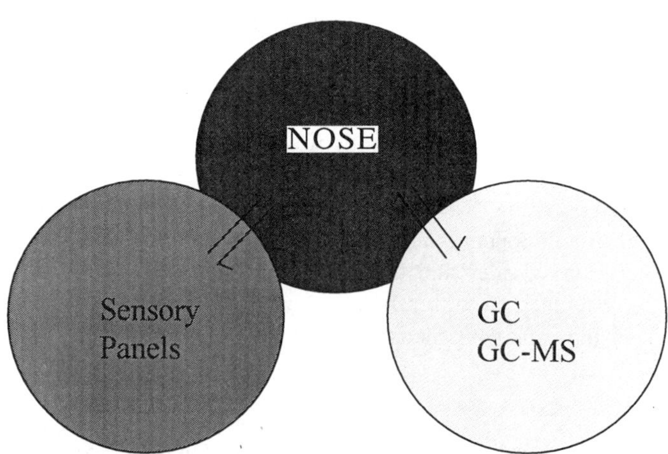

FIGURE 3 Product positioning in a QC/QA environment.

nose is that the latter cannot define what the complex vapor is or whether it is acceptable to the human. This information needs to be obtained from a human, and therefore the system can only be complementary to the human.

GC/MS gives both qualitative and quantitative information about all individual compounds present in a vapor. However, in order to determine whether individual compounds are important to humans, there also needs to be some human input. In practice, the electronic nose should accomplish a quick screening process. Samples that fail this test could then be analyzed using GC/MS to ascertain exactly what differences exist between a sample and a reference.

Current nose systems are laboratory based, and therefore process control needs to be done off-line. However, over the next few years on-line systems should become available. The main usage for this type of system is currently QC/QA applications, where a simple GO/NO GO check is required. Existing techniques are both costly and time consuming, and therefore only a limited number of checks are performed. For example, raw materials are often not checked for aroma before processing. If a taint or off-odor is present, it is likely to be present in the final product. Final product testing is normally carried out and the batch rejected. However, the faulty material may have cost the manufacturer a great deal, and it is furthermore very difficult to ascertain which supplier delivered the faulty material. An initial check of the raw material using this system would have indicated any problems, saved manufacturing costs, and pinpointed the faulty supplier.

This system could also be used in product development. For example, if a manufacturer is developing a new snack product, then fingerprints for all of the different samples used in a market survey could be obtained. One aim of the product development team would then be to match the fingerprint of their optimized product to the print or prints that consumers find acceptable. Similarly, if a manufacturer wishes to copy a competitor's product, the system could be used for aroma profiling of both products.

IV. SYSTEM DESIGN

As shown in Figure 1, the system consists of three basic components. It is important when incorporating these components into a system that the system requirements be defined. The key features of the system design are highlighted in the following section.

Having discussed the overall system design, a detailed description of the sensor array and circuit design will be given. The most important aspect of these systems is undoubtedly the sensors; these will therefore be discussed in some detail.

A. Noise

It is essential that the system be designed so that sensor performance is optimized. It is not sufficient to say that the sensors are sensitive to compound *x* at *y* concentration, and then to allow process variables into the system that could introduce "noise" that equates to levels greater than *y*. In reality the "noise" in a system is generally the limiting factor, rather than the sensors. For this type of system, "noise" can come from a number of sources, including environmental changes, electronic noise, incorrect sample handling and preparation, and system variables such as flow rates. The system described in detail concentrates on minimizing such sources of error.

B. Inertness

Ideally the system will not interfere with or alter the sample, and hence the vapor above the sample, in any way. Sensory panels take great care to ensure that samples are held in an inert environment, the most common being glass containers. To ensure this, all parts of the system that come into contact with either the sample or the vapor should be inert. Suitable materials include glass, stainless steel, and PTFE.

C. Sample Handling

Some aspects of the system design will be common to any sensor array technology employed. Also, different techniques can be adopted for obtaining the vapor above a sample and transporting the vapor to the sensor array.

Food samples may be liquid or solid and may exist as very small quantities or as large bulk materials. The system is intended for use in many varied application areas and therefore must be able to deal with samples in many different forms (Fig. 2). It should be noted that the equipment is currently available only for laboratory use and, therefore, that process monitoring would have to be done off-line.

For bulk raw material such as grain, rice, and potatoes, a large headspace already available. In such cases this headspace should be taken as the sample directly. Small liquid or solid samples should be placed into a sample vessel, which should then be sealed to allow a headspace to form. Before allowing the headspace to form, a reference point should be established, thus minimizing environmental effects. This is achieved in one such system (Fig. 4) by allowing the sample vessel to be purged with a reference gas. The equilibration time for a sample will be defined by the volatility of the different compounds, the temperature and the surface area of the sample, and the vol-

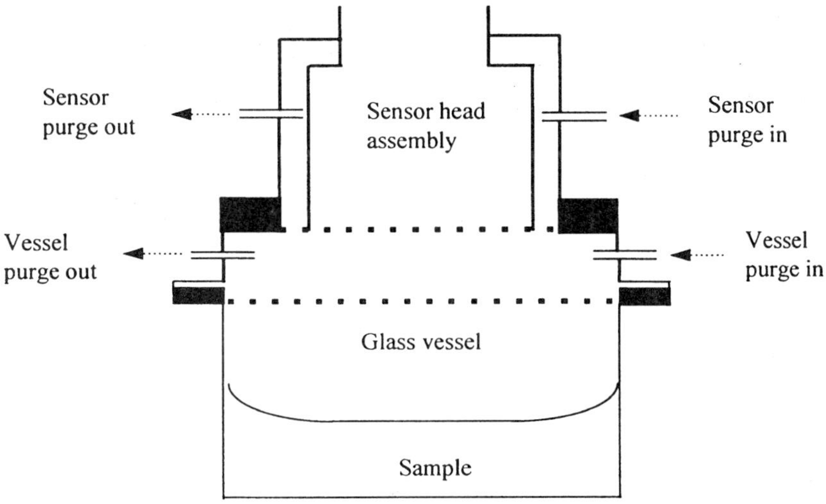

FIGURE 4 Schematic of sensor head and glass vessel.

ume of the headspace. Generally the user would be advised to ascertain the equilibration time for a sample type and then allow a little longer to ensure that if slightly less sample is used or the surface area is reduced slightly, the headspace will still have reached equilibration. This would ensure that sample handling and preparation is not a variable introducing "noise" into the system. With regard to the temperature the user could either work in a temperature-controlled environment or run at a set temperature controlled by the instrument. In some instances, like the measurement of oils, it may be beneficial to elevate the temperature to increase the volatiles. However, in the majority of cases for final product QC/QA testing, the temperature should be kept close to ambient conditions, since that is the temperature at which the consumer will generally smell the product.

The sample is placed into a glass vessel, which can be purged with any reference gas. Any headspace sample would be pumped into this vessel directly. Transferring the headspace to the sensor array can be achieved either by diffusion (i.e., statically) or by pumping the vapor to the sensors (i.e., dynamically). The system works via diffusion, where the sensory array is lowered into the headspace at the start of a test. The time for diffusion of the vapor to the sensors is less than 100 msec and is constant for the design. Therefore, there are no flowrate system variables that could introduce noise into the system.

An alternative approach, which could be adopted by the user of this system if required, is to pump the vapor from a headspace over the sensor array and out to the environment. This method is not preferred since possible system variables are introduced, primarily due to pump rate. These could result in laminar or turbulent flow in the dead volume between the input and the output, including over the sensors. As the flow characteristics are altered, the mixing of the headspace with the dead volume will also vary, which would appear as a difference in concentration with time. Even if the flow remained laminar but varied, the concentration level with time would vary. Care would also need to be taken to ensure that the previous sample vapor was not present in the dead volume.

V. SENSOR ARRAY DESIGN

The different types of sensor technologies that can be employed in an electronic NOSE will be described in the next section. The most promising to date and the type used in the equipment described in detail in this chapter are conducting polymer sensors. This type of sensor is not specific but can be designed to be highly sensitive to aroma compounds. Due to their nonspecificity, a small number of sensors can be used to monitor vapors from a large number of compounds: how small a number is difficult to quantify, although there is research (5,6) suggesting that three broad sensors would be sufficient.

Every compound present in a vapor should be detected by at least one sensor. Furthermore, if additional compound(s) are added or removed, at least one sensor must detect this. It could be argued that the more sensors are used, the more likely these criteria are to be met. In practice, such an approach will lead to systems far more complex than the user wants and a great deal of unnecessary data. Furthermore, a number of sensors may respond in an identical manner, thus giving redundant information, and many may not be sensitive to the initial or additional compound(s) from the sample.

The preferred approach is to limit the number of sensors to meet the criteria, with a few extra for safety. As more sensor types are developed, the arrays may be "tuned" more for application areas. For example, rancidity in many products is key, and therefore a few sensor types may be specifically designed for this type of application. These would be included with other sensor types, which would be suitable for monitoring the sample, e.g., nuts or potato chips.

The system described here utilizes 12 different sensor types. Testing has been carried out on many different samples to ascertain whether this is a suitable number of sensors. It has been found that often 6–8 sensors are adequate, and in all cases 12 was sufficient.

For other sensor technologies, this would probably not be the case. For example, if surface wave devices were used, then because they tend to be more specific, more sensors would need to be incorporated to meet the criteria specified.

Having established that an array of sensors is required, these need to be mounted together so that they are all exposed to the vapor at the same time. The sensor array design will be dependent upon the sensor fabrication technique adopted. The conducting polymer sensors described here in some detail are electrochemically grown individually onto silicon substrates, and, therefore, certain mounting techniques have been adopted. One method involves individual sensors soldered onto a single PCB, such that each sensor is at right angles to the main PCB. In practice, the volume of the complete sensor assembly could be reduced by mounting the sensors flat and reducing the size of the individual sensor assembly. It is anticipated that as systems evolve, design changes like these will be introduced.

Alternative sensor-manufacturing techniques include depositing all sensor types onto a single ceramic substrate. This minimizes the volume of the array but also limits the sensor-fabrication techniques available. Since the sensors are key to the performance of the system, whereas the volume of the sensor array is of less importance, individually electrochemically grown sensors are preferred. Other benefits include the ability to test sensors individually before mounting them into an array; if a sensor fails during manufacture or use, it could then be replaced without replacing the complete array.

VI. SENSORS

There are a number of different sensor technologies currently available for monitoring gases and vapors. Some of these are well established, while others are still in the research and development (R&D) phase.

All technologies that may be relevant for use in an electronic nose are briefly described here and their relative merits given. For more detailed descriptions, the reader should refer to the references cited. An indication of the sensors' relevant sensitivity and selectivity is given in Figure 5.

A. Semiconductor Gas Sensors

This type of sensor has been available for many years. One leading manufacturer is Taguch in Japan, which has produced millions of these devices for simple gas-monitoring applications. There are two main types of metallic oxide sensors (7,8): the N-type, which is responsive to oxidizing gases, and the P-

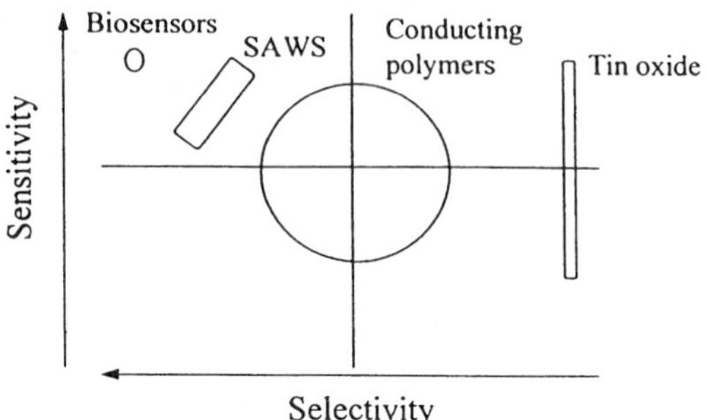

FIGURE 5 Relative sensitivity/selectivity of different sensor technologies.

type, which is responsive to reducing gases. The basic materials can also be doped to make them more responsible to a number of compounds. This type of device needs to run at an elevated temperature, typically between 300 and 600°C.

Conventional sensors are made with a platinum heater coil coated with alumina. The metal oxide material is then coated onto the alumina. As current is passed through the coil, the metal oxide heats up. The reaction between the vapor and the metal oxide causes a change in resistance at a fixed temperature. This change in resistance can be measured and related to the vapor being monitored.

More recently manufacturers have been developing planar devices (9), which consume considerably less power and are easier to manufacture in quantity. However, the basic limitations of this type of device in relation to vapor analysis remain. As stated, they primarily detect oxidizing or reducing gases, many of which are not present in a complex vapor. Adding dopants to the material is difficult and only slightly alters their selectivity to other compounds. They are, therefore, generally not sufficiently broadband to cover the range required for food products. It is also difficult to get the sensitivity down to the range required. Manufacturing sensor-to-sensor reproducibility is also difficult to achieve, particularly if dopants are added. Therefore, this type of sensor technology is generally not recommended.

B. Surface Acoustic Wave Devices

This sensor technology has been in the research and development phase for 5–10 years, and low-volume production devices have recently become available (10–12). The principle of operation is that a surface wave is generated in a material that absorbs compounds of interest. The surface wave is normally generated using a quartz resonator with interdigitated electrodes. The frequency of operation is typically between 100 MHZ and 1 GHZ, depending upon the sensitivity required from the system. When the material is not exposed to a varpor, it will have a certain resonant frequency. Upon exposure to a vapor, the material absorbs certain compounds, which primarily causes a change in the mass and hence the resonant frequency of the material. This change in resonant frequency can be monitored and related to the vapor present. Generally a reference sensor that is not exposed to the vapor would be used. Thus a difference between the reference and active sensor of typically 100 HZ with an offset of around 500 MHZ could easily be achieved. The sensitivity of this type of sensor is therefore likely to be better than that of conducting polymer sensors. However, they are also more selective, which implies that a very large number would need to be used to cover all the vapors likely to occur in food products. It is therefore anticipated that as these sensors become better established, hybrid electronic noses will become available, which include this type of sensor technology, to improve the sensitivity in certain areas.

C. Biosensors/Enzyme Sensors

These sensors are designed to measure a specific compound and therefore would not be suitable for use in isolation in the electronic nose. However, there may be cases where the user wishes to monitor a specific compound as well as the complete vapor, in which case this sensor technology would be appropriate.

Again researchers worldwide have or are investigating different types of biosensors and enzyme sensors (13–15), yet there are only a very limited number on the market. The primary reason for this is that they are living organisms and therefore tend to be unstable. Enzyme sensors can generally be stabilized more successfully than biosensors, but it is very much a problem still to be overcome.

The sensitivity of these sensors is likely to be around two orders of magnitude greater than that of conducting polymer sensors, provided that the system can be designed to optimize the sensor performance. It is anticipated that over the years, as new bio/enzyme sensors are made available, discrete sensors will be included in hybrid electronic nose.

D. Conducting Polymer Sensors

These sensors have been under development for approximately 10 years and have recently been put into production (16). This type of sensor responded to a number of different compounds and often at very low levels; therefore, they were seen as ideal candidates to be used with an electronic nose (17).

The basic material comprises a conducting polymer, counterion, and a solvent. This may be fabricated using a number of techniques, the most favorable being electrochemical deposition (see Sec. VIII). Different sensor characteristics can be achieved by altering the polymer, counterion, or solvent. Thus, by using an array of such sensors the complete vapor profile can be measured. A detailed description of the material and its interaction with the vapor is given in the following section. At this stage, this sensor technology is preferred for electronic nose application, since the sensors have been shown to be sensitive to aroma compounds at similar levels to the human as well as being nonselective.

VII. HOW CONDUCTING POLYMER SENSORS INTERACT WITH A VAPOR

Since conducting polymer sensors are used in the nose, it is important that there be some understanding as to how they interact with a complex vapor. It must, however, be recognized that, as with every new sensor technology, many years of research are needed before even guidelines can be established.

For conducting polymer sensors, every sensor type will have a different response characteristic and should be analyzed separately. In practice this is unlikely, since so many types are under development. An alternative approach would be to establish design guidelines and theoretical models for sensor materials. As sensors are developed, they should be tested with known molecules, e.g., ethanol, ammonia, etc., and the theoretical models modified where necessary.

In the vapor phase it can be shown that molecules join together to form a complex matrix. As more molecules are present, the form of the complex matrix becomes effectively impossible to predict. The addition of even a single molecule may affect the form of the matrix. Therefore, although a model may exist for the sensor interaction with individual molecules, it is not easy to predict how complex vapors will interact with the sensors. One approach when choosing an array of sensors would be to choose sensors that have different characteristics and therefore respond to a number of different types of individual molecules. This approach assumes that the complex vapor will contain compounds with similar characteristics to a number of individual molecules. In practice it has been found that this approach is acceptable for a wide range of products, from carbonated drinks, fruit and vegetable products, to complex flavor mixes.

As previously stated, each sensor is nonspecific in that a number of different compounds will interact with the polymer material. In Figure 6 the polymer material comprises a conducting polymer chain with integral cations. The anions and solvent are interspersed between the polymer chains, resulting in a clearly defined interchain distance. This two-dimensional structure will be repeated to form a three-dimensional matrix provided that a suitable fabrication technique is chosen.

Each sensor material type is unique, in that it has a different polymer, counterion, or solvent. Altering any one of these parameters will alter the response of the polymer matrix to any complex vapor.

Conduction occurs via electron transport and not ion transport. The charge carriers are associated with the cation sites of the polymer (probably polarons or bipolarons providing mobile holes for electron transport). The conductivity attained is sensitive to the presence or absence of substituents on the pyrrole rings and to their electron-donating or -withdrawing character.

In addition to the polymer chains, the conductive composite contains the counterions and at least some of the solvent used for electrode position. All three components contribute both to the inherent resistance and to the interaction of analyte species with the sensor. Some counterions and some solvents also affect the stability of sensors, so that the "sensor" is best thought of as the composite, and a good sensor is one that reproducibly recognizes analytes and has good stability.

Sensing depends on a change in conductance of the conductor compos-

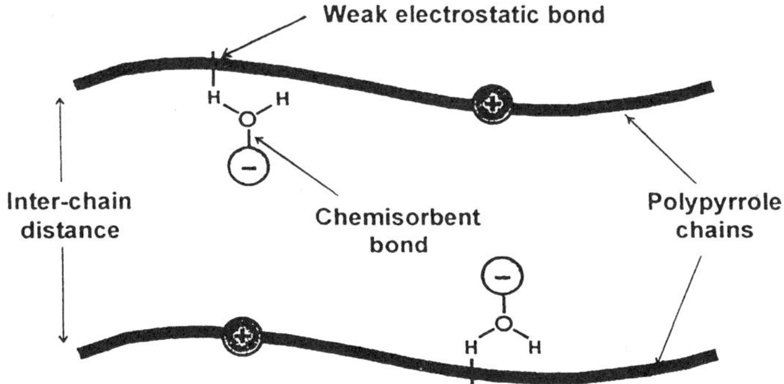

FIGURE 6 Example of bonding between the counterions and polymer chain showing that, where the anion is sufficiently small, one solvent ring exists between the ion and the polypyrrole chain.

ite on interaction (which must be reversible) with the analyte. The change may result directly from interactions between the organic vapors and the polymer, indirectly from interactions between the vapors and the solvent-counterion matrix, or both mechanisms may be operative. In any case, the sensing activity will result from a change to the "doping" of the polymer, i.e., the population of active charge carriers in its structure that contribute to the conductance.

To date there is relatively little literature (18) on the detailed microstructure of conductive polymer materials related to polypyrrole. It is known that both the counterions and the solvent exert effects in a fairly consistent manner (19) and that the polarity (or electron-donor/electron-acceptor characteristic) (20) of organic analytes helps determine what change will occur to the conductance.

VIII. ELECTROCHEMICAL DEPOSITION OF CONDUCTING POLYMERS

There are a number of different techniques that could be employed to deposit a conducting polymer material. The main requirement is that any sensor type should be reproducible.

A single-stage electrochemical deposition process should produce the same material structure every time. This technique is, therefore, described in some detail.

A three-electrode system is employed, where the polymer material is grown from solution onto the working electrode. A potential is applied to the working electrode at a fixed amplitude and temperature for a defined time. Each polymer type has a different voltage, temperature, and time profile, and this must be carefully adhered to. In practice, it is not sufficient to grow the polymer onto an electrode, since it would not be possible to monitor the small change in conductivity of the sensor material when exposed to a vapor. One technique that has been put into production is to split the working electrode by a very small gap, typically 10 μm. The resistance of the material can then simply be measured between the two electrodes.

IX. SENSOR SUBSTRATE DESIGN

The substrate design is critical in that it must be easily manufacturable and sufficiently reproducible to ensure that process variables do not effect the reproducibility or performance of the sensor material.

For the design described, two working electrodes, each typically 0.5 mm × 1 mm and separated by a 10-μm gap, are required to produce a simple electrochemically grown polymer resistance sensor. In practice, there are few processes available for depositing metalized layers 10 μm apart with a tolerance of less than 1 μm. The most widely available technique that could be applied to this application is the fabrication of integrated circuits on silicon wafers. Using this technology, separations between tracks of less than 1 μm with tolerances of 100 nm are easily achievable. This is one order of magnitude higher than required.

A design has been developed where the two working electrodes were formed on a silicon substrate. There are, however, many requirements that differ from the standard integrated circuit technology that had to be addressed before devices could be made. First, the electrode material should be inert. Second, it is necessary to make contact with the other end of each of the electrodes so that a resistance measurement can be obtained. Third, the electrodes should only be exposed where the polymer is to be grown and where the two connections are to be made. And finally, the resistance of the two electrodes should be significantly less than that of the polymer.

The final design, shown in Figure 7, comprised a 3-mm-square silicon chip with two gold electrodes. These electodes are protected with an inert material, except for a 1-mm growth window and two regions for attaching bond wires to the electrodes.

X. SENSORY SUBASSEMBLY

The individual sensor substrates are mounted onto a small PCB, and the two electrodes are wedge-bonded to the PCB tracks. These individual sensors are then soldered onto a single PCB to form an array.

XI. CIRCUIT DESIGN

Any instrument requires circuitry to convert the sensor output into digital form. Different sensor technologies require different drive and detection circuits, and digitizing these signals for software analysis may also vary.

For a system utilizing conducting polymer sensors, the change in conductance needs to be monitored. This can be done using AC or DC techniques, or indeed even at different frequencies. One of the simplest techniques is to use a constant current source to drive the sensors and monitor the change in voltage. This change in voltage relates to the change in conductance of the sensor when exposed to the vapor. A simple 12-bit analog-to-digital converter is sufficient in that the errors introduced would be significantly less than those from the rest of the system.

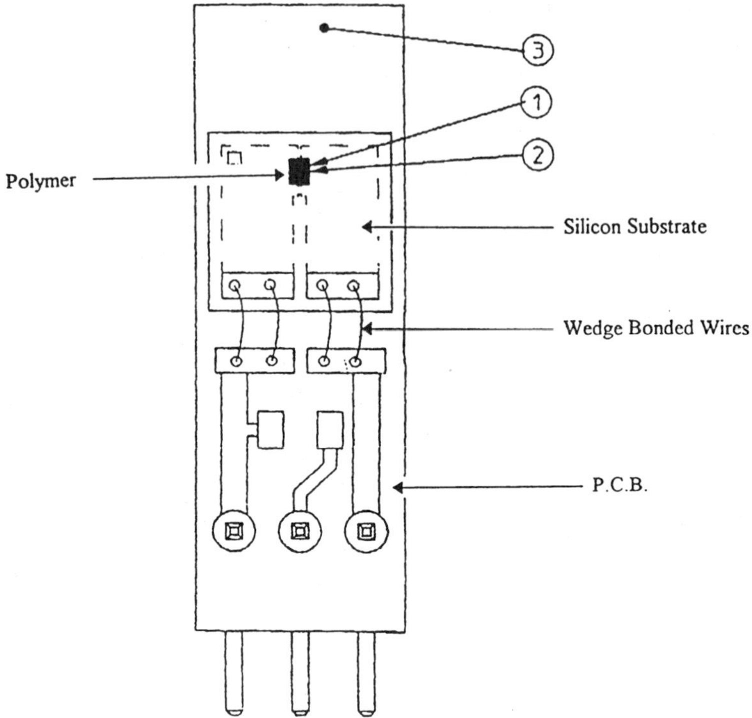

FIGURE 7 PCB sensor assembly.

System errors can and will be affected by variations in the electronic circuitry as well as connections between the sensors and the circuit. It is standard policy with any system to get the circuitry as close to the sensors as possible and to minimize the number of connectors. Future instruments will undoubtedly utilize Application Specific Integrated Circuits (ASICs) to minimize electronic noise effects. However, while this technology is still in its infancy and is expensive to design, conventional electronics and surface mount technologies will often be employed.

XII. USING AN ELECTRONIC NOSE

The design of an electronic nose has been covered in both general terms and in more detail for one specific system. Obviously each system will employ a different sample-preparation and data-acquisition technique. These will be based on parameters such as whether the system measures statically or dynamically and whether it is manual or automated. Other possible system variables such as temperature and humidity control will also be part of the data-acquisition process.

For the system described in detail in this chapter, the sample-preparation and data-acquisition methods are dependent upon the type of sample. Some guidelines for different sample types tested at room temperature are given below:

1. AQUEOUS OR LARGELY AQUEOUS SOLUTIONS
   1.1 Still aqueous solutions
   Equilibrate 5 min while purging head 5 min
   Test 1 min 10 sec
   1.2 Carbonated drinks
   Put stirrer into liquid, stir continuously
   Equilibrate for 5 min while purging head 5 min
   Test 1 min 10 sec
   1.3 Fruit/Vegetables
   Liquidize sample
   Equilibrate for 5 min while purging head for 5 min
   Test 1 min 10 sec
2. CHEMICALS
   Purge vessel for 5 min
   Equilibrate for 10 min
   Purge head for last 5 min
   Test sample for 3 min
3. DRY PRODUCTS
   Break or crush product to maximize surface area where applicable
   Purge head for last 5 min
   Test sample for 2 min
4. CONSTANT-HUMIDITY MATERIALS
   If the user wishes to keep the humidity of the sensors constant, the following procedure should be adopted. Note that one salt solution suitable for 30% RH is calcium chloride. There should be both salts and water present in the solution.
   Place salt solution into a small glass petri dish
   Place sample into the vessel, breaking or crushing if appropriate, to a depth of 20 mm
   Place salt solution on top

Purge vessel with air at the humidity level required (pumping dry air through a salt solution is sufficient) for 2 min
Equilibriate for 10 min
Purge head with the same humidity air for 5 min
Test for 2 min

It is recognized that different solids and liquids will equilibriate at differing rates, and these will vary at different temperatures. Therefore, users are requested to establish the optimum equilibration and test time for their own products using the guidelines detailed above.

The system is automated for single samples. This means that all purging, testing, and equilibration times are controlled via the PC once a sample has been loaded and the data acquisition process started.

It is also possible to test a single sample more than once. This is useful in minimizing system noise effects and seeing how a product ages over a relatively short time interval, typically 10–30 minutes. For longer-term aging effects, obviously the sample would be removed and retested at a later date.

Once the testing has been completed on a single sample, the data is stored ready for analysis.

XIII. ANALYSIS OF DATA

An electronic nose utilizes a sensor array from which a large amount of data can be obtained. It is important that different users be able to access different parts of that data. For example, if it is to be used in the laboratory for research, scientists will want to have access to all of the data and be able to manipulate it into different formats. However, if it is to be used by a nonskilled operator for QC/QA checking, then only a simple YES/NO indication is required.

Each system will acquire data in a slightly different way, but it can be assumed that all will have variations in sensor output with time for each sensors. Therefore, there should be available to the user the individual sensor outputs with time, an example of which is shown in Figure 8. Other than informing the highly skilled operator how the individual sensors responded to the vapor, this data is of little use directly.

XIV. FINGERPRINTING THE AROMA

A fingerprint can be obtained from the sensor array by taking the individual sensor outputs at any defined time during the test period. This fingerprint can be related directly to the vapor under test and can be presented in a similar

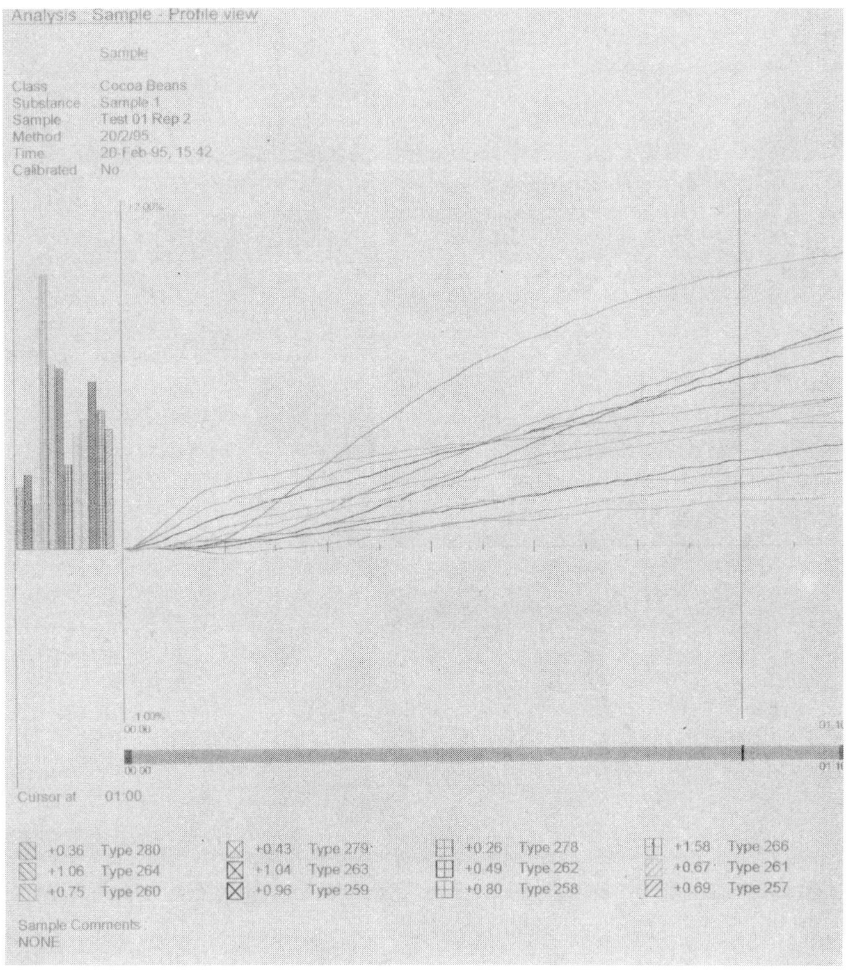

FIGURE 8 Time profile for cocoa beans.

way to sensory panel data if required. Three different visual formats are shown in Figure 9 for a 12-sensor array after 60-second exposure to cocoa beans. The first is a bar chart output and may be familiar to those who use GC equipment. The second is a polar output and would be familiar to sensory groups. The third is an offset polar, which enables positive and negative information to be presented.

The bar chart shows the output for sensors 1–12 from left to right. The

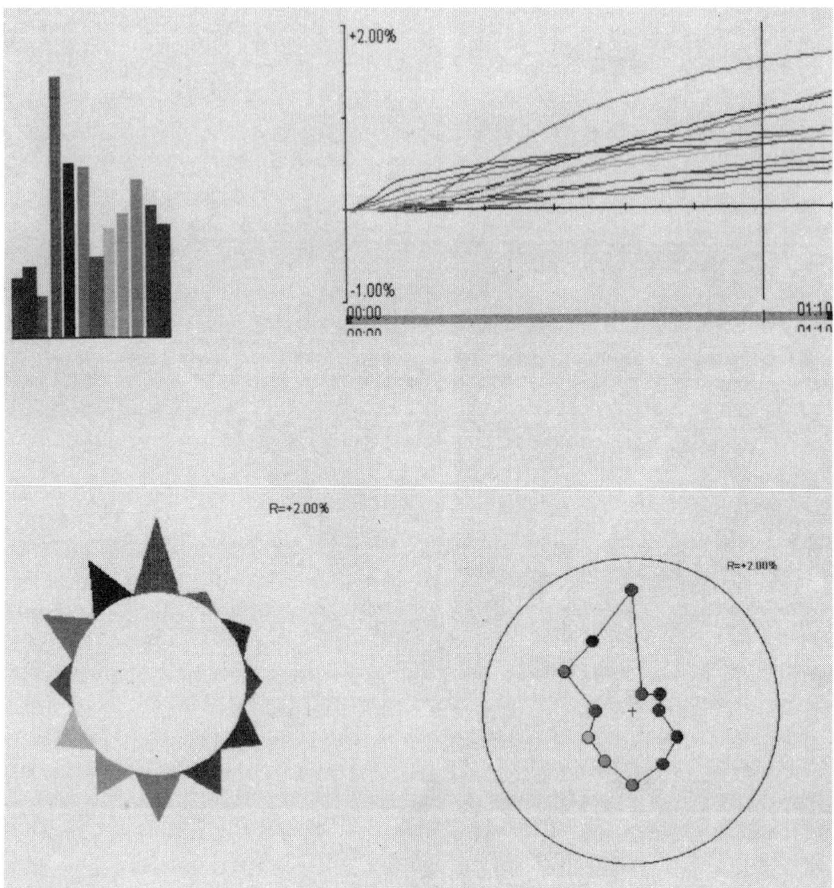

Figure 9 Three different forms of output all depicting cocoa beans at 1 minute.

spider plot shows the sensor outputs radially, with sensor 1 at 3 o'clock and then counting counterclockwise. The radius of the circle defines the magnitude of the individual sensor outputs. The offset polar also shows the individual sensor outputs with sensor 1 at 3 o'clock. In this case, the radius of the circle defines the magnitude of the sensor outputs, but if one is negative then it moves inwards on the circle, whereas if it is positive it moves outward.

For all three forms, the scale can be the sensor output directly or a normalized output, where one sensor output is set to 1 and all others are scaled accordingly. In either case the profile would look the same. However, the user will generally want to compare a sample to either a reference or a number of references. In this case a more detailed analysis is required.

XV. COMPARISON BETWEEN A SAMPLE AND A REFERENCE

Since time data for each sample tested will be available, it is possible to show the difference between any two sample types with time by subtracting one set of data from the other. Similarly a difference fingerprint can be obtained in any of the formats already described.

A. QC/QA-Type Applications

Consider the example where the user has a standard product which is being produced continuously. Initially the user would probably take a large number of samples which a sensory panel and/or GC/MS have passed as acceptable. Each of these samples would be tested on the electronic nose and the time profiles stored. The user could then set up a template to include all of the individual samples. This template could contain the average time profiles for all of the individual samples. This template could contain the average time profiles for all of the individual sensors and, assuming a gaussian distribution, the standard deviation for each sensor with time. These are shown diagramatically, in Figures 10 and 11 in the offset polar view. The user can then determine the spread that they allow for a particular product. Templates could also be generated daily, weekly, monthly, or even yearly. This would supply information as to whether there are seasonal changes to a product or if the average value or standard deviation moves erratically or slowly with time. With this information, the user may be able to modify the raw materials and/or processing accordingly.

Having established a template, the user would generally wish to compare unknown samples to it. The user can then set pass/fail limits. The limit would be set based on a combination of where failed samples sit in comparison to the average reference sample and what level of acceptable samples could be classified as failure. To determine these values, the user must first have a fair number of failed samples, as defined by a sensory panel and/or GC/MS. These samples would be tested and their outputs compared to the reference average. For each sensor the difference between the sample and average reference could be determined in terms of the number of standard deviations of the reference. For the particular system described here, this information is available to the user in a number of different formats. The aver-

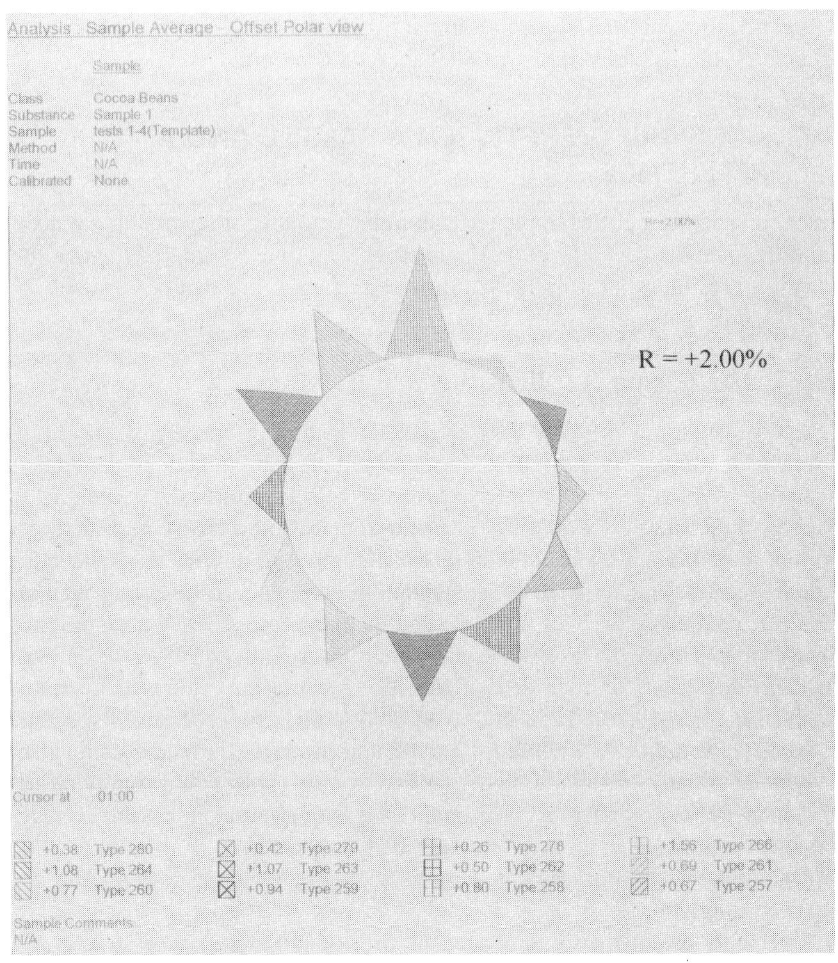

FIGURE 10 Average offset profile for cocoa beans at 1 minute.

age difference can be displayed in graphical form over the entire test period. A snapshot output can also be displayed as a bar chart polar or offset polar view. In all cases, the difference between the reference average and the sample is shown. The user can set limits for each sensor such that values are only highlighted if they exceed this value. For known failed samples, therefore, the user is able to ascertain how far they deviate from the reference.

If it is found that for all failed samples at least one sensor exhibited a

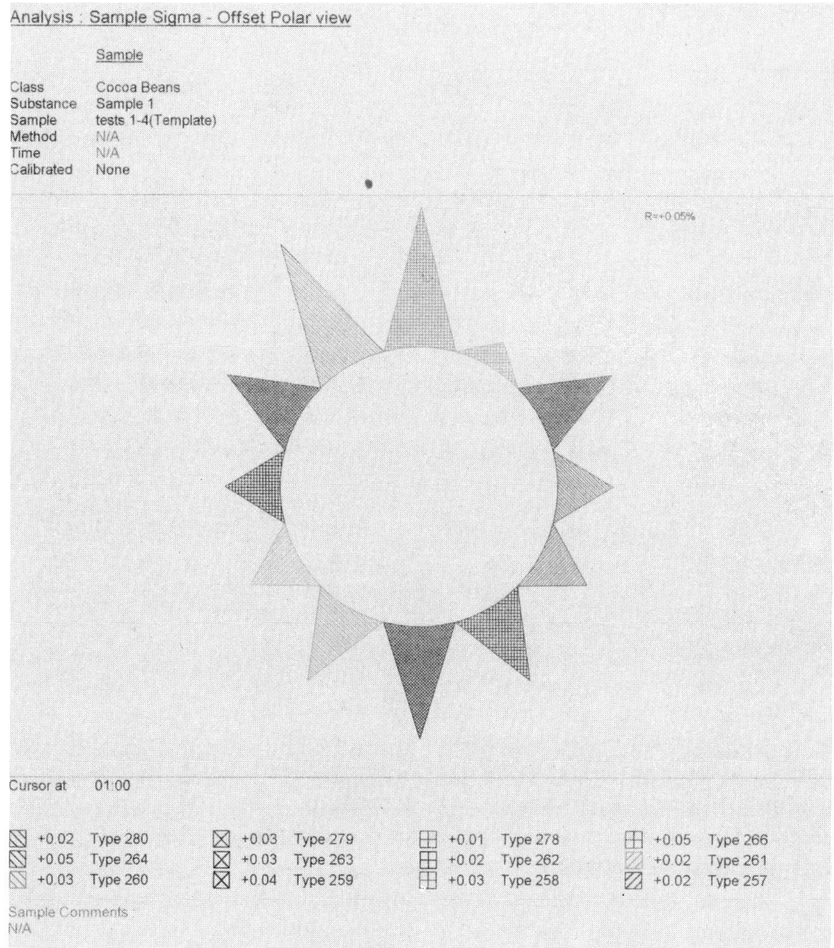

FIGURE 11 Standard deviation profile for cocoa beans at 1 minute.

difference greater than 2 standard deviations from the reference, then the user could set this value as the limit. This would mean that all failure samples should be captured together with around 5% of the acceptable samples. (Note: This technique uses the standard deviation rather than the variance formula.) If the limit was 3 standard deviations, then only around 1% of the acceptable samples would be classed as a failure.

It should be noted here that often samples are failed on a single taint,

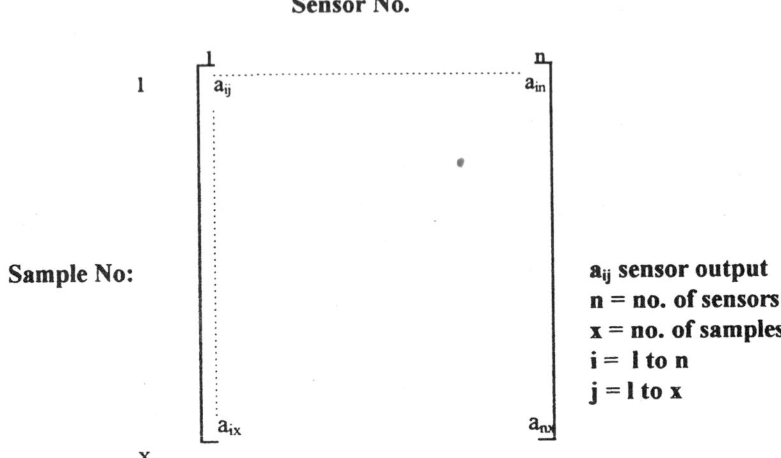

FIGURE 12 Output in matrix form for a number of samples tested using a sensor array.

which may only be detected by a single sensor. Therefore, it is entirely feasible to set the limits for failure based on the output of one sensor alone exceeding these limits.

Having established the pass/fail limit, the user can then test unknown samples and compare them to the reference in an identical manner. The system will then pick out failed samples and, depending on the limits, some acceptable samples. These will either be rejected directly or tested again using a sensory panel and/or GC/MS.

The reference template can be updated as often as the user wishes, by including those samples that pass. This will then give more comprehensive average and standard deviation information.

B. R&D/Product-Development Applications

Users in the R&D environment or in product development generally have different requirements. In their areas it is unlikely that there would be a large number of reference samples. It is more likely that these users would simply wish to compare two samples. In this case, a preferred display option may be to show the differences with respect to one of the samples. For example, test data is available for samples A and B. Taking A as the reference, the difference can be shown as a percentage of sample A for all of the sen-

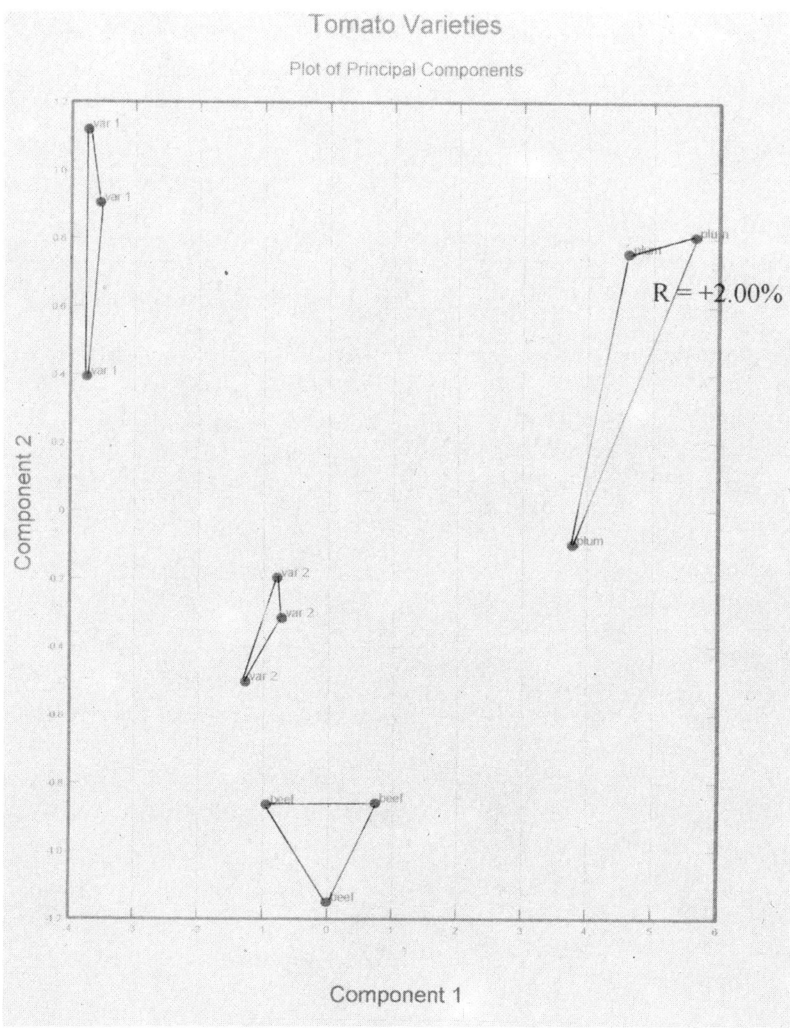

FIGURE 13 Plot of principal components of tomatoes.

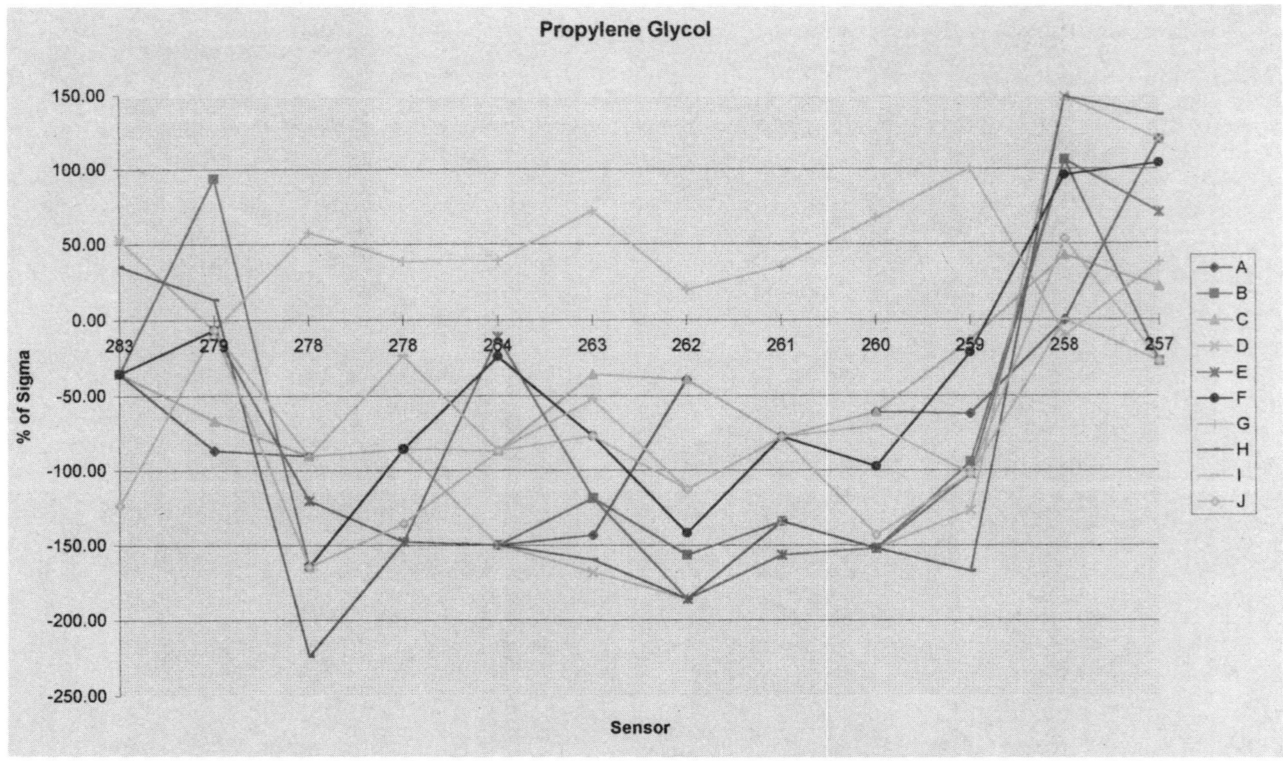

FIGURE 14 Variation in output for different samples in terms of the standard deviation of the reference.

sors. This would be a useful tool when developing a new product or when trying to match two products. Taking into account system variables, the users can set their own limits as to whether a difference is significant or not. For the system described here, a difference of 10% or greater would be significant.

XVI. COMPARISON BETWEEN A NUMBER OF SAMPLES

If the user wishes to compare a number of different samples on a single plot, then the display formats so far described would not be suitable. This application often occurs in product development and product comparison.

A. Principal Component/Cluster Analysis Techniques

The most commonly used and understood methods for multivariate analysis are principal component and cluster analysis techniques. For a detailed description of these, the user is referred to Ref. 21. Any electronic nose will have a number of sensors. Therefore, at a defined point in time any sample will produce an output vector, and for a number of samples an output matrix will be produced (Fig. 12). Using the appropriate mathematical technique, an output matrix is obtained which maximizes the variance across all the samples into principal components. Generally, provided that the data is correlated, the first two components contain more than 90% of the total variance of the system. This means that if the first two components are plotted on an *x-y* graph for each of the samples, then individual points refer to a specific sample. The user can then determine whether certain samples form clusters or whether they are all independent. An example of the form of output is shown in Figure 13. In some circumstances, three principal components may need to be plotted to obtain sufficient information: ≥90%.

Although this technique is widely used, it may not produce the correct result if there is significant variance due to noise on one or more sensor. Furthermore, it does summarize the data from *n* dimensions, where *n* is the number of sensors, down to generally two or three dimensions. Users of this analysis technique should therefore try to validate at least some of the data using other techniques, including those already described.

B. Statistical Techniques

The user could use one or two of the earlier techniques described depending upon the data available. If one sample type has a sufficient number of test runs to obtain an average and standard deviation, then all other samples could be

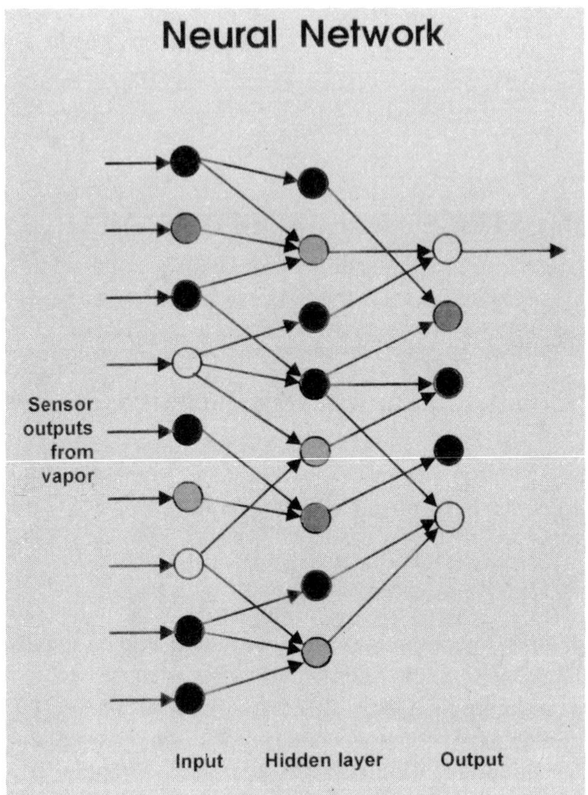

FIGURE 15 Output matrix.

plotted on a single graph with respect to the average reference sample. The x-axis would represent the different sensors and the y-axis the sample outputs as a percentage of the reference standard deviation. An example is shown in Figure 14. The user can see how close to the reference average each of the samples are loaded. All of the information is displayed, and any noise effect on the reference sample is taken into account.

If the user only has one test for each sample, then one sample could be taken as the reference and all others compared to it. In this case the x-axis would remain as the different sensors and the y-axis would be either the actual difference in output from the reference or the difference as a percentage of the reference sample. All of the data are maintained as for the previous technique.

XVII. USE OF THE TIME DATA

The analysis techniques so far described refer to a fixed point in time. As stated earlier in the chapter, the response curves for each of the sensors are dependent upon the sample. Using the techniques so far described, this information is ignored, although it may prove invaluable when looking at subtle differences between samples.

The software developed for electronic noses to date has not included such analysis as the rate of change of sensor output or the area under the curve data. However, it is perfectly feasible to use this data, and it is anticipated that as the systems develop, so too will the software to include such options.

One exception is the use of a neural network, described in the following section. It can utilize all the time information, if necessary, although it does increase both the training time and sample recognition time.

XVIII. NEURAL NETWORKS

Members of the scientific community are becoming increasingly knowledgeable in the area of neural networks. These are designed as high-power, pattern-recognition analysis packages, which can handle a large amount of input data and produce a single answer output. Their design is based on the functions of a human brain, although very much simplified.

The difference between this type of analysis technique and those previously described is that neural network does not produce a definitive answer. This is due to the fact that there are more unknowns in the system than there are equations to solve it. The user must understand this and accept that a poorly trained network is likely to produce poor results, whereas a well trained network should produce results superior to conventional analysis techniques.

In this section an overview of neural networks will be given. Details regarding neural networks have been previously reported (22).

A neural network is ideal for analyzing data from unknown samples and comparing this to data from a number of known reference samples very quickly. For example, the user may have six different products being produced at any one time. The neural network is trained using a representative number of samples for each of the different products. Once trained, the system can then take any sample data, pass them through the neural network, and produce an output, which will be the product it most closely matches to together with a confidence figure.

A number of different neural networks could be used for this task. One of the simplest, shown diagramatically in Figure 15, has been successfully used with data obtained from both an 8- and a 12-sensor array for the system described. In this case there were either 8 or 12 sensor inputs and 4–6 outputs with one hidden layer. The artificial neurons carry out a simple summation using the weighting factors from all the links connected to the neuron. An arbitrary set of weights is given to the neural network before it is trained. If the user wishes to use the time data, then the inputs could be taken as each sensor output at time $t = 10, 20, 30$, etc.

A. Training the Neural Network

The training process is one factor that will define how well the neural network will work. Data obtained from a number of tests are fed into the neural network via the input neurons. The answer for that data set is also defined, that is, which output neuron should show a value of 1. The neural network calculates the values at all the neurons in the hidden and output layer. The weighting factors are then adjusted using a back-propagation technique until the correct output is shown for that specific input set.

The training process is repeated for all of the training data. The network is said to be trained if the weighting factors are varied by no more than 10% during a training run.

Once trained, input data from a sample run where the answer is not known can be fed into the network. If the sample is the same as one of the defined references, say reference x, then there should be a single output from the network. The user would then be 100% confident that the sample was reference x. In practice, the answer from the network is seldom exact, that is, there is an output on more than one output neuron. In this case an answer, together with a percentage confidence factor, would be given. The user can then define what confidence factor would be acceptable.

If insufficient training data are available or the data vary considerably from test to test, then it is highly unlikely that a neural network could be used. Ideally hundreds to thousands of training runs should be available, whereas in practice often fewer than 100 have been used. This may be satisfactory provided the repeatability between runs for each reference type is good and there is good discrimination between the different reference types.

B. Experimental Results with a Neural Network

Neotronics has used a neural network to discriminate between three different white wines bought from a local store. The wines all had the same alcohol content, were similarly priced, and were all classed as dry. Only eight tests from each type were available, of which seven were used for training. The neural network trained well on the 21 tests. When asked to specify the wine types from the three tests not used in the training session, two of the three were specified correctly. These results indicate that more than 21 test runs should be used to train the neural network to improve the performance.

Other work has been carried out on two different types of cocoa beans. The previous findings were reiterated, in that fewer than 10 training sets for each reference type is marginal. Success rates of around 75% were obtained in each case.

C. Retraining

Many questions are asked about the use of neural networks with an electronic NOSE, primarily relating to the sensors. For example, what happens when the sensors need replacing, or start changing their characteristics due to temperature variations or aging effects?

When a sensor array is replaced, it would be extremely poor from the user's point of view if the complete system needed retraining. First, all the data gathered would be worthless, and second, effort would need to be put into obtaining new training data. This should not be a problem with the system described here. If the sensors are manufactured using the techniques described previously, their percentage response to different vapors should be identical even if the baseline resistance alters slightly. Therefore, if one sensor array is replaced with another, all the previous data should be valid.

With regard to sensor characteristics changing with temperature, it is most likely that when systems are used at different temperatures, one of the sensor inputs would be a temperature sensor. The neural network would then be trained with temperature as a variable.

Aging characteristics can be offset by adding further training data during the period of use. For example, every week the system could be tested once or twice on each reference sample, and this data could be used as training data.

XIX. APPLICATIONS FOR THE ELECTRONIC NOSE

A. Rancidity

A perennial problem in the food industry is the formation of off-flavors due to the degradation, in particular the oxidation, of fats and oils or lipids. Lipids are composed mainly of triglycerides, which consist of a glycerol background with three fatty acid groups of differing structures (see Fig. 16). It is generally accepted that the main reactions in oxidative deterioration of foods occurs between unsaturated fatty acids and oxygen. This leads to a range of aldehydes, ketones, and short-chain fatty acids, which give rise to a range of off-flavors described variously as beany, green, metallic, oily, fishy, bitter, fruity, soapy, painting, greasy, oxidized, or rancid. The problem of rancidity covers most

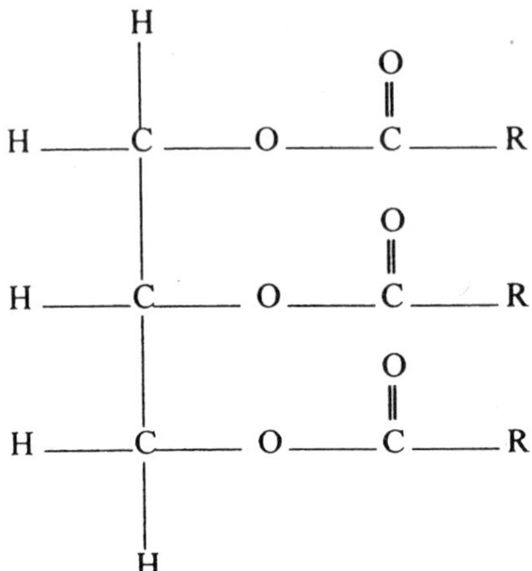

FIGURE 16 General structure of a triglyceride.

food types and needs monitoring at all stages of production from raw materials to final product. For example, nuts are used in a wide range of products from cakes to cereals. The lipids in nuts are susceptible to oxidation and can lead to a spoiled product. Detection of rancidity in the nuts prior to use is of great interest to the food industry. Figure 17 shows a difference plot comparing fresh walnuts with rancid ones. This analysis was carried out using a 10-sensor conducting polymer array. There are significant differences, with all 10 sensors showing variations between these samples. Figure 18 shows a plot of principal component 1 and principal component 2 for a range of walnut samples with varying degrees of rancidity. Clear discrimination can be seen between the groups. This system clearly offers the potential of a quick routine assessment of the degree of walnut rancidity.

B. Authenticity

Authenticity is an issue of major concern across the food industry. For example, wine is marketed based upon country and region of production and upon grape type. There is a very large difference in price between, for example, a Bulgarian country wine and a French Pamerol, making fraud a high possibility. Similar issues are of concern in the coffee industry with respect to bean types, the juice industry with respect to extraction procedure, and the spice and flavors industry with respect to country of origin. Using a 12-conducting-

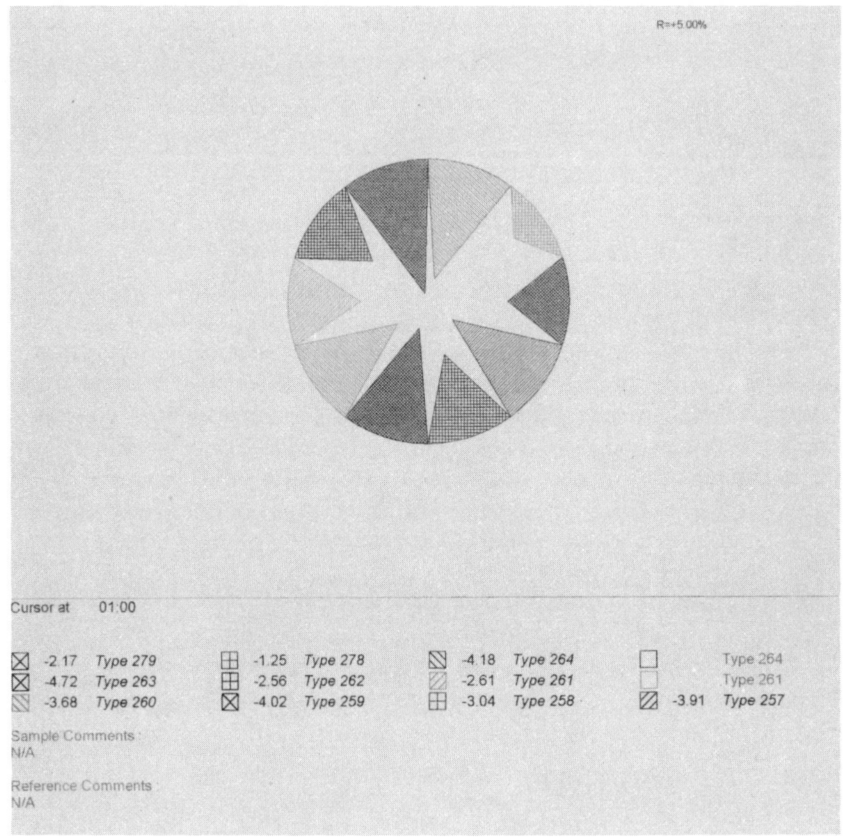

FIGURE 17 Difference between fresh and rancid walnuts.

polymer-sensor array, vanilla samples from Indonesia were compared to vanilla from Madagascar. In this case Madagascan vanilla is of a high quality and consequently commands a high price, whereas Indonesian vanilla is of a lower quality and is lower priced. Again there are clear significant differences between these samples using the nose system. Figure 19 shows a plot of principal component 1 versus principal component 2, again showing clear discrimination between the types.

C. Blending

Control of blending is a major operation carried out within the food industry. This covers tea and coffee blending, incorporation of ingredients into mixes, and

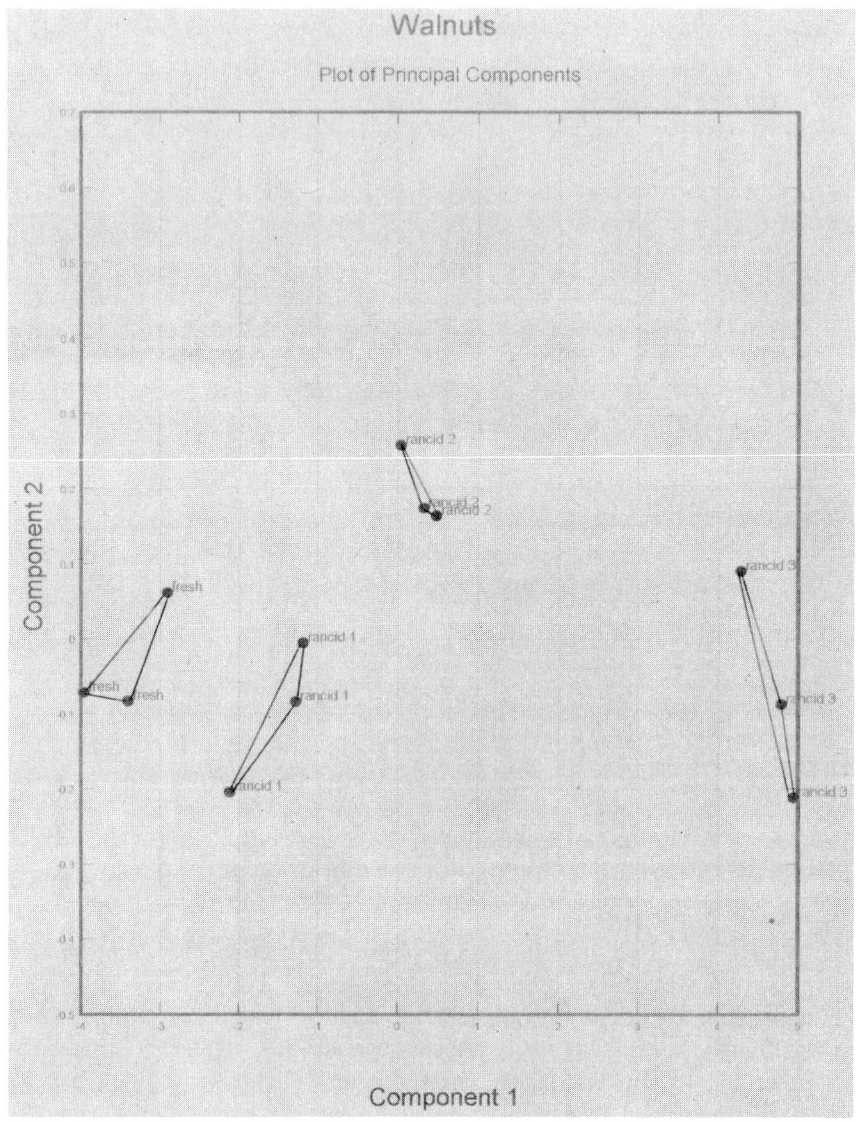

FIGURE 18 Principal component plot of walnuts with varying levels of rancidity.

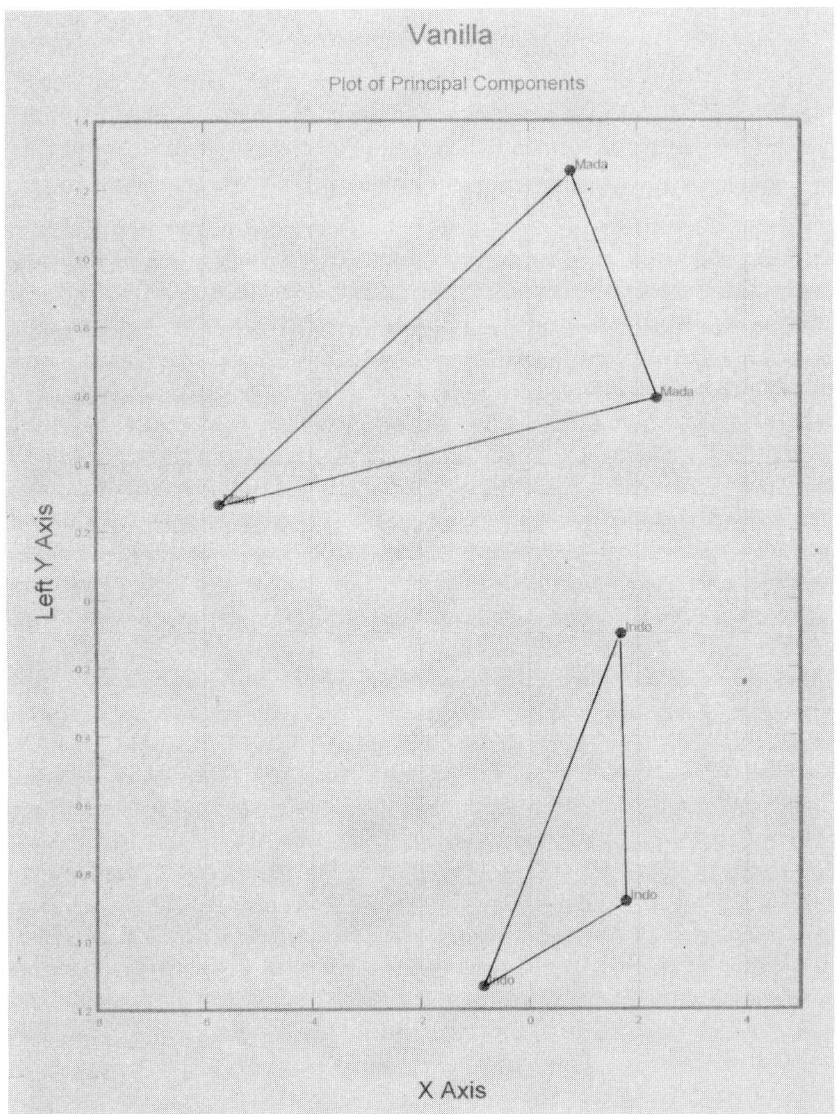

Figure 19 Differences between two types of vanilla.

addition of flavors and spices into products, etc. All of these processes require controlled blending of ingredients to ensure a consistent product. Figure 20 shows a difference plot comparing a seasoning mix with and without ginger. The difference is sown as a percentage of the seasoning with ginger. Significant differences can be seen on four sensors. Figure 21 shows a plot of principal component 1 versus principal component 2. Clear discrimination can be

Analysis : Difference Sample wrt Reference - Offset Polar view

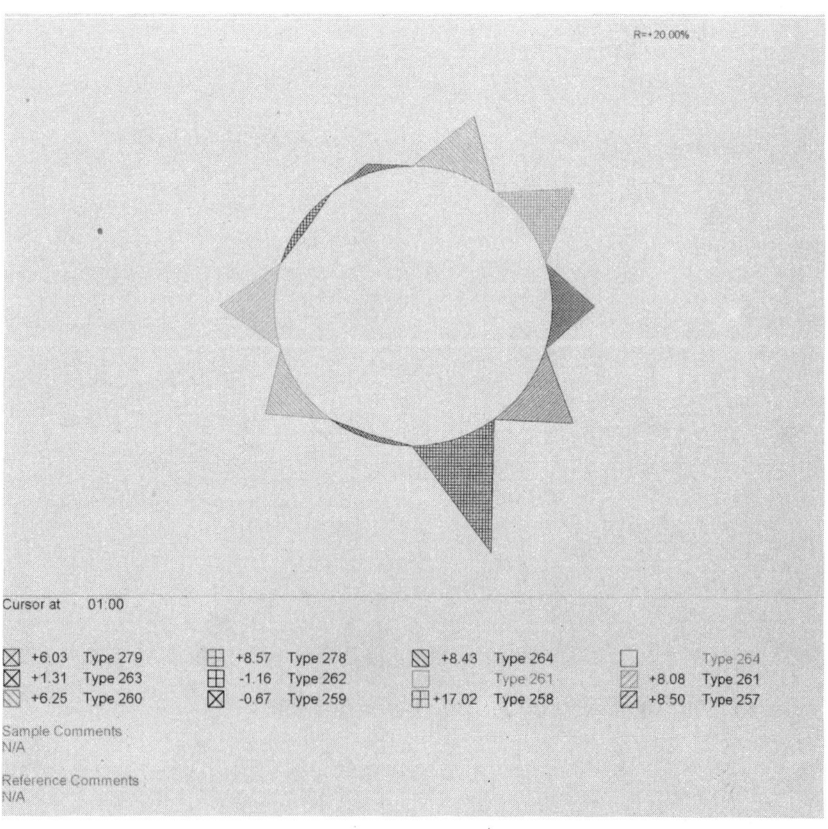

FIGURE 20 Difference between two seasonings with and without ginger.

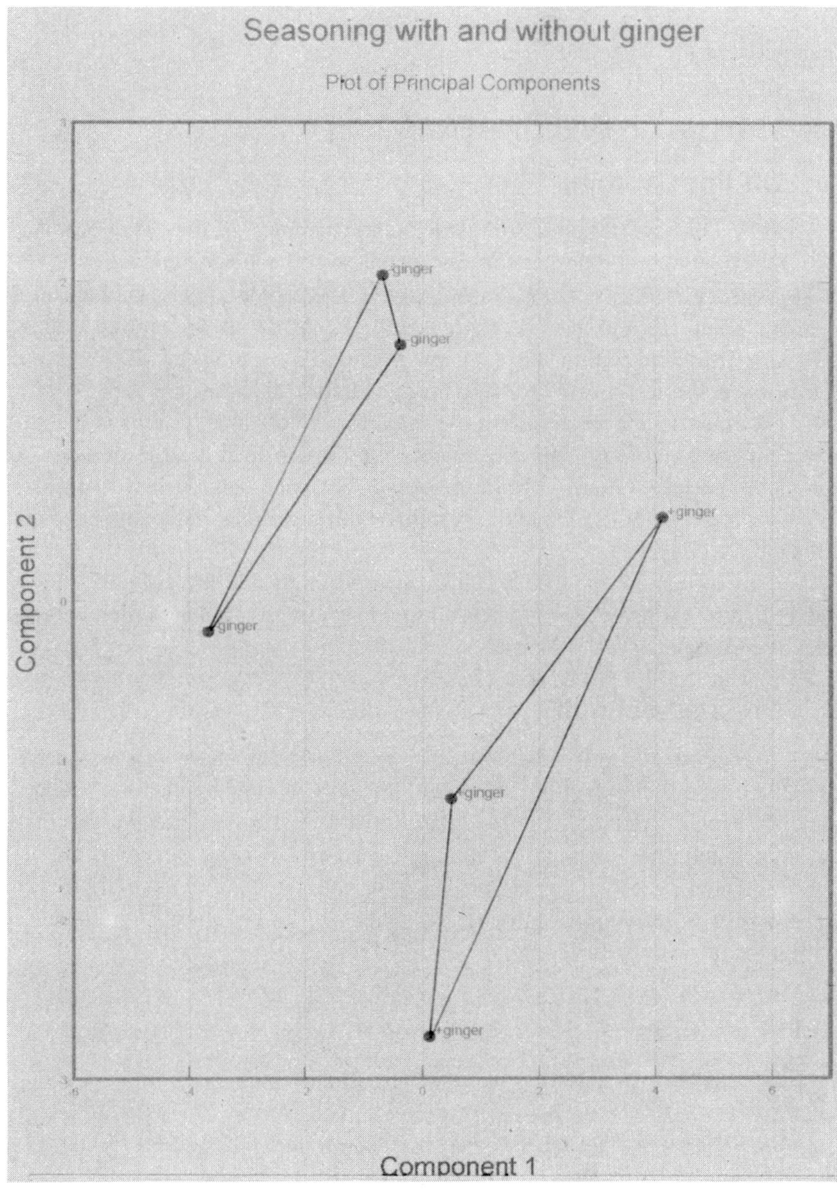

FIGURE 21 Comparison of seasonings with and without ginger using principal component analysis.

pal component 1 versus principal component 2. Clear discrimination can be seen between these samples.

XX. FUTURE DEVELOPMENTS

A. Off-line Systems

Current systems are designed for testing single samples off line. They primarily utilize conducting polymer sensors, although some are designed around tin oxide sensors. Newer systems that are in the development phase include surface wave devices and biosensors. It is envisaged that off-line systems commercially available within the next few years will combine all of the above sensor technologies in some form to produce hybrid systems.

Another development phase expected for the off-line systems is the addition of autosampling. This will enable the user to load a large number of samples, and the system will automatically test each sample in succession. The user could therefore leave the system to run overnight and analyze the results the next day.

The software will need to be developed alongside the systems. However, as industry takes up this technology, it is envisaged that some analysis packages will become the industry norm.

B. On-line Systems

Once the industry begins to accept this new technology, there will be a drive to put similar systems on-line. These systems will be more application specific and hence require dedicated software and hardware. They will need to be fully automated and may form part of a complete control system. Designers are already considering how these systems may be integrated into industrial process lines, and it is anticipated that such systems will be commercially available within the next few years.

REFERENCES

1. J. E. Moore, J. W. Johnston, and M. Rilby, The stereochemical theory of odour, *Sci Am 210:*42 (1964).
2. Contributions of topography and parallel processing to odour coding in the vertebrate olfactory pathway, *Trend Neurosci. 14:*79 (1991).
3. *Chemosensory Information Processing*, Springer, Berlin, 1990.
4. *The Cocoa Manual*, A De Zaan Publication B. V., 1993.
5. H. V. Shurmer, *Sensors + Actuators*, B, 1.48 (1990).

6. H. V. Shurmer, Analytical Processes including Analytical Communication 31, 39.
7. J. Watson and R. A. Yates, *Electronic Eng* (May):47 (1985).
8. P. T. Moseley and B. C. Tofield, *Mat. Sci. Technol.* 1:505 (1985).
9. A new SnO_2 low temperature deposition technique for integrated gas sensors. *Sensors and Actuators* B 15:63 (1993).
10. D. Arn, D. Amati, N. Blom, M. Ehrat, and H. M. Widmer, Surface acoustic wave gas sensors; developments in the chemical industry, *Sensors + Actuators* B, 8:27 (1992).
11. W. C. Quan, A. Venema, and M. J. Vellekoop, An acoustic absorption film for SAW devices, *Sensors + Actuators* A, 25–27:535 (1991).
12. M. Rapp, H. Gemmetic, J. Reichert, and A. Voigt, Analytical microsystem for organic gas detection based on SAW devices, 1994 IEEE International Ultrasonics Symposium,
13. S. P. J. Higson, S. M. Reddy, and P. M. Vadgame, Enzyme and other biosensors; evolution of a technology, *Eng. Sci. Ed. J.* (Feb.) 1994.
14. N. Matayosh, N. Muira, and N. Yamazoe, New type biosensor using solid electrolyte, *Solid State Ionics* 40/41:440 (1990).
15. Polymeric Membranes for Silicon Based Biosensors Ph Arqurnt, A. Van den Berg, D. J. Strike, N. F. De Rool, M. Koudelka—Hep Journal of Biomaterials Applications Vol 7—July 1992.
16. J. J. Miasik, A. Hooper, and B. C. Tofield, Conducting polymer gas sensors, *J. Chem. Soc. Faraday Trans.* 1, 82:1117 (1986).
17. J. W. Gardner and P. N. Bartlett, A brief history of electronic noses, *Sensors and Actuators* B, 18–19:211 (1994).
18. G. K. Chandler and D. Pletcher, The electrochemistry of conducting polymers, *Electrochemistry*, RSC Specialist Periodical Reports, Vol. 10, 1985.
19. W. Zhang and S. Dong, Effects of dopant and solvent on the properties of polypyrrole; investigations with cyclic voltammetry and electrochemical in situ conductivity, *Electrochim. Acta* 38:441 (1993).
20. Y. Kunugi, K. Nigorikawa, Y. Harima, and K. Yamashita, A selective organic vapour sensor based on simultaneous measurements of changes of mass and resistance of a polypyrrole thin film, *J. Chem. Soc. Chem. Commun.* 873 (1994).
21. B. F. J. Manly, *Multivariate Statistical Methods*, 2nd ed., Chapman and Hall,
22. J. Dayhoff, *Neural Network Architectures—An Introduction*, Van Nostrand Reinhold,

Index